Public Health
What It Is and How It Works
Third Edition

Public Health
What It Is and How It Works
Third Edition

Bernard J. Turnock, MD, MPH
Clinical Professor of Community Health Sciences
School of Public Health
University of Illinois at Chicago
Chicago, Illinois

JONES AND BARTLETT PUBLISHERS
Sudbury, Massachusetts
BOSTON   TORONTO   LONDON   SINGAPORE

World Headquarters
Jones and Bartlett Publishers
40 Tall Pine Drive
Sudbury, MA 01776
978-443-5000
info@jbpub.com
www.jbpub.com

Jones and Bartlett Publishers Canada
2406 Nikanna Road
Mississauga, ON L5C 2W6
CANADA

Jones and Bartlett Publishers International
Barb House, Barb Mews
London W6 7PA
UK

Library of Congress Cataloging-in-Publication Data

Turnock, Bernard J.
  Public health: what it is and how it works/Bernard J. Turnock.—
3rd ed.
        p.; cm.
Includes bibliographical references and index.
  ISBN 0-7637-3215-X (pbk.)
  1. Public health—United States. 2. Public health
administration—United States.
  [DNLM: 1. Public Health Administration—United States. 2. Health
Services—United States. 3. Public Health—United States. WA 540 AA1
T95p 2004] I. Title.
  RA445.T86 2004
  362.1'0973—dc22   2003020187

Production Credits

Publisher: Michael Brown
Associate Editor: Chambers Moore
Production Manager: Amy Rose
Production Assistant: Tracey Chapman
Marketing Manager: Joy Stark-Vancs
Manufacturing Buyer: Therese Bräuer
Composition: Shepherd Incorporated
Printing and Binding: Malloy, Inc.
Cover Printing: Malloy, Inc.

Printed in the United States of America
08 07 06 05 04   10 9 8 7 6 5 4 3 2 1

In loving memory of my wife Colleen's parents,

Jim and Mary Hogan,

and my mother, Jane Turnock.

Contents

Preface

The dawn of the twenty-first century provides a unique opportunity to reflect on where we have been and what we have accomplished as a nation and as a society. For public health, it is truly an opportunity to examine what we might call, for lack of a better phrase, a Century of Progress. And what a spectacular century it has been!

My grandparents were children at the turn of the last century. At that time, they lived in a young and rapidly developing nation whose 75 million people held not unreasonable hopes of a long and healthy life. They also faced an alarmingly large number of health hazards and risks that, when taken together, offered them the prospect of an average life expectancy of only about 47 years. Smallpox, tuberculosis, pneumonia, diphtheria, and a variety of diarrheal diseases were frequent, although unwelcome, visitors. It was not uncommon for families to bury several of their children before they reached adulthood.

By the time my parents were children in the 1920s and 1930s, a variety of economic, social, and scientific advances offered more than one additional decade of average life expectancy, despite even the massive social and economic disruption of the Great Depression. Still, tuberculosis, scarlet fever, whooping cough, measles, and other diseases were common. Fewer childhood deaths occurred, but many families still experienced one or more deaths among their children.

Members of the post World War II Baby Boom Generation such as me and my four siblings enjoyed the prospect of living to and even beyond age 65 and the Golden Years. When I was a child, polio was one of the few remaining childhood infectious disease threats. Some of my most vivid childhood memories are of the mass immunization programs that took place in my home town. Childhood deaths were an uncommon experience and more likely due to causes other than infectious diseases.

As the twenty-first century unfolds, more than 270 million Americans, my children and yours, now look forward to an average life expectancy of about 80 years. Today there are no fewer than 22 different conditions for which immunizations are available—11 of which are recommended for use in all children—to prevent virtually all of the conditions that threatened their parents, grandparents, and great grandparents during the twentieth century.

Today children are even being immunized against cancer through the hepatitis B immunization preparations! Overall, childhood deaths have declined more than 95% from their levels a century earlier! That means that 19 of the 20 deaths that used to occur to children in this country no longer take place!

To many of us, a century seems like a long time. In the grand scheme of things, however, it is not, and it seems even shorter when we consider how our lifetimes are so interconnected. Just look at the connections linking each of us with our grandparents and our children and even our children's children, each of whom held, hold, or my hold quite different expectations for their lives and health. These links and connections play critical roles when it comes to understanding the value and the benefits of the work of public health. At the turn of the next century, an estimated 570 million Americans will be enjoying the fruits of public health's labors over the preceding centuries. The vast majority of the people who will benefit from what public health does are yet to be born!

As someone who has spent 15 years in public health practice and another 15 years in teaching and researching the field, I have been concerned about why those who work in the field and those who benefit from its work do not better understand something so important and useful. Throughout my career as a public health physician, I have developed a profound respect for the field, the work, and the workers. I must admit, however, that even while serving as director of a large state health department, I lacked a full understanding and appreciation of this unique enterprise.

What has become clear to me is that the story of public health is not simple to tell. There is no one official at the helm, guiding it through the turbulence that is constantly encountered. There is no clear view of its intended destination and of what work needs to be done, and by whom, to get there. We cannot turn to our family physicians, elected officials, or even to distinguished public health officials, such as our Surgeon General, for vision and direction. Surely, these people play important roles, but public health is so broadly involved with the biologic, environmental, social, cultural, behavioral, and service utilization factors associated with health that no one is accountable for addressing everything. Still, we all share in the successes and failures of our collective decisions and actions, making us all accountable to each other for the results of our efforts. My hope is that this book will present a broad view of the public health system and deter current and future public health workers from narrowly defining public health in terms of only what they do. At its core, the purpose of this book is to describe public health simply and clearly in terms of what it is, what it does, how it works, and why it is important to all of us.

Although there is no dearth of fine books in this field, there is most certainly a shortage of understanding, appreciation, and support for public health and its various manifestations. Many of the current texts on public health attempt to be comprehensive in covering the field without the benefit of a conceptual framework understandable to insiders and outsiders alike. The dynamism and complexity of the field suggest that public health texts are likely to become even larger and more comprehensive as the field advances. In contrast, this book aims to present the essentials of public health, with an emphasis on comprehensibility, rather than comprehensiveness. It presents fundamental concepts but links those concepts to practice in the real world.

These are essential topics for public health students early in their academic careers, and they are increasingly important for students in the social and political sciences and other health professions, as well. This book is intended as much for public health practitioners, however, as it is for students. It represents the belief that public health cannot be adequately taught through a text, that it needs to be learned through exploration and practice of its concepts and methods. In that light, this book should be viewed as a framework for learning and understanding public health, rather than the definitive catalog of its principles and practices. Its real value will be its ability to encourage thinking "outside the book."

The first four chapters cover topics of interest to general audiences. Basic concepts underlying public health are presented in Chapter 1, including definitions, historical highlights, and unique features of public health. This and subsequent chapters focus largely on public health in the United States, although information on global public health and comparisons among nations appear in Chapters 2 and 3. Health and illness and the various factors that influence health and quality of life are discussed in Chapter 2. This chapter also presents data and information on health status and risk factors in the United States and introduces a method for analyzing health problems to identify their precursors. Chapter 3 addresses the overall health system and its intervention strategies, with a special emphasis on trends and developments that are important to public health. It highlights interfaces between public health and a rapidly changing health system. Chapter 4 examines the organization of public health responsibilities in the United States by reviewing its legal basis and the current structure of public health agencies at the federal, state, and local levels. Together, these four chapters serve as a primer on what public health is and how it relates to health interests in modern America.

The final five chapters flesh out the skeleton of public health introduced in the first half of the book. They examine how public health does what it does, addressing issues of the inner workings of public health that are critical for the more serious students of the field. Chapter 5 reviews the core functions of public health and both how and how well these are currently being addressed. This chapter identifies key processes or practices that operationalize public health's core functions and tools that have been developed to improve public health practice. Chapter 6 builds on the governmental structure of American public health (from Chapter 4) and examines other inputs of the public health system, including human, informational, and fiscal resources. Outputs of the public health system, in the form of programs and services, are the subject of Chapter 7. Evidence-based public health practice is examined in terms of its population-based community prevention services and clinical preventive services, and an approach to program planning and evaluation for public health interventions is presented. Chapter 8 examines the emergency preparedness and response roles of public health, including the opportunities afforded by increased public health expectations and a substantial influx of federal funding. The final chapter looks to the future of public health as it embarks upon a new century, building on the lessons learned from the preceding century. Emerging problems, opportunities afforded by the expansion of collaborations and partnerships, and obstacles impeding public health responses are also examined in the concluding chapter.

Each chapter includes a variety of figures, tables, and exhibits to illustrate the concepts and provide useful resources for public health practitioners. A glossary of public health terminology is provided for the benefit of those unfamiliar with some of the commonly used terms, as well as to convey the intended meaning for terms that may have several different connotations in practice. At the end of each chapter are discussion questions and exercises, many of which involve Internet-based resources that complement the topics presented and provide a framework for thought and discussion. These allow the text to be used more flexibly in public health courses at various levels, using different formats for learners at different levels of their training and careers.

Together, the chapters present a systems approach to public health, grounded in a conceptual model that characterizes public health by its mission, functions, capacity, processes, and outcomes. This model is the unifying construct for this text. It provides a framework for examining and questioning the wisdom of our current investment strategy that directs 100 times more resources toward medical services than it spends for population-based prevention strategies—even though treatment strategies contributed only 5 of the 30 years of increased life expectancy at birth that have been achieved in the United States since 1900.

Whatever wisdom might be found in this book has filtered through to me from my mentors, colleagues, co-workers, and friends. For those about to toil in this vineyard of challenge and opportunity, this is meant to be a primer on public health in the United States. It is a book that seeks to reduce the vast scope, endless complexities, and ever-expanding agenda to a format simple enough to be understood by first-year students and state health commissioners alike.

Internet-based resources for courses based on this text are available at: http://publichealth.jbpub.com/turnock/

Acknowledgments

Many people have shaped the concepts and insights provided in this text. This book evolved from an introductory course on public health concepts and practice that I have been teaching at the University of Illinois at Chicago School of Public Health since 1991. During that time, more than 2,000 current and aspiring public health professionals have influenced the material included in this book. Their enthusiasm and expectations have challenged me to find ways to make this subject interesting and valuable to learners at all levels of their careers.

Many parts of this book rely heavily on the work of public health practitioners and public health practice organizations. The Public Health Practice Program Office (PHPPO) at the Centers for Disease Control and Prevention deserves special acknowledgment for its contributions, especially those of Ed Baker (former Director of PHPPO) and Paul Halverson. The contributions and collaborations of Bill Dyal, formerly with PHPPO, are readily apparent throughout this text. Other valuable contributions came from public health colleagues, including John Lumpkin, Chris Atchison, Laura Landrum, Judith Munson, and Patrick Lenihan. In several chapters, I have drawn on the work of two public health agencies at which I have worked during my career, the Illinois Department of Public Health and the Chicago Department of Public Health. The influence of some outstanding public health figures who have served as mentors and role models—Jean Pakter, Paul Peterson, Quentin Young, George Pickett, and C. Arden Miller—is also apparent in this book.

Lloyd Novick provided early encouragement and support for this undertaking, as well as useful suggestions on the scope and focus of this text. Mike Brown, Chambers Moore, and Tracey Chapman at Jones & Bartlett Publishers have consistently provided valuable suggestions and guidance. Arden Handler has long been my colleague and collaborator on many public health capacity-building projects. I am grateful for the many and varied contributions from all of these sources.

Chapter 1

What Is Public Health?

The passing of one century and the arrival of another afford a rare opportunity to look back at where public health has been and forward to the challenges that lie ahead. Imagine a world 100 years from now where life expectancy is 30 years more and infant mortality rates are 95 percent lower than they are today. The average human life span would be more than 107 years, and less than one of every 2,000 infants would die before their first birthday. These seem like unrealistic expectations and unlikely achievements; yet, they are no greater than the gains realized during the twentieth century in the United States.

In 1900 few envisioned the century of progress in public health that lay ahead. Yet by 1925 public health leaders such as C.E.A. Winslow were noting a nearly 50 percent increase in life expectancy (from 36 years to 53 years) for residents of New York City between the years 1880 and 1920.[1] Accomplishments such as these caused Winslow to speculate what might be possible through widespread application of scientific knowledge. With the even more spectacular achievements over the rest of the twentieth century, we all should wonder what is possible in the century that has just begun.

The year 2003 will be remembered for many things, but it is unlikely that many people will remember it as a spectacular year for public health in the United States. No major discoveries, innovations, or triumphs set the year 2003 apart from other years in recent memory. Yet, on closer examination, maybe there were! Like the story of the wise man who invented the game of chess for his king and asked for payment by having the king place one grain of wheat on the first square of the chessboard, two on the second, four on the third, eight on the fourth, and so on, the small victories of public health over the past century have resulted in cumulative gains so vast in scope that they are difficult to comprehend.

In the year 2003 there were nearly 900,000 fewer cases of measles reported than in 1941, 200,000 fewer cases of diphtheria than in 1921, more than 250,000 fewer cases of whooping cough than in 1934, and 21,000 fewer cases of polio than in 1951.[2] The early years of the new century witnessed 50 million fewer smokers than would have been expected, given trends in tobacco use through 1965. More than 2 million Americans were alive that otherwise

1

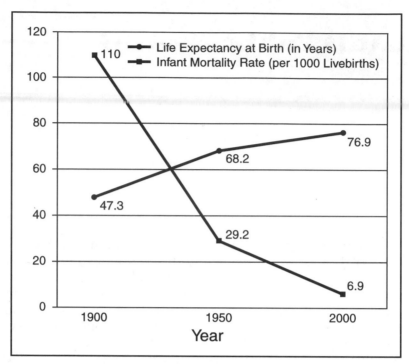

Figure 1–1 Life Expectancy at Birth and Infant Mortality Rate, United States, 1900, 1950, and 2000. *Source:* Adapted from National Center for Health Statistics, *Health United States 2002*. Public Health Service, Hyattsville MD, 2002.

would have died from heart disease and stroke, and nearly 100,000 Americans were alive as a result of automobile seat belt use. Protection of the United States blood supply had prevented more than 1.5 million hepatitis B and hepatitis C infections and more than 50,000 human immunodeficiency virus (HIV) infections, as well as more than $5 billion in medical costs associated with these three diseases.[3] Today average blood lead levels in children are less than one-third of what they were a quarter century ago. This catalog of accomplishments could be expanded many times over. Figure 1–1 summarizes this progress, as reflected in two of the most widely followed measures of a population's health status—life expectancy and infant mortality.

These results did not occur by themselves. They came about through decisions and actions that represent the essence of what public health is. It is the story of public health and its immense value and importance in our lives that is the focus of this text. With this impressive litany of accomplishments, it would seem that public health's story would be easily told. For many reasons, however, it is not. As a result, public health remains poorly understood by its prime beneficiary—the public—as well as many of its dedicated practitioners. Although public health's results, as measured in terms of improved health status, diseases prevented, scarce resources saved, and improved quality of life, are more apparent today than ever before, society seldom links the activities of public health with its results. This suggests that the public health community must more effectively communicate what public health is and what it does, so that its results can be readily traced to their source.

This chapter is an introduction to public health that links basic concepts to practice. It considers three questions:

- What is public health?
- Where did it come from?
- Why is it important in the United States today?

To address these questions, this chapter begins with a sketch of the historical development of public health activities in the United States. It then examines several definitions and characterizations of what public health is and explores some of its unique features. Finally, it offers insights into the value of public health in biologic, economic, and human terms.

Taken together, the topics in this chapter provide a foundation for understanding what public health is and why it is important. A conceptual framework that approaches public health from a systems perspective is introduced to identify the dimensions of the public health system and facilitate an understanding of the various images of public health that coexist in the United States today. We will see that, as in the story of the blind men examining the elephant, various sectors of our society have mistaken separate components of public health for the entire system. Later chapters will more thoroughly examine and discuss the various components and dimensions of the public health system.

A BRIEF HISTORY OF PUBLIC HEALTH IN THE UNITED STATES

Early Influences on American Public Health

Although the complete history of public health is a fascinating saga in its own right, this section presents only selected highlights. Suffice it to say that when ancient cultures perceived illness as the manifestation of supernatural forces, they also felt that little in the way of either personal or collective action was possible. For many centuries disease was synonymous with epidemic. Diseases, including horrific epidemics of infectious diseases such as the Black Death (plague), leprosy, and cholera, were phenomena to be accepted. It was not until the so-called Age of Reason and the Enlightenment that scholarly inquiry began to challenge the "givens" or accepted realities of society. Eventually the expansion of the science and knowledge base would reap substantial rewards.

With the advent of industrialism and imperialism, the stage was set for epidemic diseases to increase their terrible toll. As populations shifted to urban centers for purpose of commerce and industry, public health conditions worsened. The mixing of dense populations living in unsanitary conditions and working long hours in unsafe and exploitative industries with wave-after-wave of cholera, smallpox, typhoid, tuberculosis, yellow fever, and other diseases was a formula for disaster. Such disaster struck again and again across the globe, but most seriously and most often at the industrialized seaport cities that provided the portal of entry for diseases transported as stowaways alongside commercial cargo. The experience, and subsequent susceptibility, of different cultures to these diseases partly explains how relatively small bands of Europeans were able to overcome and subjugate vast Native American cultures. Seeing the Europeans unaffected by scourges such as smallpox served to reinforce beliefs that these light-skinned visitors were supernatural figures, unaffected by natural forces.[4]

The British colonies in North America and the fledgling United States certainly bore their share of the burden. American diaries of the seventeenth and eighteenth centuries chronicle one infectious disease onslaught after another. These epidemics left their mark on families, communities, and even history. For example, the national capital had to be moved out of Philadelphia due to a devastating yellow fever epidemic in 1793. This epidemic also prompted the city to develop its first board of health in that same year.

The formulation of local boards of distinguished citizens, the first boards of health, was one of the earliest organized responses to epidemics. This response was revealing in that it represented an attempt to confront disease collectively. Because science had not yet determined that specific microorganisms were the causes of epidemics, avoidance had long been the primary tactic used. Avoidance meant evacuating the general location of the epidemic until it subsided or isolating diseased individuals or those recently exposed to diseases on the basis of a mix of fear, tradition, and scientific speculation. Several developments, however, were swinging the pendulum ever closer to more effective counteractions.

The work of public health pioneers such as Edward Jenner, John Snow, and Edwin Chadwick illustrates the value of public health, even when its methods are applied amidst scientific uncertainty. Well before Koch's postulates established scientific methods for linking bacteria with specific diseases and before Pasteur's experiments helped to establish the germ theory, both Jenner and Snow used deductive logic and common sense to do battle with smallpox and cholera, respectively. In 1796 Jenner successfully used vaccination for a disease that ran rampant through communities across the globe. This was the initial shot in a long and arduous campaign that, by the year 1977, had totally eradicated smallpox from all of its human hiding places in every country in the world. The potential for its reemergence through the actions of terrorists is a topic left to a later chapter of this text.

Snow's accomplishments even further advanced the art and science of public health. In 1848 Snow traced an outbreak of cholera to the well water drawn from the pump at Broad Street and helped to prevent hundreds, perhaps thousands, of cholera cases. In 1854 he demonstrated that another large outbreak could be traced to one particular water company that drew its water from the Thames River, downstream from London, and that another company that drew its water upstream from London was not linked with cholera cases. In both efforts, Snow's ability to collect and analyze data allowed him to determine causation, which, in turn, allowed him to implement corrective actions that prevented additional cases. All of this occurred without benefit of the knowledge that there was an odd-shaped little bacterium that was carried in water and spread from person to person by hand-to-mouth contact!

England's General Board of Health conducted its own investigations of these outbreaks and concluded that air, rather than contaminated water, was the cause.[5] Its approach, however, was one of collecting a vast amount of information and accepting only that which supported its view of disease causation. Snow, on the other hand, systematically tested his hypothesis by exploring evidence that ran contrary to his initial expectations.

Chadwick was a more official leader of what has become known as the *sanitary movement* of the latter half of the nineteenth century. In a variety of official capacities, he played a major part in structuring government's role and responsibilities for protecting the public's health. Due to the growing concern over the social and sanitary conditions in England, a National Vaccination Board was established in 1837. Shortly thereafter, Chadwick's *Report on an Inquiry into the Sanitary Conditions of the Laboring Population of Great Britain* articulated a framework for broad public actions that served as a blueprint for the growing sanitary movement. One result was the establishment in 1848 of a General Board of Health. Interestingly, Chadwick's interest in public health had its roots in Jeremy Bentham's utilitarian movement. For Chadwick, disease was viewed as causing poverty, and poverty was responsible for the great social ills of the time, including societal disorder and high taxation to provide for the general welfare.[6] Public health efforts were necessary to reduce poverty and its wider social effects. This view recognizes a link between poverty and health that differs somewhat from current views. Today, it is more common to consider poor health as a result of poverty, rather than as its cause.

Chadwick was also a key participant in the partly scientific, partly political debate that took place in British government as to whether deaths should be attributed to clinical conditions or to their underlying factors, such as hunger and poverty. It was Chadwick's view that pathologic, as opposed to less proximal social and behavioral, factors should be the basis for classifying deaths.[6] Chadwick's arguments prevailed, although aspects of this debate continue to the present day. William Farr, sometimes called the *father of modern vital statistics,* championed the opposing view.

In the latter half of the nineteenth century, as sanitation and environmental engineering methods evolved, more effective interventions became available against epidemic diseases. Further, the scientific advances of this period paved the way for modern disease control efforts targeting specific microorganisms.

Growth of Local and State Public Health Activities in the United States

In the United States, Lemuel Shattuck's *Report of the Sanitary Commission of Massachusetts* in 1850 outlined existing and future public health needs for that state and became America's blueprint for development of a public health system. Shattuck called for the establishment of state and local health departments to organize public efforts aimed at sanitary inspections, communicable disease control, food sanitation, vital statistics, and services for infants and children. Although Shattuck's report closely paralleled Chadwick's efforts in Great Britain, acceptance of his recommendations did not occur for several decades. In the latter part of the century, his farsighted and far-reaching recommendations came to be widely implemented. With greater understanding of the value of environmental controls for water and sewage and of the role of specific control measures for specific diseases (including quarantine, isolation, and vaccination), the creation of local health agencies to carry out these activities supplemented—and, in some cases, supplanted—local boards of health.

These local health departments developed rapidly in the seaports and other industrial urban centers, beginning with a health department in Baltimore in 1798, because these were the settings where the problems were reaching unacceptable levels. An illustration of such local public health efforts is presented in Appendix 1-A, which traces public health activities in Chicago from 1835 through 2003. The history summarized in this appendix parallels that of other American cities through the nineteenth and twentieth centuries.

Because infectious and environmental hazards are no respecters of local jurisdictional boundaries, states began to develop their own boards and agencies after 1870. These agencies often had very broad powers to protect the health and lives of state residents, although the clear intent at the time was that these powers be used to battle epidemics of infectious diseases. In later chapters we will revisit these powers and duties because they serve as both a stimulus and a limitation for what can be done to address many contemporary public health issues and problems.

Federal Public Health Activities in the United States

This sketch of the development of public health in the United States would be incomplete without a brief introduction to the roles and powers of the federal government. Federal health powers, at least as enumerated in the U.S. Constitution, are minimal. It is surprising to some to learn that the word *health* does not even appear in the Constitution. As a result of not being a power granted to the federal government (such as defense, foreign diplomacy, international and interstate commerce, or printing money), health became a power to be exercised by states or reserved to the people themselves.

Two sections of the Constitution have been interpreted over time to allow for federal roles in health, in concert with the concept of the so-called implied powers necessary to carry out explicit powers. These are the ability to tax in order to provide for the "general welfare" (a phrase appearing in both the preamble and body of the Constitution) and the specific power to regulate commerce, both international and interstate. These opportunities allowed the federal government to establish a beachhead in health, initially through the Marine Hospital Service (eventually to become the Public Health Service). After the ratification of the Sixteenth Amendment in 1916, authorizing a national income tax, the federal government acquired the ability to raise vast sums of money, which could then be directed toward promoting the general welfare. The specific means to this end were a variety of grants-in-aid to state and local governments. Beginning in the 1960s, federal grant-in-aid programs designed to fill gaps in the medical care system nudged state and local governments further and further into the business of medical service provision. Fed-

Exhibit 1-1 Major Eras in Public Health History in the United States

Prior to 1850	Battling Epidemics
1850–1949	Building State and Local Infrastructure
1950–1999	Filling Gaps in Medical Care Delivery
After 1999	Preparing for and Responding to Community Health Threats

eral grant programs for other social, substance abuse, mental health, and community prevention services soon followed. The expansion of federal involvement into these areas, however, was not accomplished by these means alone.

Prior to 1900, and perhaps not until the Great Depression, Americans did not believe that the federal government should intervene in their social circumstances. Social values shifted dramatically during the Depression, a period of such great social insecurity and need that the federal government was now permitted—indeed, expected—to intervene. Later chapters will expand on the growth of the federal government's influence on public health activities and its impact on the activities of state and local governments.

To explain more easily the broad trends of public health in the United States it is useful to delineate distinct eras in its history. One simple scheme, illustrated in Exhibit 1-1, uses the years 1850, 1950, and 2000 as approximate dividers. Prior to 1850, the system was characterized by recurrent epidemics of infectious diseases, with little in the way of collective response possible. During the sanitary movement in the second half of the nineteenth century and first half of the twentieth century, science-based control measures were organized and deployed through a public health infrastructure that was developing in the form of local and state health departments. After 1950 gaps in the medical care system and federal grant dollars acted together to increase public provision of a wide range of health services. That increase set the stage for the current reexamination of the links between medical and public health practice. Some retrenchment from the direct service provision role has occurred since about 1990. As we will examine in subsequent chapters, a new era for public health that seeks to balance community-driven public health practice with preparedness and response for public health emergencies lies ahead.

IMAGES AND DEFINITIONS OF PUBLIC HEALTH

The historical development of public health activities in the United States provides a basis for understanding what public health is today. Nonetheless, the term *public health* evokes several different images among the general public and those dedicated to its improvement. To some, the term describes a broad social enterprise or system.

To others, the term describes the professionals and workforce whose job it is to solve certain important health problems. At a meeting in the early 1980s to plan a community-wide education and outreach campaign to encourage early prenatal care in order to reduce infant mortality, a community relations

Exhibit 1–2 Images of Public Health

- Public Health: The System and Social Enterprise
- Public Health: The Profession
- Public Health: The Methods (Knowledge and Techniques)
- Public Health: Governmental Services (Especially Medical Care for the Poor)
- Public Health: The Health of the Public

director of a large television station made some comments that reflected this view. When asked whether his station had been involved in infant mortality reduction efforts in the past, he responded, "Yes, but that's not our job. If you people in public health had been doing your job properly, we wouldn't be called on to bail you out!" Obviously, this man viewed public health as an effort of which he was not a part.

Still another image of public health is that of a body of knowledge and techniques that can be applied to health-related problems. Here, public health is seen as what public health does. Snow's investigations exemplify this perspective.

Similarly, many people perceive public health primarily as the activities ascribed to governmental public health agencies. For the majority of the public, this latter image represents public health in the U.S., resulting in the common view that public health primarily involves the provision of medical care to indigent populations. Since 2001, however, public health has also emerged as a front line defense against bioterrorism and other threats to personal security and safety.

A final image of public health is that of the intended results of these endeavors. In this image, public health is literally the health of the public, as measured in terms of health and illness in a population.

This chapter will focus primarily on the first of these images, public health as a social enterprise or system. Later chapters will examine each of the other images of public health. It is important to understand what people mean when they speak of public health. As presented in Exhibit 1–2, the profession, the methods, the governmental services, the ultimate outcomes, and even the broad social enterprise itself are all commonly encountered images of what public health is today.

With varying images of what public health is, we would expect no shortage of definitions. There have been many, and it serves little purpose to try to catalog all of them here. Three definitions, each separated by a generation, provide important insights into what public health is; these are summarized in Exhibit 1–3.

In 1988 the prestigious Institute of Medicine (IOM) provided a useful definition in its landmark study of public health in the United States, *The Future of Public Health*. The IOM report characterized public health's mission as "fulfilling society's interest in assuring conditions in which people can be healthy."[7] This definition directs our attention to the many conditions that influence health and wellness, underscoring the broad scope of public health

Exhibit 1–3 Selected Definitions of Public Health

- "the science and art of preventing disease, prolonging life and promoting health and efficiency through organized community effort"[8]
- "Successive re-definings of the unacceptable"[9]
- "fulfilling society's interest in assuring conditions in which people can be healthy"[7]

Source: Data from Institute of Medicine, National Academy of Sciences, *The Future of Public Health,* © 1988, National Academy Press; C.E.A. Winslow. The Untilled Field of Public Health, *Modern Medicine,* Vol. 2, pp. 183–191, © 1920; and G. Vickers, What Sets the Goals of Public Health?, *Lancet,* Vol. 1, pp. 599–604, © 1958.

---

and legitimizing its interest in social, economic, political, and medical care factors that affect health and illness. The definition's premise that society has an interest in the health of its members implies that improving conditions and health status for others is acting in our own self-interest. The assertion that improving the health status of others provides benefits to all is a core value of public health.

Another core value of public health is reflected in the IOM definition's use of the term *assuring.* Assuring conditions in which people can be healthy means vigilantly promoting and protecting everyone's interests in health and well-being. This value echoes the wisdom in the often-quoted African aphorism that "it takes a village to raise a child." Former Surgeon General David Satcher, the first African-American to head this country's most respected federal public health agency, the Centers for Disease Control and Prevention (CDC), once described a visit to Africa in which he met with African teenagers to learn firsthand of their personal health attitudes and behaviors. Satcher was struck by their concerns over the rapid urbanization of the various African nations and the changes that were affecting their culture and sense of community. These young people felt lost and abandoned; they questioned Satcher as to what CDC, the U.S. government, and the world community were willing to do to help them survive these changes. As one young man put it, "Where will we find our village?" Public health's role is one of serving us all as our village, whether we are teens in Africa or adults in the United States. The IOM report's characterization of public health advocated for just such a social enterprise and stands as a bold philosophical statement of mission and purpose.

The IOM report also sought to define the boundaries of public health by identifying three core functions of public health: assessment, policy development, and assurance. In one sense, these functions are comparable to those generally ascribed to the medical care system involving diagnosis and treatment. Assessment is the analogue of diagnosis, except that the diagnosis, or problem identification, is made for a group or population of individuals. Similarly, assurance is analogous to treatment and implies that the necessary remedies or interventions are put into place. Finally, policy development is an intermediate role of collectively deciding which remedies or interventions are most appropriate for the problems identified (the formulation of a treatment plan is the medical system's analogue). These core functions broadly describe what public health does (as opposed to what it is) and will be examined more thoroughly in later chapters.

The concepts embedded in the IOM definition are also reflected in Winslow's definition, developed more than 80 years ago. His definition describes both what public health does and how this gets done. It is a comprehensive definition that has stood the test of time in characterizing public health as

> . . . the science and art of preventing disease, prolonging life and promoting health and efficiency through organized community effort for the sanitation of the environment, the control of communicable infections, the education of the individual in personal hygiene, the organization of medical and nursing services for the early diagnosis and preventive treatment of disease, and for the development of the social machinery to insure everyone a standard of living adequate for the maintenance of health, so organizing these benefits as to enable every citizen to realize his birthright of health and longevity.[8]

There is much to consider in Winslow's definition. The phrases, "science and art," "organized community effort," and "birthright of health and longevity" capture the substance and aims of public health. Winslow's catalog of methods illuminates the scope of the endeavor, embracing public health's initial targeting of infectious and environmental risks, as well as current activities related to the organization, financing, and accountability of medical care services. His allusion to the "social machinery necessary to insure everyone a standard of living adequate for the maintenance of health" speaks to the relationship between social conditions and health in all societies.

There have been many other attempts to define public health, although these have received less attention than either the Winslow or IOM definitions. Several build on the observation that, over time, public health activities reflect the interaction of disease with two other phenomena that can be roughly characterized as science and social values: (1) what do we know, and (2) what do we choose to do with that knowledge?

A prominent British industrialist, Geoffrey Vickers, provided an interesting addition to this mix a half century ago while serving as Secretary of the Medical Research Council. In identifying the forces that set the agenda for public health, Vickers noted, "The landmarks of political, economic and social history are the moments when some condition passed from the category of the given into the category of the intolerable. I believe that the history of public health might well be written as a record of successive re-definings of the unacceptable."[9]

The usefulness of Vickers' formulation lies in its focus on the delicate and shifting interface between science and social values. Through this lens, we can view a tracing of public health over history, facilitating an understanding of why and how different societies have reacted to health risks differently at various points in time and space. In this light, the history of public health is one of blending knowledge with social values to shape responses to problems that require collective action after they have crossed the boundary from the acceptable to the unacceptable.

Each of these definitions offers important insights into what public health is and what it does. Individually and collectively, they describe a social enterprise that is both important and unique, as we will see in the section that follows.

PUBLIC HEALTH AS A SYSTEM

So what is public health? Maybe no single answer will satisfy everyone. There are, in fact, several views of public health that must be considered. One or more of them may be apparent to the inquirer. The public health described in this chapter is a broad social enterprise, more akin to a movement, that seeks to extend the benefits of current knowledge in ways that will have the maximum impact on the health status of a population. It does so by identifying problems that call for collective action to protect, promote, and improve health, primarily through preventive strategies. This public health is unique in its interdisciplinary approach and methods, its emphasis on preventive strategies, its linkage with government and political decision making, and its dynamic adaptation to new problems placed on its agenda. Above all else, it is a collective effort to identify and address the unacceptable realities that result in preventable and avoidable health and quality of life outcomes, and it is the composite of efforts and activities that are carried out by people and organizations committed to these ends.

With this broad view of public health as a social enterprise, the question shifts from what public health is to what these other images of public health represent and how they relate to each other. To understand these separate images of public health, a conceptual model would be useful. Surprisingly, an understandable and useful framework to tie these pieces together has been lacking. Other enterprises have found ways to describe their complex systems, and, from what appears to be an industrial production model, we can begin to look at the various components of our public health system.

This framework brings together the mission and functions of public health in relation to the inputs, processes, outputs, and outcomes of the system. Exhibit 1–4 provides general descriptions for the terms used in this framework. It is sometimes easier to appreciate this model when a more familiar industry, such as the automobile industry, is used as an example. The mission or purpose might be expressed as meeting the personal transportation needs of the population. This industry carries out its mission by providing passenger cars to its customers; this characterizes its function. In this light, we can now examine the inputs, processes, outputs, and outcomes of the system set up to carry out this function. Inputs would include steel, rubber, plastic, and so forth, as well as the workers, know-how, technology, facilities, machinery, and support services necessary to allow the raw materials to become automobiles. The key processes necessary to carry out the primary function might be characterized as designing cars, making or acquiring parts, assembling parts into automobiles, moving cars to dealers, and selling and servicing cars after

Exhibit 1–4 Dimensions of the Public Health System

- Capacity (Inputs):
  the resources and relationships necessary to carry out the core functions and essential services of public health; these include human resources, information resources, fiscal and physical resources, and appropriate relationships among the system components.
- Process (Practices and Outputs):
  those collective practices or processes that are necessary and sufficient to assure that the core functions and essential services of public health are being carried out effectively, including the key processes that identify and address health problems and their causative factors and the interventions intended to prevent death, disease, and disability, and to promote quality of life.
- Outcomes (Results):
  indicators of health status, risk reduction, and quality-of-life enhancement; outcomes are long-term objectives that define optimal, measurable future levels of health status; maximum acceptable levels of disease, injury, or dysfunction; or prevalence of risk factors.

Source: Adapted from Public Health Practice Program Office, 1990, the Centers for Disease Control and Prevention.

purchase. No doubt this is an incomplete listing of this industry's processes; it is oversimplified here to make the point. In any event, these processes translate the abstract concept of getting cars to people into the operational steps necessary to carry out this basic function. The outputs of these processes are cars located where people can purchase them. The outcomes include satisfied customers and company profits.

Applying this same general framework to the public health system is also possible but may not be so obvious to the general public. The mission and functions of public health are well described in the IOM report's framework. The core functions of assessment, policy development, and assurance are considerably more abstract functions than making cars but still can be made operational through descriptions of their key steps or practices.[10,11] The inputs of the public health system include its human, organizational, informational, fiscal, and other resources. These resources and relationships are structured to carry out public health's core functions through a variety of processes that can also be termed *essential public health practices or services*. These processes include a variety of interventions that result from some of the more basic processes of assessing health needs and planning effective strategies.[12] These outputs or interventions are intended to produce the desired results, which, with public health, might well be characterized as health or quality-of-life outcomes. Figure 1–2 illustrates these relationships.

In this model, not all components are as readily understandable and measurable as others. Several of the inputs are easily counted or measured, including human, fiscal, and organizational resources. Outputs are also generally easy to recognize and count; e.g., prenatal care programs, number of immunizations provided, health messages on the dangers of tobacco, and so on. Health outcomes are also readily understood in terms of mortality, mor-

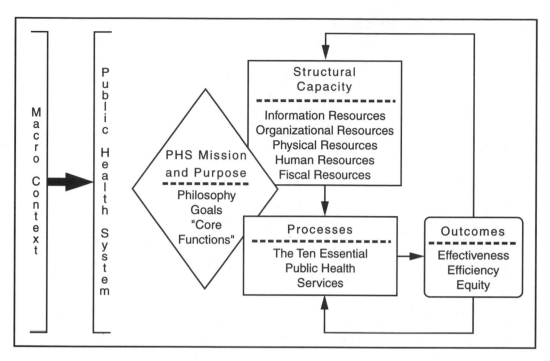

Figure 1–2 Conceptual Framework of the Public Health System as a Basis for Measuring System Performance. *Source:* Handler A, Issel M and Turnock BJ. A conceptual framework to measure performance of the public health system. *Amer J Pub Health* 2001; 91 (8), 1235–1239. © 2001, American Public Health Association.

bidity, functional disability, time lost from work or school, and even more sophisticated measures, such as years of potential life lost and quality-of-life years lost. The elements that are most difficult to understand and visualize are the processes or essential services of the public health system. Although this is an evolving field, there have been efforts to characterize these operational aspects of public health. By such efforts, we are better able to understand public health practice, to measure it, and to relate it to its outputs and outcomes. A national work group was assembled by the U.S. Public Health Service in 1994 in an attempt to develop a consensus statement of what public health is and does in language understandable to those both inside and outside the field of public health. Exhibit 1–5 presents the result of that process in a statement entitled "Public Health in America."[13] The conceptual framework identified in Figure 1–2 and the narrative representation in the "Public Health in America" statement are useful models for understanding the public health system and how it works, as we will see throughout this text.

This framework attempts to bridge the gap between what public health is, what it does (purpose/mission and functions, Figure 1–2), and how it does what it does (through its capacity, processes, and outcomes). It also allows us to examine the various components of the system so that we can better appreciate how the pieces fit together. Later chapters will refer back to this model as the capacity, processes (including outputs), and outcomes are presented in greater depth.

Exhibit 1–5 Public Health in America

Vision:
Healthy People in Healthy Communities
Mission:
*Promote Physical and Mental Health
and Prevent Disease, Injury, and Disability*

Public Health
- Prevents epidemics and the spread of disease
- Protects against environmental hazards
- Prevents injuries
- Promotes and encourages healthy behaviors
- Responds to disasters and assists communities in recovery
- Assures the quality and accessibility of health services

Essential Public Health Services
- Monitor health status to identify community health problems
- Diagnose and investigate health problems and health hazards in the community
- Inform, educate, and empower people about health issues
- Mobilize community partnerships to identify and solve health problems
- Develop policies and plans that support individual and community health efforts
- Enforce laws and regulations that protect health and ensure safety
- Link people with needed personal health services and assure the provision of health care when otherwise unavailable
- Assure a competent public health and personal health care work force
- Evaluate effectiveness, accessibility, and quality of personal and population-based health services
- Research for new insights and innovative solutions to health problems

Source: Reprinted from Essential Public Health Services Working Group of the Core Public Health Functions Steering Committee, 1994, U.S. Public Health Service.

UNIQUE FEATURES OF PUBLIC HEALTH

Several unique features of public health individually and collectively serve to make understanding and appreciation of this enterprise difficult (Exhibit 1–6). These include the underlying social justice philosophy of public health; its inherently political nature; its ever-expanding agenda, with new problems and issues being assigned over time; its link with government; its grounding in a broad base of biologic, physical, quantitative, social, and behavioral sciences; its focus on prevention as a prime intervention strategy; and the unique bond and sense of mission that links its proponents.

Social Justice Philosophy

It is vital to recognize the social justice orientation of public health and even more critical to understand the potential for conflict and confrontation that it generates. Social justice is said to be the foundation of public health. The concept first emerged around 1848, a time that might be considered the birth of

Exhibit 1–6 Selected Unique Features of Public Health

- Basis in social justice philosophy
- Inherently political nature
- Dynamic, ever-expanding agenda
- Link with government
- Grounding in the sciences
- Use of prevention as a prime strategy
- Uncommon culture and bond

modern public health. Social justice argues that public health is properly a public matter and that its results in terms of death, disease, health, and well-being reflect the decisions and actions that a society makes, for good or for ill.[14] Justice is an abstract concept that determines how each member of a society is allocated his or her fair share of collective burdens and benefits. Societal benefits to be distributed may include happiness, income, or social status. Burdens include restrictions of individual action and taxation. Justice dictates that there is fairness in the distribution of benefits and burdens; injustices occur when persons are denied some benefit to which they are entitled or when some burden is imposed unduly. If access to health services, or even health itself, is considered to be a societal benefit (or if poor health is considered to be a burden), the links between the concepts of justice and public health become clear. Market justice and social justice represent two forms of modern justice.

Market justice emphasizes personal responsibility as the basis for distributing burdens and benefits. Other than respecting the basic rights of others, individuals are responsible primarily for their own actions and are free from collective obligations. Individual rights are highly valued, whereas collective responsibilities are minimized. In terms of health, individuals assume primary responsibility for their own health. There is little expectation that society should act to protect or promote the health of its members beyond addressing risks that cannot be controlled through individual action.

Social justice argues that significant factors within the society impede the fair distribution of benefits and burdens.[15] Examples of such impediments include social class distinctions, heredity, racism, and ethnism. Collective action, often leading to the assumption of additional burdens, is necessary to neutralize or overcome those impediments. In the case of public health, the goal of extending the potential benefits of the physical and behavioral sciences to all groups in the society, especially when the burden of disease and ill health within that society is unequally distributed, is largely based on principles of social justice. It is clear that many modern public health (and other public policy) problems disproportionately affect some groups, usually a minority of the population, more than others. As a result, their resolution requires collective actions in which those less affected take on greater burdens, while not commensurately benefiting from those actions. When the necessary collective actions are not taken, even the most important public policy problems remain unsolved, despite periodically becoming highly visible.[15] This scenario reflects responses to such intractable American problems as inadequate housing, poor public education systems, unemployment, racial discrimination, and poverty. However, it is also true for public health problems such as tobacco-related illnesses, infant mortality, substance abuse, mental health services, long-term care, and environmental pollution. The failure to effect comprehensive national health reform in 1994 is an example of this phenomenon. At that time, middle-class Americans deemed the modest price tag of health reform to be excessive, refusing to pay more out of their own pockets when they perceived that their own access and services were not likely to improve.

These and similar examples suggest that a critical challenge for public health as a social enterprise lies in overcoming the social and ethical barriers that prevent us from doing more with the tools already available to us.[15] Extending the frontiers of science and knowledge may not be as useful for improving public health as shifting the collective values of our society to act on what we already know. Recent public health successes, such as public attitudes toward smoking in both public and private locations and operating motor vehicles after alcohol consumption, provide evidence in support of this assertion. These advances came through changes in social norms, rather than through bigger and better science.

Inherently Political Nature

The social justice underpinnings of public health serve to stimulate political conflict. Public health is both public and political in nature. It serves populations, which are composites of many different communities, cultures, and values. Politics allows for issues to be considered, negotiated, and finally determined for populations. At the core of political processes are differing values and perspectives as to both the ends to be achieved and the means for achieving those ends. Advocating causes and agitating various segments of society to identify and address unacceptable conditions that adversely affect health status often lead to increased expectations and demands on society, generally through government. As a result, public health advocates appear at times as anti-government and anti-institutional. Governmental public health agencies seeking to serve the interests of both government and public health are frequently caught in the middle. This creates tensions and conflict that can put these agencies at odds with governmental leaders on the one hand and external public health advocates on the other.

Expanding Agenda

A third unique feature of public health is its broad and ever-increasing scope. Traditional domains of public health interest include biology, environment, lifestyle, and health service organization. Within each of these domains are many factors that affect health status; in recent decades, many new public policy problems have been moved onto the public health agenda as their predisposing factors have been identified and found to fall into one or more of these domains.

The assignment of new problems to the public health agenda is an interesting phenomenon. For example, prior to 1900 the primary problems addressed by public health were infectious diseases and related environmental risks. After 1900 the focus expanded to include problems and needs of children and mothers to be addressed through health education and maternal and child health services as public sentiment over the health and safety of children increased. In the middle of the century, chronic disease prevention and medical care fell into public health's realm as an epidemiologic revolution began to identify causative agents for chronic diseases and links between use of health services and health outcomes. Later, substance abuse, mental illness, teen pregnancy, long-term care, and other issues fell to public health, as did several emerging problems, most notably the epidemics of violence and HIV infections, including acquired immune deficiency syndrome (AIDS). The public health agenda expanded even further as a result of the recent national dialogue over health reform and how health services will be organized and managed. Bioterrorism preparedness is an even more recent addition to this agenda amidst heightened concerns and expectations after the events of September 11, 2001 and the anthrax attacks the following month.

Link with Government

A fourth unique facet of public health is its link with government. Although public health is far more than the activities of federal, state, and local health departments, many people think only of governmental public health agencies when they think of public health. Government does play a unique role in seeing that the key elements are in place and that public health's mission gets addressed. Only government can exercise the enforcement provisions of our public policies that limit the personal and property rights of individuals and corporations in areas such as retail food establishments, sewage and water systems, occupational health and safety, consumer product safety, infectious disease control, and drug efficacy and safety. Government also can play the convener and facilitator role for identifying and prioritizing health problems that might be addressed through public resources and actions. These roles derive from the underlying principle of beneficence, in that government exists to improve the well-being of its members. Beneficence often involves a balance between maximizing benefits and minimizing harms on the one hand and doing no harm on the other.

Two general strategies are available for governmental efforts to influence public health. At the broadest level, governments can modify public policies that influence health through social and environmental conditions, such as policies for education, employment, housing, public safety, child welfare, pollution control, workplace safety, and family support. In line with the IOM report's definition of public health, these actions seek to ensure conditions in which people can be healthy. Another strategy of government is to directly provide programs and services that are designed to meet the health needs of the population. It is often easier to garner support for relatively small-scale programs directed toward a specific problem (such as tuberculosis or HIV infections) than to achieve consensus around broader health and social issues. This strategy is basically a "command-and-control" approach, in which government attempts to increase access to and utilization of services largely through deployment of its own resources rather than through working with others. A variation of this strategy for government is to ensure access to health care services through public financing approaches (Medicare and Medicaid are prime examples) or through specialized delivery systems (such as the Veterans Administration facilities, the Indian Health Service, and federally funded community health centers).

Whereas the United States has generally opted for the latter of these strategies, other countries have acted to place greater emphasis on broader social policies. Both the overall level of investment for and relative emphasis between these strategies contribute to the widely varying results achieved in terms of health status indicators among different nations (to be discussed in Chapter 2).

Many factors dictate the approaches used by a specific government at any point in time. These factors include history, culture, the structure of the government in question, and current social circumstances. There are also several underlying motivations that support government intervention. For paternalistic reasons, governments may act to control or restrict the liberties of individuals to benefit a group, whether or not that group seeks these benefits. For utilitarian reasons, governments intervene because of the perception that the state as a whole will benefit in some important way. For equality considerations, governments act to ensure that benefits and burdens are equally distributed among individuals. For equity considerations, governments justify interventions in order to distribute the benefits of society in proportion to need. These motivations reflect the views of each society as to whether health itself or merely access to health services is to be considered a right of individuals and populations within that society. Many societies, including the United States, act through government to ensure equal access to a broad array of preventive and treatment services. Equity in health status for all groups within the society may not be an explicit aspiration, however, even where efforts are in place to ensure equality in access. Even more important for achieving equity in health status are concerted efforts to improve health status in population groups with the greatest disadvantage, mechanisms to monitor health status and contributing factors across all population groups, and participation of disadvantaged population groups in the key political decision-making processes within the society.[16] To the extent that equity in health status among all population groups does not guide actions of a society's government, these other elements will be only marginally effective.

As noted previously, the link between government and public health makes for a particularly precarious situation for governmental public health agencies. The conflicting value systems of public health and the wider community generally translate into public health agencies having to document their failure in order to make progress. It is said that only the squeaky wheel gets the grease; in public health, it often takes an outbreak, disaster, or other tragedy to demonstrate public health's value. Since 1985 increased funding for basic public health protection programs quickly followed outbreaks related to bacteria-contaminated milk in Illinois, tainted hamburgers in Washington state, and contaminated public water supplies in Milwaukee. Following concerns over preparedness of public health agencies to deal with bioterrorism and other public health threats, a massive infusion of federal funding occurred.

The assumption and delegation of public health responsibilities are quite complex in the United States, with different patterns in each of the 50 states (to be described in Chapter 4). Over recent decades, the concept of a governmental presence in health has emerged and gained widespread acceptance within the public health community. This concept characterizes the role of local government, often, but not necessarily always, operating through its official health agencies, which serve as the residual guarantors that needed services will actually be there when needed. In practice it means that, no matter how duties are assigned locally, there is a presence that ensures that health needs are identified and considered for collective action. We will return to this concept and how it is operationalized in Chapter 5.

Grounded in Science

One of the most unique aspects of public health—and one that continues to separate public health from many other social movements—is its grounding in science.[17] This relationship is clear for the medical and physical sciences that govern our understanding of the biologic aspects of humans, microorganisms, and vectors, as well as the risks present in our physical environments. However, it is also true for the social sciences of anthropology, sociology, and psychology that affect our understanding of human culture and behaviors influencing health and illness. The quantitative sciences of epidemiology and biostatistics remain essential tools and methods of public health practice. Often five basic sciences of public health are identified: epidemiology, biostatistics, environmental science, management sciences, and behavioral sciences. These constitute the core education of public health professionals.

The importance of a solid and diverse scientific base is both a strength and weakness of public health. Surely there is no substitute for science in the modern world. The public remains curiously attracted to scientific advances, at least in the physical and biologic sciences, and this base is important to market and promote public health interventions. For many years epidemiology has been touted as the basic science of public health practice, suggesting that public health itself is applied epidemiology. Modern public health thinking views epidemiology less as the basic science of public health than as one of many contributors to a complex undertaking. In recent decades knowledge from the social sciences has greatly enriched and supplemented the physical and biologic sciences. Yet these are areas less familiar to and perhaps less well appreciated by the public, making it difficult to garner public support for newer, more behaviorally mediated public health interventions. The old image of public health based on the scientific principles of environmental sanitation and communicable disease control is being superseded by a new image of public health approaches more grounded in what the public perceives to be "softer" science. This transition, at least temporarily, threatens public understanding and confidence in public health and its methods.

Focus on Prevention

If public health professionals were pressed to provide a one word synonym for public health, the most frequent response would probably be *prevention*. In general, prevention characterizes actions that are taken to reduce the possibility that something will happen or in hopes of minimizing the damage that may occur if it does happen. Prevention is a widely appreciated and valued concept that is best understood when its object is identified. Although prevention is considered by many to be the purpose of public health, the specific intentions of prevention can vary greatly. Prevention can be aimed at deaths, hospital admissions, days lost from school, consumption of human and fiscal resources, and many other ends. There are as many targets for prevention as there are various health outcomes and effects to be avoided.

Prevention efforts often lack a clear constituency because success results in unseen consequences. Because these consequences are unseen, people are less likely to develop an attachment for or support the efforts preventing them. Advocates for such causes as mental health services, care for individuals with developmental disabilities, and organ transplants often make their presence felt. However, few state capitols have seen candlelight demonstrations by thousands of people who did not get diphtheria. This invisible constituency for prevention is partly a result of the interdisciplinary nature of public health. With no predominant discipline, it is even more difficult for people to understand and appreciate the work of public health. From one perspective, the undervaluation of public health is understandable; the majority of the beneficiaries of recent and current public health prevention efforts have not yet been born! Despite its lack of recognition, prevention as a strategy has been remarkably successful and appears to offer great potential for future success, as well. Later chapters will explore this potential in greater depth.

Uncommon Culture

The final unique feature of public health to be discussed here appears to be both a strength and weakness. The tie that binds public health professionals is neither a common preparation through education and training nor a common set of work experiences and work settings. Public health is unique in that the common link is a set of intended outcomes toward which many different sciences, arts, and methods can contribute. As a result, public health professionals include anthropologists, sociologists, psychologists, physicians, nurses, nutritionists, lawyers, economists, political scientists, social workers, laboratorians, managers, sanitarians, engineers, epidemiologists, biostatisticians, gerontologists, disability specialists, and dozens of other professions and disciplines. All are bound to common ends, and all employ somewhat different perspectives from their diverse education, training, and work experiences. "Whatever it takes to get the job done" is the theme, suggesting that the basic task is one of problem solving around health issues. This aspect of public health is the foundation for strategies and methods that rely heavily on collaborations and partnerships.

This multidisciplinary and interdisciplinary approach is unique among professions, calling into question whether public health is really a profession at all. There are several strong arguments that public health is not a profession. There is no minimum credential or training that distinguishes public health professionals from either other professionals or nonprofessionals. Only a tiny proportion of those who work in organizations dedicated to improving the health of the public possesses one of the academic public health degrees (the master's of public health degree and several other master's and doctoral degrees granted by schools of public health and other institutions). With the vast majority of public health workers not formally trained in public health, it is difficult to characterize its workforce as a profession. In many respects it is more reasonable to view public health as a movement than as a profession.

VALUE OF PUBLIC HEALTH

How can we measure the value of public health efforts? This question is addressed both directly and indirectly throughout this text. Later chapters will examine the dimensions of public health's value in terms of lives saved and diseases prevented, as well as in dollars and cents. Nonetheless, some initial information will set the stage for greater detail later.

Public opinion polls conducted in recent years suggest that public health is highly valued in the United States.[18] The overwhelming majority of the public rated a variety of key public health services as "very important." Specifically,

- 91 percent of all adults believe that prevention of the spread of infectious diseases such as tuberculosis, measles, flu, and AIDS is very important
- 88 percent also believe that conducting research into the causes and prevention of disease is very important
- 87 percent believe that immunization to prevent diseases is very important
- 86 percent believe that ensuring that people are not exposed to unsafe water, air pollution, or toxic waste is very important
- 85 percent believe that it is very important to work to reduce death and injuries from violence
- 68 percent believe that it is important to encourage people to live healthier lifestyles, to eat well, and not to smoke
- 66 percent believe that it is important to work to reduce death and injuries from accidents at work, in the home, and on the streets

In a related poll conducted in 1999, the Pew Charitable Trusts found that 46 percent of all Americans thought that "public health/protecting populations from disease" was more important than "medicine/treating people who are sick." Almost 30 percent thought medicine was more important than public health; 22 percent said both were equally important, and 3 percent had no opinion. Public opinion surveys suggest that public health's contributions to health and quality of life have not gone unnoticed. Other assessments of the value of public health support this contention.

In 1965 McKeown concluded that "health has advanced significantly only since the late eighteenth century and until recently owed little to medical advances."[19] This conclusion is bolstered by more recent studies that found public health's prevention efforts are responsible for 25 years of the nearly 30-year improvement in life expectancy at birth in the United States since 1900. This bold claim is based on evidence that only 5 years of the 30-year improvement are the result of medical care.[20] Of these 5 years, medical treatment accounts for 3.7 years, and clinical preventive services (such as immunizations and screening tests) account for 1.5 years. The remaining 25 years have resulted largely from prevention efforts in the form of social policies, community actions, and personal decisions. Many of these decisions and actions targeted infectious diseases affecting infants and children early in the century. Later in the century, gains in life expectancy have also been achieved through reductions in chronic diseases affecting adults.

Many notable public health achievements have occurred during the twentieth century. Each chapter of this text will highlight one or more of these achievements to illustrate the value of public health to American society in the twenty-first century by telling the story of its accomplishments in the preceding century. The first of these chronicles the prevention and control of infectious diseases in twentieth-century America (see "Public Health Achievements in Twentieth-Century America: Prevention and Control of Infectious Disease," later in this chapter).

The value of public health in our society can be described in human terms as well as by public opinion, statistics of infections prevented, and values in dollars and cents. A poignant example dates from the 1950s, when the United States was in the midst of a terrorizing polio epidemic (Exhibit 1–7). Few communities were spared during the periodic onslaughts of this serious disease during the first half of the twentieth century in America. Public fear was so great that public libraries, community swimming pools, and other group activities were closed during the summers when the disease was most feared. Biomedical research had discovered a possible weapon against epidemic polio in the form of the Salk vaccine, however, which was developed in 1954 and licensed for

---

Exhibit 1–7 The Value of Public Health: Fear of Polio, United States, 1950s

"I can remember no experience more horrifying than watching by the bedside of my five-year-old stricken with polio. The disease attacked his right leg, and we watched helplessly as his limb steadily weakened. On the third day, the doctor told us that he would survive and that paralysis was the worst he would suffer. I was grateful, although I continued to agonize about whether my wife and unborn child would be affected. What a blessing that no other parent will have to endure the terror that my wife and I and thousands of others shared that August."—Morton Chapman, Sarasota, Florida

Source: Reprinted from *For a Healthy Nation: Returns on Investments in Public-Health,* 1994, U.S. Public Health Service.

Example

Public Health Achievements in Twentieth-Century America: Prevention and Control of Infectious Diseases

Prior to 1900, infectious diseases represented the most serious threat to the health of populations across the globe. The twentieth century witnessed a dramatic shift in the balance of power in the centuries-long battle between humans and microorganisms. Changes in both science and social values contributed to the assault on microbes, setting into motion the forces of organized community efforts to improve the health of the public. This approach served as a model for later public health initiatives targeting other major threats to health and well-being.

Deaths from infectious diseases have declined markedly in the United States during the twentieth century (Figure 1–3). This decline contributed to a sharp drop in infant and child mortality and to the 29.2-year increase in life expectancy. In 1900, 30.4 percent of all deaths occurred among children aged less than 5 years; in 1997, that percentage was only 1.4 percent. In 1900, the three leading causes of death were pneumonia, tuberculosis (TB), and diarrhea and enteritis, which (together with diphtheria) caused one-third of all deaths. Of these deaths, 40 percent were among children aged less than 5 years. In 1997, heart disease and cancers accounted for 54.7 percent of all deaths, with 4.5 percent attributable to pneumonia, influenza, and HIV infection. Despite this overall progress, one of the most devastating epidemics in human history occurred during the twentieth century—the 1918 influenza pandemic that resulted in 20 million deaths, including 500,000 in the United States, in less than 1 year. These total more than have died in as short a time during any war or famine in the world. HIV infection, first recognized in 1981, has caused a pandemic that is still in progress, affecting 33 million people and causing an estimated 13.9 million deaths. These episodes illustrate the volatility of infectious disease death rates and the unpredictability of disease emergence.

Public health action to control infectious diseases is based on the nineteenth-century discovery of microorganisms as the cause of many serious diseases (e.g., cholera and TB). Disease control resulted from improvements in sanitation and hygiene, the discovery of antibiotics, and the implementation of universal childhood vaccination programs. Scientific and technologic advances played a major role in each of these areas and are the foundation for today's disease surveillance and control systems. Scientific findings also have contributed to a new understanding of the evolving relation between humans and microbes.

At the beginning of the twentieth century, infectious diseases were widely prevalent in the United States and exacted an enormous toll on the population (Table 1–1). In 1900, for example, 21,064 smallpox cases

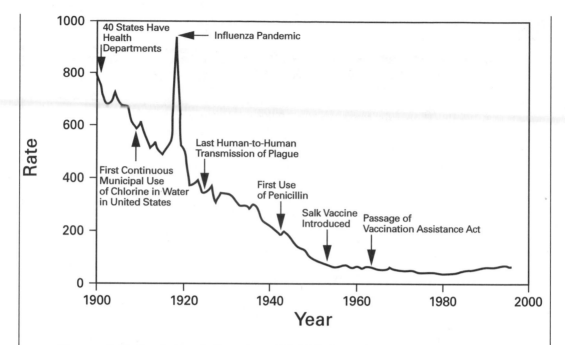

Figure 1–3 Crude Death Rate (per 100,000) for Infectious Diseases—United States, 1900–1996. *Source:* Reprinted from Public Health Achievements, United States, 1900–1999; Control of Infectious Diseases, *Morbidity and Mortality Weekly Report,* Vol. 48, No. 29, pp. 621–629, the Centers for Disease Control and Prevention, 1999.

were reported, and 894 patients died. In 1920, there were 469,924 measles cases reported, and 7,575 patients died; 147,991 diphtheria cases were reported, and 13,170 patients died. In 1922, the total number of pertussis cases reported was 107,473, and 5,099 patients died.

The nineteenth-century shift in population from country to city that accompanied industrialization and immigration led to overcrowding in poor housing served by inadequate or nonexistent public water supplies and waste-disposal systems. These conditions resulted in repeated outbreaks of cholera, dysentery, TB, typhoid fever, influenza, yellow fever, and malaria.

By 1900, however, the incidence of many of these diseases had begun to decline because of public health improvements, implementation of which continued into the twentieth century. Local, state, and federal efforts to improve sanitation and hygiene reinforced the concept of collective "public health" action (e.g., to prevent infection by providing clean drinking water). By 1900, of the 45 states, 40 had established health departments. The first county health departments were established in 1908. From the 1930s through the 1950s, state and local health departments made substantial progress in disease prevention activities, including sewage disposal, water treatment, food safety, organized solid waste disposal, and public education about hygienic

Table 1–1 Baseline 20th-Century Annual Morbidity and 1998 Provisional Morbidity from Nine Diseases with Vaccines Recommended before 1990 for Universal Use for Children, United States

Disease	Baseline 20th-Century Annual Morbidity	1998 Morbidity (Provisional)	Percent Decrease
Smallpox	48,164	0	100%
Diphtheria	175,885	1	100%
Pertussis	147,271	6,279	95.7%
Tetanus	1,314	34	97.4%
Poliomyelitis (paralytic)	16,316	0	100%
Measles	503,282	89	100%
Mumps	152,209	606	99.6%
Rubella	47,745	345	99.3%
Congenital rubella syndrome	823	5	99.4%
Haemophilus influenzae type b infection	20,000	54	99.7%

Source: Reprinted from Public Health Achievements, United States, 1900–1999: Impact of Vaccines Universally Recommended for Children, *Morbidity and Mortality Weekly Report*, Vol. 48, No. 12, pp. 243–248, the Centers for Disease Control and Prevention, 1999.

practices (e.g., food handling and hand washing). Chlorination and other treatments of drinking water began in the early 1900s and became widespread public health practices, further decreasing the incidence of water-borne diseases. The incidence of TB also declined as improvements in housing reduced crowding and TB control programs were initiated. In 1900, of every 100,000 U.S. residents, 194 died from TB; most were residents of urban areas. In 1940 (before the introduction of antibiotic therapy), TB remained a leading cause of death, but the crude death rate had decreased to 46 per 100,000 persons.

Animal and pest control also contributed to disease reduction. Nationally sponsored, state-coordinated vaccination and animal-control programs eliminated dog-to-dog transmission of rabies. Malaria, once endemic throughout the southeastern United States, was reduced to negligible levels by the late 1940s; regional mosquito-control programs played an important role in these efforts. Plague also diminished; the U.S. Marine Hospital Service (which later became the Public Health Service) led quarantine and ship inspection activities and rodent-and vector-control operations. The last major rat-associated outbreak of plague in the United States occurred during 1924–1925 in Los Angeles. This outbreak included the last identified instance of human-to-human transmission of plague (through inhalation of infectious respiratory droplets from coughing patients) in this country.

In 1900, few effective treatment and preventive measures existed to prevent infectious diseases. Although the first vaccine against smallpox was developed in 1796, more than 100 years later, its use had not been widespread enough to control the disease fully. Four other vaccines— against rabies, typhoid, cholera, and plague—had been developed late in the nineteenth century but were not used widely by 1900.

Since 1900, vaccines have been developed or licensed against 21 other diseases. Ten of these vaccines have been recommended for use only in selected populations at high risk because of area of residence, age, medical condition, or risk behaviors. The other 11 have been recommended for use in all U.S. children.

During the twentieth century, substantial achievements have been made in the control of many vaccine-preventable diseases. Smallpox has been eradicated, poliomyelitis caused by wild-type viruses has been eliminated, and measles and *Haemophilus influenzae* type b (Hib) invasive disease among children aged less than 5 years have been reduced to record low numbers of cases.

National efforts to promote vaccine use among all children began with the appropriation of federal funds for polio vaccination after introduction of the vaccine in 1955. Since then, federal, state, and local governments and public and private health-care providers have collaborated to develop and maintain the vaccine-delivery system in the United States. Dramatic declines in morbidity have been reported for the nine vaccine-preventable diseases for which vaccination was universally recommended for use in children before 1990 (excluding hepatitis B, rotavirus, and varicella). Morbidity associated with smallpox and polio caused by wild-type viruses has declined 100 percent and nearly 100 percent for each of the other seven diseases.

Penicillin was developed into a widely available medical product that provided quick and complete treatment of previously incurable bacterial illnesses, with a wider range of targets and fewer side effects than sulfa drugs. Discovered fortuitously in 1928, penicillin was not developed for medical use until the 1940s, when it was produced in substantial quantities and used by the U.S. military to treat sick and wounded soldiers.

Technologic changes that increased capacity for detecting, diagnosing, and monitoring infectious diseases included development early in the century of serologic testing and, more recently, the development of molecular assays based on nucleic acid and antibody probes. The use of computers and electronic forms of communication enhanced the ability to gather, analyze, and disseminate disease surveillance data.

During the last quarter of the twentieth century, molecular biology has provided powerful new tools to detect and characterize infectious pathogens. The use of nucleic acid hybridization and sequencing techniques has made it possible to characterize the causative agents of previously unknown diseases (e.g., hepatitis C, human ehrlichiosis, hantavirus pulmonary syndrome, AIDS, and Nipah virus disease). Molecular tools have enhanced capacity to track the transmission of new threats and find new ways to prevent and treat them. Had AIDS emerged 100 years ago, when laboratory-based diagnostic methods were in their infancy, the disease might have remained a mysterious syndrome for many decades. Moreover, the drugs used to treat HIV-infected persons and prevent perinatal transmission (e.g., replication analogues and protease inhibitors) were developed based on a modern understanding of retroviral replication at the molecular level.

Source: Adapted from Public Health Achievements, United States, 1900–1999: Impact of Vaccines Universally Recommended for Children, *Morbidity and Mortality Weekly Report,* Vol. 48, No. 12, pp. 243–248, the Centers for Disease Control and Prevention, 1999; and Public Health Achievements, United States, 1900–1999: Control of Infectious Diseases, *Morbidity and Mortality Weekly Report,* Vol. 48, No. 29, pp. 621–629, the Centers for Disease Control and Prevention, 1999.

use one year later. A massive and unprecedented campaign to immunize the public was quickly undertaken, setting the stage for a triumph of public health. The real triumph came in a way that might not have been expected, however, because soon into the campaign, isolated reports of vaccine-induced polio were identified in Chicago and California. Within two days of the initial case reports, action by governmental public health organizations at all levels resulted in the determination that these cases could be traced to one particular manufacturer. This determination was made only a few hours before the same vaccine was to be provided to hundreds of thousands of California children. The result was prevention of a disaster and rescue of the credibility of an immunization campaign that has virtually cut this disease off at its knees. The campaign proceeded on schedule and, five decades later, wild poliovirus has been eradicated from the western hemisphere.

Similar examples have occurred throughout history. The battle against diphtheria is a case in point. A major cause of death in 1900, diphtheria infections are virtually unheard of today. This achievement cannot be traced solely to advances in bacteriology and the antitoxins and immunizations that were deployed against this disease. Neither was it defeated by brilliant political and programmatic initiatives led by public health experts. It was the confluence of scientific advances and public perception of the disease itself that resulted in diphtheria's demise as a threat to entire populations. These forces shaped public health policies and the effectiveness of intervention strategies. In the end, diphtheria made some practices and politics possible, while it constrained others.[21] The story is one of science, social values, and public health.

CONCLUSION

Public health evokes different images for different people, and, even to the same people, it can mean different things in different contexts. The intent of this chapter has been to describe some of the common perceptions of public health in the United States. Is it a complex, dynamic, social enterprise, akin to a movement? Or is it best characterized as a goal of the improved health outcomes and health status that can be achieved by the work of all of us, individually and collectively? Or is public health some collection of activities that move us ever closer toward our aspirations? Or is it the profession that includes all of those dedicated to its cause? Or is public health merely what we see coming out of our official governmental health agencies—a strange mix of safety-net medical services for the poor and a variety of often-invisible community prevention services?

Although it is tempting to consider expunging the term *public health* from our vocabularies because of the baggage associated with these various images, this would do little to address the obstacles to accomplishing our central task because public health encompasses all of these images and perhaps more!

Based on principles of social justice, inherently political in its processes, addressing a constantly expanding agenda of problems inextricably linked with government, grounded in science, and emphasizing preventive strategies, and with a work force bound by common aspirations, public health is unique in many ways. Its value, however, transcends its uniqueness. Public health efforts have been major contributors to recent improvements in health status and can contribute even more as we approach a new century with new challenges.

By carefully examining the various dimensions of the public health system in terms of its inputs, practices, outputs, and outcomes, we can gain insights into what it does, how it works, and how it can be improved. Better results do not come from setting new goals; they come from understanding and improving the processes that will then produce better outputs, in turn leading to better outcomes. This theme of understanding the public health system and public health practice as a necessary step toward its improvement will recur throughout this text.

DISCUSSION QUESTIONS AND EXERCISES

1. What definition of public health best describes public health in the twenty-first century?
2. To what extent has public health contributed to improvement in health status and quality of life over history?
3. What historical phenomena are most responsible for the development of public health responses?
4. Which features of public health make it different from other fields? Which features are most unique and distinctive? Which is most important?
5. Because of your interest in a public health career, a producer working at a local television station has asked you to provide input into the development of a video explaining public health to the general public. What themes or messages would you suggest for this video? How would you propose presenting or packaging these messages?
6. There is little written in history books about public health problems and responses, suggesting that these issues have had little impact on history. Consider the European colonization of the Americas, beginning in the sixteenth century. How was it possible for Cortez and other European figures to overcome immense Native American cultures with millions of people? What role, if any, did public health themes and issues play?

7. Choose a relatively recent (within the last 3 years) occurrence/ event that has drawn significant media attention to a public health issue or problem (e.g., bioterrorism, contaminated meat products, tobacco settlement, hurricane, flooding). Have different under- standings of what public health is influenced public, as well as gov- ernmental responses to this event? If so, in what ways?

8. Review the history of public health activities in Chicago from 1834 to 2003 in Appendix 1-A and describe how public health strategies and interventions have changed over time in the United States. What influences were most responsible for these changes? Does this suggest that public health functions have changed over time, as well?

9. Access the National Library of Medicine website <http://www.nlm. nih.gov> and conduct an online literature search of key words related to the definition, development, and current status of public health. Indicate the parameters used in this search and the general contents of the most useful article that you found.

10. Examine each of the websites listed below and become familiar with their general contents. Which ones are most useful for provid- ing information and insights related to the question, "What is pub- lic health?" Why? Are there other websites you would suggest adding to this list?

   - American Public Health Association <http://www.apha.org>
   - Association of State and Territorial Health Officials <http://www.astho.org>
   - National Association of County and City Health Officials <http://www.naccho.org>
   - Public Health Foundation <http://www.phf.org>
   - U.S. Department of Health and Human Services <http://www.dhhs.gov> and its various Public Health Service Agencies (Centers for Disease Control and Prevention <http://www.cdc.gov>, Food and Drug Administration <http://www.fda.gov>, Health Resources and Services Administration <http://www.hrsa.dhhs.gov>, National Institutes of Health <http://www.nih.gov>, Agency for Healthcare Research and Quality <http://www.ahrq.gov>, etc.)
   - U.S. Environmental Protection Agency <http://www.epa.gov>
   - State health departments, available through the ASTHO Website
   - Local health departments, available through the NACCHO, other national organizations, and state health department Websites
   - Association of Schools of Public Health <http://www.asph.org> and individual schools, available through the ASPH Website

REFERENCES

1. Winslow CEA. Public health at the crossroads. *Am J Public Health*. 1926;16:1075–1085.
2. Hinman A. Eradication of vaccine-preventable diseases. *Ann Rev Public Health*. 1999;20:211–229.
3. *For a Healthy Nation: Returns on Investment in Public Health*. Washington, DC: U.S. Public Health Service (PHS); 1994.
4. McNeil WH. *Plagues and Peoples*. New York: Doubleday; 1977.
5. Paneth N, Vinten-Johansen P, Brody H. A rivalry of foulness: Official and unofficial investigations of the London cholera epidemic of 1854. *Am J Public Health*. 1998;88:1545–1553.
6. Hamlin C. Could you starve to death in England in 1839? The Chadwick-Farr controversy and the loss of the "social" in public health. *Am J Public Health*. 1995;85:856–866.
7. Institute of Medicine, National Academy of Sciences. *The Future of Public Health*. Washington, DC: National Academy Press; 1988.
8. Winslow CEA. The untilled field of public health. *Mod Med*. 920;2:183–191.
9. Vickers G. What sets the goals of public health? *Lancet*. 1958;1:599–604.
10. Baker EL, Melton RJ, Stange PV, et al. Health reform and the health of the public. *JAMA*. 1994;272:1276–1282.
11. Harrell JA, Baker EL. The essential services of public health. *Leadership Public Health*. 1994;3(3):27–30.
12. Handler A, Issel LM, Turnock BJ. A conceptual framework to measure performance of the public health system. *Am J Public Health*. 2001;91(8):1235–1239.
13. Public Health Functions Steering Committee. *Public Health in America*. Washington, DC: PHS; 1995.
14. Krieger N, Brin AE. A vision of social justice as the foundation of public health: Commemorating 150 years of the spirit of 1848. *Am J Public Health*. 1998;88:1603–1606.
15. Beauchamp DE. Public health as social justice. *Inquiry*. 1976;13(1):3–14.
16. Susser M. Health as a human right: An epidemiologist's perspective on public health. *Am J Public Health*. 1993;83:418–426.
17. Afifi AA, Breslow L. The maturing paradigm of public health. *Ann Rev Public Health*. 1994;15:223–235.
18. Harris Polls. *Public Opinion about Public Health, United States. 1999*.
19. McKeown T. *Medicine in Modern Society*. London, England: Allen & Unwin; 1965.
20. Bunker JP, Frazier HS, Mosteller F. Improving health: Measuring effects of medical care. *Milbank Q*. 1994;72:225–258.
21. Hammonds EM. *Childhood's Deadly Scourge: The Campaign to Control Diphtheria in New York City, 1880–1930*. Baltimore, MD: Johns Hopkins University Press; 1999.

Selected History of Public Health Activities in Chicago, 1834–2003

1834	A temporary board of health was formed to fight the threat of cholera.
1835	Chicago Board of Health established by the state legislature to secure the general health of the inhabitants because of the threat of cholera epidemic. Chicago, then a town, had an estimated 3,265 residents.
1837	Chicago incorporated as a city of 4,170 residents. Three health commissioners and a health officer named to inspect marketplaces, prepare death certificates, construct a pesthouse, visit persons suffering from infectious diseases in their homes, and board vessels in the harbor to check on the health of crews.
1841	Vital statistics start in a limited way with collection of data (age, sex, disease) related to deaths; an ordinance requiring reports of death was passed but not enforced for several years.
1846	A committee of the Chicago Medical Society reported the mortality rates through 1850.
1848	First cooperative effort of the medical profession and city officials to prevent the spread of smallpox as physicians volunteer to vaccinate the poor without charge.
1849	Cholera brought to Chicago by the emigrant boat John Drew from New Orleans, killing one in 36 of the entire population. A district health officer was appointed for each city block.
1851	A new city charter provided greater powers in health matters to the City Council. In the mid-1850s, with the city free from smallpox and cholera, the powers of the Board of Health were reduced accordingly.
1855	Sewerage became an issue; Board of Sewerage Commissioners was appointed and the first sewers were constructed the following year. The quarantine placard introduced with signs reading "Smallpox Here" after 30 die of the disease.
1857	The financial depression of 1857 caused the Board of Health to be viewed as a luxury; it was abolished and its duties were transferred to the Police Department. New permanent City Hospital completed at cost of $75,000. (Later taken over by Cook County Hospital as one of its earlier buildings.)

1862   Smallpox outbreak caused the City Council to appoint a Health Officer to work with the Police Department, but severely circumscribed tenure and duties rendered the position meaningless.

1867   A new Board of Health was established in response to the 1866 cholera outbreak with authority independent of the City Council and Police Department.

1868   Meat inspection initiated at Union Stock Yards.

1869   The Board of Health required vaccination of all children.

1870   First milk ordinance making it illegal to sell skim milk unless so labeled.

1871   Help given to refugees of Chicago Fire; camps of homeless inspected; and controls initiated for food supply and epidemic prevention. Birth and death records lost in the fire.

1872   In aftermath of the Great Fire, death rate increased 32.6 percent to 27.6 deaths per 1,000 persons. Smallpox attacked 2,382 and killed 655. Fatalities among children under five were the highest ever recorded. (For the period 1843 to 1872, children under five accounted for half of all deaths occurring in the city.)

1876   The health functions of city government were reorganized under a department of health, and Commissioner of Health position was established.

1877   Commissioner of Health required the reporting of contagious diseases by physicians, a move opposed by many physicians.

1885   A cholera and typhoid epidemic kills 90,000 Chicagoans when a heavy storm washes sewage into Lake Michigan, the city's source of drinking water.

1888   Chicago Visiting Nurse Association was founded.

1889   Drainage and plumbing regulations issued, and five women inspectors of tenements appointed.

1890   Garbage disposal was placed under the direction of a general sanitary officer in the health department.

1892   Full milk inspection starts. Laws requiring reporting of communicable diseases existed; however, doctors argued they should receive payments for reporting as they received under state law for reporting births. Without this reimbursement, many physicians refused to comply and were prosecuted.

1893   Bacteriological laboratory opens to conduct microscopic examinations of milk samples and examine throat cultures for diphtheria. A "Boil the Water" crusade against typhoid was conducted.

1893/94 Last smallpox epidemic to cause great loss of life (1,033 died in its second year). Vigorous vaccination efforts (1,084,500 given) result in a reduction of cases to seven in 1897. During this period, the department was the first to proclaim the superiority of hermetically sealed glycerinated vaccine. Circulars distributed on hot weather care of babies in one of the first public education efforts. The Health Department began publishing a Monthly Statement of Mortality.

1895   The first diphtheria antitoxin issued, and a corps of antitoxin administrators appointed. Daily analysis of water supply inaugurated.

1896   Medical school inspections inaugurated—the second city in the U.S. to do so. Rules regulating the practice of midwifery were promulgated.

1899   Campaign against infant mortality enlists support of a voluntary corps of 73 physicians.

1900   Sanitary engineers reverse the flow of the Chicago River to prevent a recurrence of epidemics, giving the city the world's only river that runs backward. Department publishes a study reporting that the average span of life in Chicago more than doubled in a generation.

1901   Ordinance passed prohibiting spitting in public places. The Health Department began publishing State of the City's Health every week in the newspapers; Monthly Statement of Mortality was discontinued.

1902   Milk Commission of Chicago was established to ensure pasteurized milk was made available for needy children; dairy inspections were started with the salaries of two dairy inspectors initially paid for by the Chicago Civic Federation. Fourth of July "Don'ts" were first promulgated to prevent accidents.

1903   A Tuberculosis Committee of the Visiting Nurse Association was established; it reorganized in 1906 as the Chicago Tuberculosis Institute.

1905   The 39th Street intercepting sewer opens, resulting in a marked decrease in typhoid deaths.

1906   City Council passed an ordinance providing for the licensing and control of restaurants.

1907   Chicago Tuberculosis Institute opened dispensaries for the diagnosis and treatment of TB cases.

1908   Full communicable disease program inaugurated, and 100 physicians sent to congested districts during July and August to instruct mothers in baby care. Forty nurses loaned to the department by the Visiting Nurses Association of Chicago to help in a scarlet fever epidemic. They were so effective that the City Council appropriated funds to hire the department's first nurses to work in maternal and child welfare and communicable and venereal diseases.

1909   Chicago became first city in the United States to adopt a compulsory milk pasteurization ordinance. Public health nurses from the Board of Health, Visiting Nurse Association, and United Charities collaborate to become "finders of sick infants" and referred these babies and their mothers to tent camps where treatment was provided and hygiene classes held.

1910   Municipal Social Hygiene Clinic established, and dispensaries required to report venereal diseases. New milk standards applied to ice cream. Health Department nurses were assigned to conduct intensive follow-up on babies in hospital wards where infant death rates were high; the Infant Welfare Society was organized as the successor to the Milk Commission.

1911   Common drinking cups and common roller towels prohibited by ordinance.

1912   Sterilization of Chicago's water begins, and within four years the entire supply is being treated, causing a dramatic decline in the city's typhoid fever rate—from second highest among the 20 largest U.S. cities in 1881 to the lowest by 1917.

1915   The Eastland, a lake excursion boat docked at the Clark Street bridge, rolls over while loaded with passengers; 812 die, 300 more than the Titanic. Dental services provided in Chicago public schools following a three-year introductory pilot program funded by a local philanthropist. The Municipal Tuberculosis Sanitarium opened.

1916   Policy initiated to hospitalize all cases of infantile paralysis (polio) after 34 patients died out of 254 afflicted.

1917   Municipal Contagious Disease Hospital established. New health ordinances range from requiring the reporting and treatment of venereal diseases to requiring the screening of residence, stables, and barns against fleas. Immunization against diphtheria with von Behring's toxin-antitoxin starts in public schools and institutions.

1918   Influenza becomes a reportable disease with the pandemic of influenza reaching Chicago, to cause 381 deaths on one day (October 17) alone.

1919   Department wins its first case in the prosecution of landlords for failure to provide sufficient heat to tenants.

1920   The right of the department to quarantine carriers of contagion was upheld in the Superior Court of Cook County.

1922   New Health Commissioner began a campaign against venereal disease, proposing education and distribution of prophylactic outfits in brothels; opposition from medical profession was based more on moral than medical grounds.

1923   Committee appointed on prenatal care in the first concerted effort to coordinate the activities of all agencies doing prenatal work in the city. Inspection of summer camps for children inaugurated. Venereal disease clinics were established at the Cook County Jail and House of Correction.

1924   Venereal disease prevention literature distributed to 500,000 homes in Chicago.

1925   Department institutes a regular schedule of home visits by nurses during the first six months of an infant's life. Conferences inaugurated for care of preschool children. Order installation of sanitary types of drinking fountains.

1927   Health Commissioner was forced to resign when mayor directs that the Health Department include political literature with information about baby care being distributed to all Chicago mothers.

1930   Intensive campaign against diphtheria results in 400,219 injections being given in three months.

1932   Staff of 300 nurses carried throughout the city on buses to give diphtheria inoculations. Physicians sent to the homes of mothers unable to take children to welfare stations for shots. After campaign, cases drop to 154 with nine deaths, compared to 1,266 cases with 68 deaths the previous year.

1933   Outbreak of amebic dysentery among out-of-town guests who came to the Century of Progress (1,409 cases and 98 deaths scattered in 43 states, the Territory of Hawaii, and three Canadian provinces) in the first recognized waterborne epidemic of the disease in a civilian population. Cause traced to water contamination through faulty plumbing.

1934   A plumbing survey for cross-connections in hotels and mercantile buildings begun to prevent future amebic dysentery outbreaks. As a result of drinking from contaminated water supply at the Union Stock Yards fire on May 19, 69 persons contract typhoid fever, 11 of whom die.

1935   Ordinance passed requiring that only Grade A milk and milk products can be sold in Chicago. A premature-infant welfare program initiated. A mother's milk station starts operating to supply breast milk to premature, sick, or debilitated infants whose parents could not afford this expense.

1936   Summer brings 210 deaths from sunstroke and exhaustion compared to 11 from the same cause in 1935. With 1,000 premature infants under supervision, two additional premature stations open, making 31 conferences available each week.

1937   Chicago public schools open three weeks late because of a polio scare. Chicago Syphilis Control Project established with the emphasis on breaking the chain of infection.

1942   Chicago Intensive Treatment Center for venereal disease launches an effort so successful that it wins a War Department commendation in 1943 and records a declining VD rate following World War II demobilization, in contrast to soaring rates in other large cities.

1946   Chicago-Cook County health survey undertaken by US Public Health Service, including an audit of all city and county facilities conducted by outside experts. Various recommendations made, including more food inspection staff, establishment of district health centers, restructuring of the Board of Health with an executive director and deputies in charge of engineering, preventive medicine, and district health services.

1947   Mental Health section for Health Department was approved.

1948   A federal grant of $46,270 is made available through the state to subsidize a psychiatric program. Comprehensive food ordinance adopted by the City Council.

1952   Chicago counts 1,203 cases of polio, including 82 deaths and hundreds of persons with paralysis. Frightened parents keep their youngsters out of movies and swimming pools. Beaches close. Insect and rodent control program starts.

1955   Chicago is one of the first cities in the U.S. to introduce Salk vaccine after it is pronounced safe and effective against the polio virus on April 12.

1956   With warning signs of an approaching polio epidemic, mass inoculations of Salk vaccine given in all parts of the city with department
staff working in vacant stores, garages, street corners, from the backs
of trucks, and in park fieldhouses. Chicago takes the lead among
major American cities in introducing a water fluoridation program,
which reduces tooth decay among children.

1957   Nursing Home Section and Hospital Inspection Unit initiated.

1958   A section for chronic illness is activated, with mental health as one of
its activities.

1959   First Community Mental Health Center started on South Side.

1960   Bureau of Institutional Care consolidates nursing home and hospital
inspection services.

1961   Division of Adult Health and Aging begins consolidating activities of
chronic diseases, cardiovascular diseases, diabetes, cervical cancer,
rheumatic heart fever, and nutrition. A lead poison survey begins on
Chicago's West Side.

1962   Mental Health division, with more than 15 community-based mental
health centers, is established in the Health Department.

1965   Family planning initiated in limited number of clinics.

1966   Testing for sickle cell initiated; citywide lead poisoning screening and
treatment began.

1968   Planning for Comprehensive Neighborhood Health Centers in 4 areas
began in cooperation with Chicago Model Cities program.

1970   First Model Cities Neighborhood Health Center opened in Uptown. A
record 1.2 million inoculations were provided for Chicago children in
immunization drive.

1973   Englewood Neighborhood Health Center opened. 40 hospitals
approved as trauma centers in accordance with state statute on emergency medical services.

1974   Women, Infant and Children (WIC) supplemental nutrition program
initiated. Senior citizen clinic and new hypertension center open
while plans were unveiled to phase out the TB Sanitarium.

1975   City Council revised the municipal code to delineate the duties of the
9-member Board of Health as a policy making body and the Department of Health as the agency administering health programs and
enforcing regulations. Outpatient TB services were decentralized to 5
health centers.

1976   Health Department formed interdisciplinary committee on child
abuse with representatives from health, law enforcement, and welfare
agencies.

1981   Chicago Alcohol Treatment Center comes under jurisdiction of
Health Department only to be closed several years later with its funding used to support community-based providers of substance abuse
treatment services. Refugee health program was initiated.

1983   Chicago Area AIDS Task Force was established and the Health Department creates an AIDS Activity Office.

1984   Partnerships in Health program was initiated with hospitals to assure continuity of care for Health Department patients.

1985   Health Department sponsors city's first major pastoral conference on religion and health.

1986   Infant mortality reduction strategic plan developed.

1987   The first child lead poisoning death in nearly a decade leads to the establishment of the Mayor's Task Force on Lead Poisoning.

1989   Health Department coordinates development of Chicago AIDS Strategic Plan through a multidisciplinary advisory council of 125 individuals.

1990   Chicago/Cook County Health Care Summit produces plan to improve local delivery of health services, calling for ambulatory care reforms, restructuring of inpatient care, and changes in system financing. As a result, the Chicago and Cook County Ambulatory Care Council is established to assess health needs and undertake initiatives.

1991   Epidemiology Office is established in the Health Department.

1995   Extreme heat conditions in Chicago during July result in 514 heat-related deaths. Violence Prevention Office is established.

1997   City Council passes Managed Care Consumer Protection ordinance, calling for the Health Department to create an Office of Managed Care—the nation's first municipal effort to monitor the managed care industry.

1998   Health Department coordinates development of Chicago Violence Prevention Strategic Plan, developed by more than 150 participants.

1999   Chicago Turning Point Partnership convenes to develop a plan to strengthen the public health infrastructure in Chicago.

2001   Bioterrorism Preparedness unit established.

2002   Health Department receives federal grant for bioterrorism preparedness and response.

2003   Chicago participates in national bioterrorism response exercise involving top officials of city, state, and federal government (TOPOFF-2).

Sources: 150 Years of Municipal Health Care in the City of Chicago: Board of Health, Department of Health 1835–1985. Chicago Department of Health, 1985; Medicine in Chicago: 1850–1950, chapter in *The Social and Scientific Development of a City*, TN Bonner; *The Rise and Fall of Disease in Illinois*, Illinois Department of Public Health, 1927.

Chapter 2

Understanding and Measuring Health

The twenty-first century began much like its predecessor did, with immense opportunities to advance the public's health through actions to assure conditions favorable for health and quality of life. All systems direct their efforts toward certain outcomes; they track progress by ensuring that these outcomes are clearly defined and measurable. In public health, this calls for clear definitions and measures of health and quality of life in populations. That task is the focus of this chapter. Key questions to be addressed are:

- What is health?
- What factors influence health and illness?
- How can health status and quality of life be measured?
- What do current measures tell us about the health status and quality of life of Americans at the beginning of the twenty-first century?
- How can this information be used to develop effective public health interventions and public policy?

The relevance of these questions resides in their focus on factors that cause or influence particular health outcomes. Efforts to identify and measure key aspects of health and factors influencing health have relied on traditional approaches over the past century, although there are signs that this pattern may be changing. The key questions identified above will be addressed slightly out of order, for reasons that should become apparent as we proceed.

HEALTH IN THE UNITED STATES

Many important indicators of health status in the U.S. have improved considerably over the past century, although there is evidence that health status could be even better than it is. At the turn of the twentieth century, nearly 2 percent of the U.S. population died each year. The crude mortality rate in 1900 was about 1,700 deaths per 100,000 population. Life expectancy at birth was 47 years. Additional life expectancy at age 65 was another 12 years. Medicine and health care were largely proprietary in 1900 and of questionable benefit to health. More extensive information on the health status of the population at that time would be useful, but very little exists.

Indicators of health status improved in the U.S. throughout the twentieth century.[1] Between 1900 and 2000, the crude mortality rate was cut nearly in half to 872 per 100,000. By the year 2000 life expectancy at birth was nearly 77 years and life expectancy at age 65 was another 18 years.

The leading causes of death also changed dramatically over the twentieth century, as demonstrated in Figure 2–1. In 1900 the ten leading causes of death were: influenza and pneumonia; tuberculosis; diarrhea and related diseases; heart disease; stroke; chronic nephritis; accidents; cancer; perinatal conditions; and diphtheria. By the year 2000 tuberculosis, gastroenteritis, and diphtheria dropped off the list of the top 10 killers, and deaths from influenza and pneumonia fell from first to seventh position on the list. Diseases of aging and other chronic conditions superseded these infectious disease processes as changes in the age structure of the population, especially the increase in persons over age 65, resulted in higher overall crude rates for heart disease and cancer and the appearance of diabetes, Alzheimer's disease, chronic kidney conditions, and septicemia on the modern list of the top ten killers.

But changes in crude death rates only partly explain the gains in life expectancy realized for all age groups over the twentieth century. On an age-adjusted basis, improvements were even more impressive. Age-adjusted mortality fell about 75 percent between 1900 and 2000. Over the course of the entire twentieth century, infant and child mortality rates fell 95 percent, adolescent and young adult mortality rates dropped 80 percent, rates for adults aged 25–64 fell 60 percent, and rates for older adults (over age 65) declined 35 percent.

During the second half of the twentieth century, overall age-adjusted mortality fell about 50 percent (Figure 2–2) while infant mortality rates declined more than 75 percent. During that period mortality rates among children and young adults (ages 1–24 years) and adults 45–64 years were reduced by more than one-half. Mortality among adults 25–44 fell more than 40 percent and rates for elderly persons (age 65 and over) fell about one-third.

Gains for adult age groups in recent decades have outstripped those for younger age groups, a trend that began about 1960 as progress accelerated toward reduction of mortality from injuries and certain major chronic diseases that largely affected adults (earlier reductions for children also left little room for further improvements). Table 2–1 demonstrates changes in the age-adjusted frequency of selected major causes of death over the second half of the twentieth century. Dramatic reductions in the death rates for heart disease, stroke, unintentional injuries, influenza and pneumonia, and infant mortality have been joined by more recent reductions in rates for HIV infections, liver diseases, and suicide. Age-adjusted death rates have increased for diabetes, Alzheimer's disease, and chronic lung and kidney conditions, signaling the new morbidities associated with longer life spans. Homicide rates have improved somewhat over the past decade but reflect a substantial increase since 1950.

Table 2–1 also demonstrates the considerable disparities that exist for many of the major causes of death. Differences among races are notable, but there are also significant differences by gender for the various causes of death. These differences are often dramatic and run from top to bottom through the chain of causation. Disparities are found not only in indicators

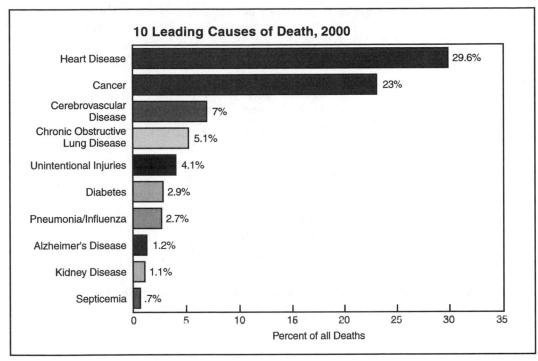

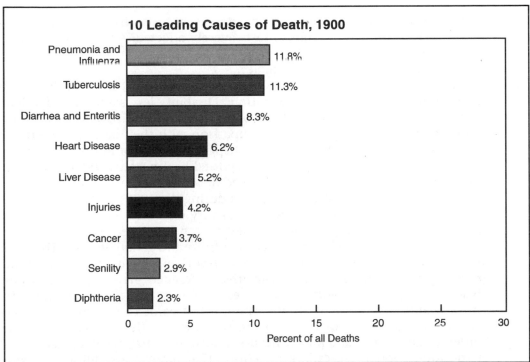

Figure 2–1 The 10 Leading Causes of Death as a Percentage of All Deaths in the United States, 1900 and 2000. *Source:* Adapted from U.S. Department of Health and Human Services. *Healthy People 2010: Understanding and Improving Health.* Washington DC; DHHS-PHS; 2000 and *Health United States 2002.* Public Health Service: Hyattsville MD; 2002.

Table 2–1 Year 2000 Age-Adjusted Death Rates (per 100,000 Population) for Selected Leading Causes of Death, Percent of all 2000 Deaths, Percentage Rate Change from 1950 to 2000, and 2000 Ratio by Sex and Race, United States

Cause of Death	Percent of 2000 Deaths	Year 2000 Rate	Percent Change in Rates 1950–2000	Male to Female 2000 Ratio	Black to White 2000 Ratio
Diseases of the heart	29.6	257.9	−56.0	1.5	1.3
Malignant neoplasms	23.0	201.0	+3.7	1.5	1.3
Cerebrovascular disease	7.0	60.8	−66.4	1.0	1.4
Chronic lung disease	5.1	44.3	x	1.4	0.7
Accidents & adverse effects	4.1	35.5	−54.5	2.3	1.1
Diabetes	2.9	25.2	+9.1	1.2	2.2
Influenza & pneumonia	2.7	23.7	−50.7	1.3	1.1
Suicide	1.2	10.6	−19.7	4.5	0.5
Chronic liver disease & cirrhosis	1.1	9.6	−15.0	2.2	1.0
Homicide	0.7	6.1	+19.6	3.3	5.7

Notes: Rates age-adjusted to the 2000 U.S. population; x = 1950 comparison rate not available, although believed to be much lower than 2000 rate.

Source: Health United States 2002. Public Health Service; Hyattsville MD, 2002.

of poor health outcomes, such as mortality, but also in the levels of risk factors in the population groups most severely affected. A poignant example of these disparities is reflected in the 12-year difference in life expectancy between white females and black males.

There is also evidence that health is improving and that disability levels are declining in the population over time. Disability levels among individuals aged 55–70 years who were offspring of the famous Framingham Heart Study cohort were substantially lower, in comparison with their parents' experience at the same age.[2] In addition, fewer offspring had chronic diseases or perceived their health as fair or poor. Self-reported health status and activity limitations due to chronic conditions changed little during the 1990s, and injuries with lost workdays have steadily declined during the 1990s.

In sum, U.S. health indicators tell two very different tales. By many measures, the American population has never been healthier. By others, much more needs to be done for specific racial, ethnic, and gender groups. The gains in health status over the past century have not been shared equally by all subgroups of the population. In fact, relative differences have been increasing. This widening gap in health status creates both a challenge and a dilemma for future health improvement efforts. The greatest gains can be made through closing these gaps and equalizing health status within the population. Yet the burden of greater risk and poorer health status resides in a relatively small part of the total population, calling for efforts that target those minorities with increased resources. An alternative approach is to continue current strategies and resource deployment levels. Although this may continue the steady overall improvement among all groups in the population, it is likely to continue or worsen existing gaps. In the early years of the new century, the major health challenge facing the United States appears to be less related to the need to improve population-wide health outcomes than the need to eliminate or reduce disparities. This challenges the nation's commitment to its principles of equality and social justice. However, addressing inequalities in measures of health and quality of life requires a greater understanding of health and the measures used to describe it than afforded by death rates and life expectancies.

HEALTH, ILLNESS, AND DISEASE

The relationship between outcomes and the factors that influence them is complex, often confounded by different understandings of the concepts in question and how they are measured. Health is difficult to define and more difficult yet to measure. For much of history, the notion of health has been negative. This was due in part to the continuous onslaught of epidemic diseases. With disease a frequent visitor, health became the disease-free state. One was healthy by exclusion.

However, as knowledge of disease increased and methods of prevention and control improved, health was more commonly considered from a positive perspective. The World Health Organization (WHO) seized this opportunity in its 1946 constitution, defining health as not merely the absence of disease but a state of complete physical, mental, and social well-being.[3] This definition of health emphasizes that there are different, complexly-related forms of wellness and illness, and suggests that a wide range of factors can influence the health of individuals and groups. It also suggests that health is not an absolute concept.

Although health and well-being may be synonyms, health and disease are not necessarily opposites. Most people view health and illness as existing along a continuum and as opposite and mutually exclusive states. However, this simplistic, one-dimensional model of health and illness does not comport very well with the real world. A person can have a disease or injury and still be healthy or at least feel well. There are many examples, but certainly Olympic wheelchair racers would fit into this category. It is also possible for someone without a specific disease or injury to feel ill or not well. If health and illness are not mutually exclusive, then they exist in separate dimensions, with wellness and illness in one dimension and the presence or absence of disease or injury in another.

These distinctions are important because disease is a relatively objective, pathologic phenomenon, whereas wellness and illness represent subjective experiences. This allows for several different states to exist: wellness without disease or injury, wellness with disease or injury, illness with disease or injury, and illness without physical disease or injury. This multidimensional view of health states is consistent with the WHO delineation of physical, mental, and social dimensions of health or well-being. Health or wellness is more than the absence of disease alone. Furthermore, one can be physically but not mentally and socially well.

With health measurable in several different dimensions, the question arises as to whether there is some maximum or optimal end point of health or well-being or whether health is something that can always be improved through changes in its physical, mental, and social facets. The latter alternative suggests that the goal should be a minimal acceptable level of health, rather than a state of complete and absolute health. Due in part to these considerations, WHO revised its definition in 1978 calling for a level of health that permits people to lead socially and economically productive lives.[4] This shifts the focus of health from an end in itself to a resource for everyday life, linking physical to personal and social capacities. It also suggests that it will be easier to identify measures of illness than of health.

Disease and injury are often viewed as phenomena that may lead to significant loss or disability in social functioning, making one unable to carry out one's main personal or social functions in life, such as parenting, schooling, or employment. In this perspective, health is equivalent to the absence of disability; individuals able to carry out their basic functions in life are healthy. This characterization of health as the absence of significant functional disabilities is perhaps the most common one for this highly sought state. Still, this definition is negative in that it defines health as the absence of disability.

In attempting to measure health, both quantity and quality become important considerations. However, it is not always easy to answer the questions: How much? Compared with what? For example, physical health for a 10-year-old child carries a much different expectation than physical health for an 80-year-old. It is reasonable to conclude that the natural processes of aging lead to gradual diminution of functional reserve capacity and that this is normal and not easily prevented. Thus, our perceptions of normal functioning are influenced by social and cultural factors.

The concept of well-being advanced in the WHO definition goes beyond the physical aspects of health that are the usual focus of measurements and comparisons. Including the mental and social aspects of well-being or health legitimizes the examination of factors that affect mental and social health. Together, these themes suggest that we need to consider carefully what we are measuring in order to understand what these measures are telling us about health, illness, and disease states in a population and the factors that influence these outcomes.

MEASURING HEALTH

The availability of information on health outcomes suggests that measuring the health status of populations is a simple task. However, although often interesting and sometimes even dramatic, the commonly used measures of health status fail to paint a complete picture of health. Many of the reasons are obvious. The commonly used measures actually reflect disease and mortality, rather than health itself. The longstanding misperception that health is the absence of disease is reinforced by the relative ease of measuring disease states, in comparison with states of health. Actually, the most commonly used indicators focus on a state that is neither health nor disease—namely, death.

Despite the many problems with using mortality as a proxy for health, mortality data are generally available and widely used to describe the health status of populations. This is ironic because such data only indirectly describe the health status of living populations. Unfortunately, data on morbidity (illnesses, injuries, and functional limitations of the population) are neither as available nor as readily understood as are mortality data. This situation is improving, however, as new forms and sources of information on health conditions become more readily available. Sources for information on morbidities and disabilities now include medical records from hospitals, managed care organizations, and other providers, as well as information derived from surveys, businesses, schools, and other sources. Assessments of the health status of populations are increasingly utilizing measures from these sources. Chapter 6 will further describe data and information sources for use in public health. An excellent compilation of data and information on both health status and health services, *Health United States,*[1] is published annually by the National Center for Health Statistics. Much of the data used in this chapter is derived from this source.

Mortality-Based Measures

Although mortality-based indicators of health status are both widely used and useful, there are some important differences in their use and interpretation. The most commonly used are crude mortality, age-specific and age-adjusted mortality, life expectancy, and years of potential life lost (YPLL). Although all are based on the same events, each provides somewhat different information as to the health status of a population.

Crude mortality rates count deaths within the entire population and are not sensitive to differences in the age distribution of different populations. The mortality comparisons presented earlier in Figure 2–2 illustrate the limitations of using crude death rates to compare the mortality experience of the U.S. population late in the twentieth century with that of the year 1950. On the basis of these data, we might conclude that mortality rates in the United States had declined about 20 percent since 1950. However, because there was a greater proportion of the late twentieth-century population in the higher age categories, these are not truly comparable populations. The 20 percent reduction actually understates the differences in mortality experience over the twentieth century. Because differences in the age characteristics of the two populations are a primary concern, we look for methods to correct or adjust for the age factor. Age-specific and age-adjusted rates do just that.

Age-specific mortality rates relate the number of deaths to the number of persons in a specific age group. The infant mortality rate is probably the best known example, describing the number of deaths of live-born infants occurring in the first year of life per 1,000 live births. Public health studies often use age-adjusted mortality rates to compensate for different mixes of age groups within a population, for example, a high proportion of children or elderly. Age-adjusted rates are calculated by applying age-specific rates to a standard population (we now use the 2000 U.S. population). This adjustment permits

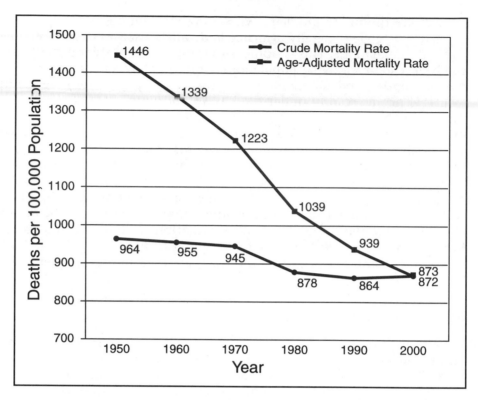

Figure 2–2 Crude and Age-Adjusted Mortality Rates, United States 1950–2000. *Source:* Adapted from National Center for Health Statistics. *Health United States 2002.* Hyattsville MD; PHS; 2002.

more meaningful comparisons of mortality experience between populations with different age distribution patterns. Differences between crude and age-adjusted mortality rates can be substantial, such as those in Figure 2–2. The explanation is simply that the population at the end of the twentieth century had a greater proportion of persons in older age groups than the 1900 or 1950 populations. Using crude rates, the improvement between 1950 and 2000 was about 20 percent; age-adjusted rates showed a 40 percent improvement.

Life expectancy, also based on the mortality experience of a population, is a computation of the number of years between any given age (e.g., birth or age 45) and the average age of death for that population. Together with infant mortality rates, life expectancies are commonly used in comparisons of health status among nations. These two mortality-based indicators are often perceived as general indicators of the overall health status of a population. Infant mortality and life expectancy measures for the United States are mediocre, in comparison with those of other developed nations. Figure 2–3 presents international comparisons of life expectancy by gender for the United States and selected other countries for 1995.

Life Expectancy by Country

FEMALE				MALE	
Country		Years of Life Expectancy	Country		Years of Life Expectancy
	Japan	82.9		Japan	76.4
	France	82.6		Sweden	76.2
	Switzerland	81.9		Israel	75.3
	Sweden	81.6		Canada	75.2
	Spain	81.5		Switzerland	75.1
	Canada	81.2		Greece	75.1
	Australia	80.9		Australia	75.0
	Italy	80.8		Norway	74.9
	Norway	80.7		Netherlands	74.6
	Netherlands	80.4		Italy	74.4
	Greece	80.3		England and Wales	74.3
	Finland	80.3		France	74.2
	Austria	80.1		Spain	74.2
	Germany	79.8		Austria	73.5
	Belgium	79.8		Singapore	73.4
	England and Wales	79.6		Germany	73.3
	Israel	79.3		New Zealand	73.3
	Singapore	79.0		Northern Ireland	73.1
	United States	78.9		Belgium	73.0
				Cuba	73.0
				Costa Rica	73.0
				Finland	72.8
				Denmark	72.8
				Ireland	72.5
				United States	72.5

Source: World Health Organization, United Nations, Centers for Disease Control and Prevention, National Center for Health Statistics, National Vital Statistics System, 1990-1995 and unpublished data.

Figure 2–3 Life Expectancy at Birth by Gender and Ranked by Selected Countries, 1995. *Source:* Reprinted from *Healthy People 2010: Understanding and Improving Health,* U.S. Department of Health and Human Services, Public Health Service, 2000.

Table 2–2 Age-Adjusted Years of Potential Life Lost (YPLL) Before Age 75 by Cause of Death and Ranks for YPLL and Number of Deaths, U.S. 2000

Causes of Death	YPLL	Rank by YPLL	Rank by Number of Deaths
Cancer	1,698,500	1	2
Heart disease	1,270,700	2	1
Unintentional injuries	1,052,500	3	5
Suicide	343,300	4	11
Homicide	274,200	5	14
Cerebrovascular diseases	226,500	6	3
Chronic obstructive lung disease	190,700	7	4
Diabetes mellitus	181,200	8	6
HIV infections	178,900	9	18
Chronic liver disease and cirrhosis	141,700	10	12

Notes: Years lost before age 75 per 100,000 population under 75 years of age.

Source: Adapted from National Center for Health Statistics. *Health United States 2002.* Hyattsville MD; PHS; 2002.

Years of potential life lost (YPLL) is a mortality-based indicator that places greater weight on deaths that occur at younger ages. Years of life lost before some arbitrary age (often age 65 or 75) are computed and used to measure the relative impact on society of different causes of death. If age 65 is used as the threshold for calculating YPLL, an infant death would contribute 65 YPLL, and a homicide at age 25 would contribute 40 YPLL. A death due to stroke at age 70 would contribute no years of life lost before age 65, and so on. Until relatively recently, age 65 was widely used as the threshold age. With life expectancies now exceeding 75 years at birth, YPLL calculations using age 75 as the threshold have become more common. Table 2–2 presents data on YPLL before age 75, illustrating the usefulness of this approach in providing a somewhat different perspective as to which problems are most important in terms of their magnitude and impact. The use of YPLL ranks cancer, HIV/AIDS, and various forms of injury-related deaths higher than does the use of crude numbers or rates. Conversely, the use of crude rates ranks heart disease, stroke, pneumonia, diabetes, and chronic lung and liver diseases higher than does the use of YPLL. Four of the top ten causes of death, as determined by the number of deaths, do not appear in the list of the top ten causes of YPLL.

Each of these different mortality indicators can be examined for various racial and ethnic subpopulations to identify disparities among these groups. For example, age-adjusted rates of YPLL before age 75 for 2000 ranged from 6,284 per 100,000 population for Hispanics to 7,029 for whites and 13,177 per 100,000 for blacks. The rate for all groups was 7,694 per 100,000. The large disparity for blacks is attributable primarily to differences in infant mortality, homicide, and HIV infection deaths.

Morbidity, Disability, and Quality Measures

Mortality indicators can also be combined with other health indicators that describe quality considerations to provide a measure of the span of healthy life. These indicators can be an especially meaningful measure of health status in a population because they also consider morbidity and disability from conditions that impact on functioning but do not cause death (e.g., cerebral palsy, schizophrenia, arthritis). A commonly used measure of aggregate disease burden is the disability-adjusted life year or DALY. Other variants on this theme are span-of-healthy-life indicators (called years of healthy life [YHL]) that combine mortality data with self-reported health status and activity limitation data acquired through the National Health Interview Survey. In 1998, an average of 11.5 years of life (when life expectancy was 76.7 years at birth) involved limitations of major life activities, such as self-care (bathing, grooming, cooking, etc.), recreation, work, and school. The 65-year span of healthy life presents a better, although not precise, picture of health status and quality of life. This indicator is illustrated in Figure 2–4, with 1998 data identifying disparities among blacks, whites, and Hispanics in both the number of healthy years of life and the percentage of healthy years

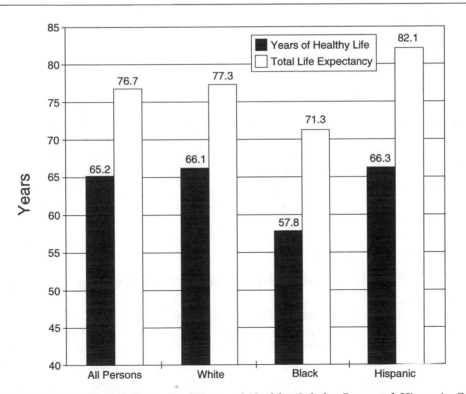

Figure 2–4 Total Life Expectancy and Years of Healthy Life by Race and Hispanic Origin, United States, 1998. *Source:* CDC/NCHS National Vital Statistics System and National Health Interview Survey[29]

in comparison with life expectancy. Hispanics had the greatest life expectancy at 82.1 years, of which 66.3 (81 percent) were years of healthy life. In contrast, blacks had 11 fewer years in life expectancy (71.3 years), but the same proportion (81 percent) were healthy years. Life expectancy for whites was 77.3 years, with a higher percentage of healthy years (86 percent) than Hispanics or blacks. These differences illustrate different forms of disparities among these groups with blacks experiencing higher mortality (lower life expectancy) and Hispanics carrying a greater burden of disease prevalence (higher number of unhealthy life years) than the white population. Among the mortality-related measures discussed here, span of healthy life comes closest to measuring health in terms of the ability to function normally.

Though less frequently encountered, indicators of morbidity and disability are also quite useful in measuring health status. Figure 2–5 presents information on both morbidity and disability for children in terms of the prevalence of specific childhood diseases (here, the percentage of children 0–17 years old who have ever had these conditions) and the relationship between these conditions and self-reported health and activity status (a measure of disability).

Both prevalence (the number or rate of cases at a specific point or period in time) and incidence (the number or rate of new cases occurring during a specific period) are widely used measures of morbidity. One of the earliest systems for reporting on diseases of public health significance is the national notifiable disease-reporting system for specific diseases. This system operates through the collaboration of local, state, and federal health agencies. Although initially developed to track the incidence of communicable diseases, this system has steadily moved toward collecting information on noninfectious conditions, as well as important risk factors.

Increasingly, information on self-reported health status and on days lost from work or school due to acute or chronic conditions is collected through surveys of the general population. The National Center for Health Statistics also conducts ongoing surveys of health providers on complaints and conditions requiring medical care in outpatient settings. These surveys provide direct information on self-reported health status and illuminate some of the factors, such as household income levels depicted in Figure 2–6, that are associated with health status.

INFLUENCES ON HEALTH

In 1996 public health surveillance in the United States took a historic step, reflecting changes in national morbidity and mortality patterns, as well as in the ability to identify specific factors that result in disease and injury. At that time the Centers for Disease Control and Prevention (CDC) added prevalence of cigarette smoking to the list of diseases and conditions to be reported by states to CDC.[5] This action marked the first time that a health behavior, rather than an illness or disease, was considered nationally reportable—a groundbreaking step for surveillance efforts. How the focus of public health efforts shifted from conventional disease outcomes to reporting on underlying causes amenable to public health intervention is an important story. That story is

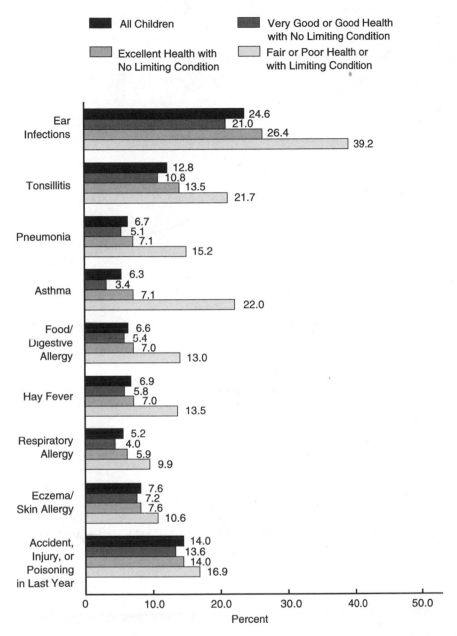

Figure 2–5 Percentage of Children 0–17 Years of Age Who Have Had Selected Childhood Diseases, by Child's Health and Limitation Status, United States, 1988. *Source:* Reprinted from M.J. Coiro, N. Zill, and B. Bloom, Health of Our Nation's Children, *Vital Health Statistics,* Vol. 10, No. 191, National Center for Health Statistics, 1994.

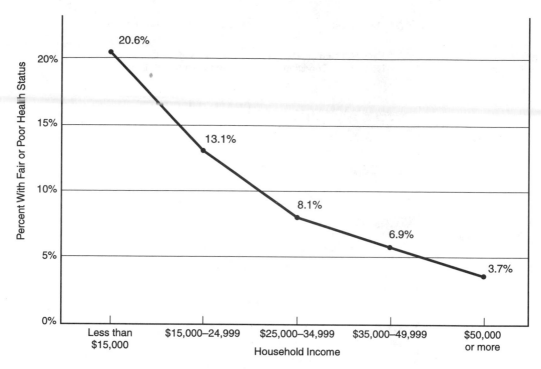

Figure 2–6 Percentage of Persons with Fair or Poor Perceived Health Status by Household Income, United States, 1995. *Source:* Reprinted from *Healthy People 2010; Understanding and Improving Health,* U.S. Department of Health and Human Services, Public Health Service, 2000.

closely linked to one of the most important and most bitterly contested public health achievements of the twentieth century, the recognition of tobacco use as a major health hazard. "Public Health Achievements in Twentieth-Century America: Tobacco Use," chronicles this story, providing important lessons for public health efforts in the twenty-first century seeking to improve measures of health status and quality of life.

Example

Public Health Achievements in Twentieth-Century America: Tobacco Use

Initial suspicions that tobacco use was harmful for humans were confirmed by epidemiologic studies in the mid-twentieth century, stimulating new interest in measures of health, illness, and their related factors. By the time the prevalence of tobacco use, a risk behavior, became a reportable condition in the 1990s, the use of a wide variety of measures of health had become common place in public health practice.

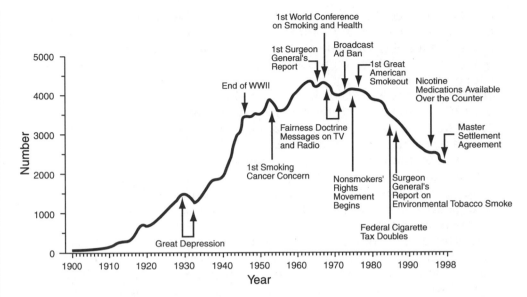

Figure 2–7 Annual Adult Per Capita Cigarette Consumption and Major Smoking and Health Events—United States, 1900–1998. *Source:* Reprinted from Achievements in Public Health, United States, 1990–1999: Tobacco Use, *Morbidity and Mortality Weekly Report,* Vol. 48, No. 43, pp. 986–993, the Centers for Disease Control and Prevention, 1999.

Smoking—once a socially accepted behavior—is the leading preventable cause of death and disability in the United States. During the first decades of the twentieth century, lung cancer was rare; however, as cigarette smoking became increasingly popular, first among men and later among women, the incidence of lung cancer became epidemic (Figure 2–7). In 1930 the lung cancer death rate for men was 4.9 per 100,000; in 1990 the rate had increased to 75.6 per 100,000. Other diseases and conditions now known to be caused by tobacco use include heart disease, atherosclerotic peripheral vascular disease, laryngeal cancer, oral cancer, esophageal cancer, chronic obstructive pulmonary disease, intrauterine growth retardation, and low birth weight. During the latter part of the twentieth century, the adverse health effects from exposure to environmental tobacco smoke also were documented. These include lung cancer, asthma, respiratory infections, and decreased pulmonary function.

Large epidemiologic studies conducted in the 1940s and 1950s linked cigarette smoking and lung cancer. In 1964 on the basis of approximately 7,000 articles relating to smoking and disease, the Advisory Committee to the U.S. Surgeon General concluded that cigarette smoking is a cause of lung and laryngeal cancer in men, a probable cause of lung cancer in women, and the most important cause of chronic bronchitis in both sexes. The committee stated that "cigarette smoking is a health hazard of sufficient importance in the United States to warrant appropriate remedial action." Substantial public health efforts to reduce the prevalence of tobacco use began shortly after the risk was described in 1964. With the subsequent decline in smoking, the incidence of smoking-related cancers (including cancers of the lung, oral cavity, and pharynx) has also declined (with the exception of lung cancer among women). In addition, age-adjusted death rates per 100,000 persons (standardized to the 1940 population) for heart conditions (i.e., coronary heart disease) have decreased from 307.4 in 1950 to 134.6 in 1996. During 1964–1992, approximately 1.6 million deaths caused by smoking were prevented.

Early in the twentieth century, several events coincided that contributed to increases in annual per capita consumption, including the introduction of blends and curing processes that allowed the inhalation of tobacco, the invention of the safety match, improvements in mass production, transportation that permitted widespread distribution of cigarettes, and use of mass media advertising to promote cigarettes. Cigarette smoking among women began to increase in the 1920s, when targeted industry marketing and social changes reflecting the liberalization of women's roles and behavior led to the increasing acceptability of smoking among women. Annual per capita cigarette consumption increased from 54 cigarettes in 1900 to 4,345 cigarettes in 1963, then decreased to 2,261 in 1998. Some decreases correlate with events, such as the first research suggesting a link between smoking and cancer in the 1950s, the 1964 Surgeon General's report, the 1968 Fairness Doctrine, and increased tobacco taxation and industry price increases during the 1980s (Figure 2–7).

An important accomplishment of the second half of the twentieth century has been the reduction of smoking prevalence among persons aged greater than or equal to 18 years from 42.4 percent in 1965 to 24.7 percent in 1997, with the rate for men (27.6 percent) higher than for women (22.1 percent) (Figure 2–8). The percentage of adults who never smoked increased from 44 percent in the mid-1960s to 55 percent in 1997. In 1998 tobacco use varied within and among racial/ethnic groups. The prevalence of smoking was highest among American Indians/Alaska Natives and second highest among black and Southeast Asian men. The prevalence was lowest among Asian American and Hispanic women. Smokeless tobacco use has changed little since 1970, with a 5 percent prevalence in 1970 and a 6 percent prevalence in 1991 among men, and 2 percent and 1 percent, respectively, for women. The prevalence of smokeless tobacco use is highest among high school males, with prevalence being 20 percent among white males, 6 percent among Hispanics males, and 4 percent among black males. Prevalence of use tends to be lower in the northeastern region and higher in the southern region of the United States. Total consumption of cigars decreased from 8 million in 1970 to 2 million in 1993 but increased 68 percent to 3.6 million in 1997.

Reductions in smoking result from many factors, including scientific evidence of the relation among disease, tobacco use, and environ-

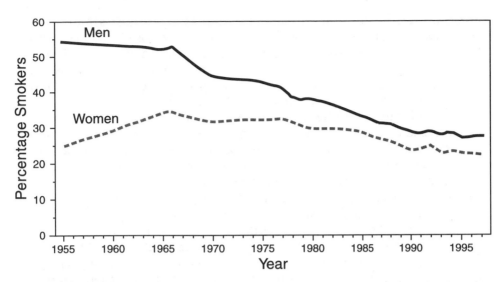

Figure 2–8 Trends in Cigarette Smoking among Persons ≥18 years, by Sex—United States, 1955–1997. *Source:* Reprinted from Achievements in Public Health, United States, 1900–1999: Tobacco Use, *Morbidity and Mortality Weekly Report,* Vol. 48, No. 43, pp. 986–993, the Centers for Disease Control and Prevention, 1999.

mental exposure to tobacco; dissemination of this information to the public; surveillance and evaluation of prevention and cessation programs; campaigns by advocates for nonsmokers' rights; restrictions on cigarette advertising; counter advertising; policy changes (i.e., enforcement of minors' access laws, legislation restricting smoking in public places, and increased taxation); improvements in treatment and prevention programs; and an increased understanding of the economic costs of tobacco.

The cigarette itself has changed. When cigarettes were first associated with lung cancer in the early 1950s, most U.S. smokers smoked unfiltered cigarettes. With a growing awareness of the danger of smoking came the first filter, which was designed to reduce the tar inhaled in the smoke. Later, low-tar cigarettes were marketed; however, many smokers compensated by smoking more intensely and by blocking the filter's ventilation holes. Adenocarcinoma has replaced squamous cell carcinoma as the leading cause of lung cancer-related death in the United States. This increase in adenocarcinoma parallels the changes in cigarette design and smoking behavior.

Changes in the social norms surrounding smoking can be documented by examining changes in public policy, including availability of Fairness Doctrine counter advertising messages on television and radio and increased restrictions on tobacco advertising, beginning with the ban on broadcast advertising in 1971. Cigarette advertising no longer appears on television or billboards, and efforts to restrict sales and marketing to adolescents have increased. Indoor air policies switched from favoring smokers to favoring nonsmokers. Smoking is no longer permitted on airplanes, and many people, including 12.5 percent of adult smokers with children, do not smoke at home. Now, 42 states have restrictions on smoking at government work sites, and 20 states have restrictions at private work sites.

One of the most effective means of reducing the prevalence of tobacco use is by increasing federal and state excise tax rates. A 10 percent increase in the price of cigarettes can lead to a 4 percent reduction in the demand for cigarettes. This reduction is the result of people smoking fewer cigarettes or quitting altogether. Studies show that low income, adolescent, Hispanic, and non-Hispanic black smokers are more likely than others to stop smoking in response to a price increase.

The November 1998 Master Settlement Agreement marked the end of the twentieth century with an unprecedented event. Although admitting no wrongdoing, the tobacco companies signed an agreement with the attorneys general of 46 states. This agreement settled lawsuits totaling $206 billion; however, the agreement did not require that any of the state money be spent for tobacco use prevention and control.

Source: Adapted from Achievements in Public Health, 1990–1999: Tobacco Use, *Morbidity and Mortality Weekly Report,* Vol. 48, No. 43, pp. 986–993, the Centers for Disease Control and Prevention, 1999.

Risk Factors

The recognition of tobacco use as a major health hazard was no simple achievement, partly because many factors directly or indirectly influence the level of a health outcome in a given population. For example, greater per capita tobacco use in a population is associated with higher rates of heart disease and lung cancer, and lower rates of early prenatal care are associated with higher infant mortality rates. Because these factors are part of the chain of causation for health outcomes, tracking their levels provides an early indication as to the direction in which the health outcome is likely to change. These factors increase the likelihood or risk of particular health outcomes occurring and can be characterized broadly as risk factors.

The types and number of risk factors are as varied as the influences themselves. Depending on how these factors are lumped or split, traditional categories include biologic factors (from genetic endowment to aging), environmental factors (from food, air, and water to communicable diseases), lifestyle factors (from diet to injury avoidance and sexual behaviors), psychosocial factors (from poverty to stress, personality, and cultural factors), and use of and access to health-related services. Some recent refinements of this framework differentiate several outcomes of interest, including disease, functional capacity, prosperity, and well-being that can be influenced by various risk factors (Figure 2–9). These various components are often interrelated (e.g., stress, a social environmental factor, may stimulate individual responses, such as

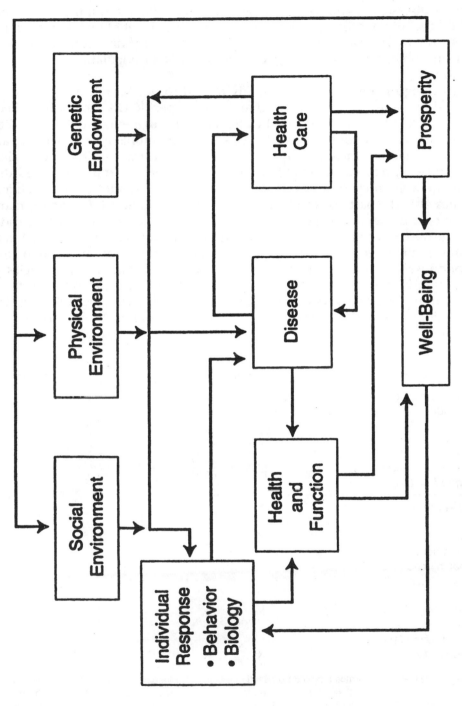

Figure 2-9 Determinants of Health. *Source:* Reprinted from *Social Science and Medicine,* Vol. 31, No. 12, R. G. Evans and G. L. Stoddard, Producing Health, Consuming Health Care, p. 1359, Copyright 1990 with permission from Elsevier Science.

57

tobacco or illicit drug use, which, in turn, influence the likelihood of disease, functional capacity, and well-being). In addition, variations in one outcome, such as disease, may influence changes in others, such as well-being, depending on the mix of other factors present. This complex set of interactions draws attention to general factors that can result in many diseases, rather than focusing on specific factors that contribute little to population-wide health outcomes.

Although many factors are causally related to health outcomes, some are more direct and proximal causes than others. Specific risk factors have been clearly linked to specific adverse health states through epidemiologic studies. For example, numerous studies have linked unintentional injuries with a variety of risk factors, including the accessibility to firearms and the use of alcohol, tobacco, and seat belts. Tobacco, hypertension, overnutrition, and diabetes are well-known risk factors for heart disease. Epidemiologic research and studies over the past 50 years have identified behavioral risk factors for many common diseases and conditions,[6] as shown in Table 2–3. In recent decades the prevalence of obesity has doubled in virtually all gender, age, racial, and ethnic groups. Ongoing behavioral risk factor surveys (often through telephone interviews) are conducted by governmental public health agencies to track trends in the prevalence of many important risk behaviors within the population. These surveys document that the health-related behaviors of tens of millions of Americans place them at risk of developing chronic disease and injuries.

Table 2–3 Selected Behavioral Risk Factors Related to Leading Causes of Deaths in the U.S., 2000

Cause of Death and Percentage of All Deaths	Smoking	High Fat/ Low Fiber	Sedentary Lifestyle	High Blood Pressure	Elevated Cholesterol	Obesity	Alcohol Use
Heart disease (30%)	X	X	X	X	X	X	X
Cancer (23%)	X	X	X			X	X
Stroke (7%)	X	X		X	X	X	
Chronic lung disease (5%)	X						
Unintentional injuries (4%)	X						X
Pneumonia & influenza (3%)	X						
Diabetes (3%)		X	X			X	
HIV infection (1%)							
Suicide (1%)							X
Chronic liver disease (1%)							X
Atherosclerosis (1%)	X	X	X		X		

Source: Causes and Percent Deaths adapted from National Center for Health Statistics. *Health United States 2002.* Hyattsville, MD; PHS; 2002. Risk Factors Related to Causes adapted from Brownson et al., *Chronic Disease Epidemiology and Control,* 2nd edition. Washington, DC; American Public Health Association; 1998 and Surgeon General's *Report on Nutrition and Health,* 1988.

Despite the recent emphasis on behavioral factors, risk factors in the physical environment remain important influences on health. Air pollution, for example, is directly related to a wide range of diseases, including lung cancer, pulmonary emphysema, chronic bronchitis, and bronchial asthma. National standards exist for many of the most important air pollutants and are tracked to determine the extent of these risks in the general population. The proportion of the U.S. population residing in counties that have exceeded national standards for these pollutants suggests that air pollution risks, like behavioral risks, affect tens of millions of Americans.[7] Environmental risks are ubiquitous and growing in the U.S. Estimates from CDC are that 22–30 million people drink water from private wells, 40–45 million people are exposed to extreme heat; 150 million people are exposed to environmental tobacco smoke; and 65 million people reside in homes built before 1950, when lead paint was banned for residential use.

Behavioral and environmental risk factors are clearly germane to public health interest and efforts. Focusing on these factors provides a different perspective of the enemies of personal and public health than that conveyed by disease-specific incidence or mortality data. Such a focus also promotes rational policy development and interventions. Unfortunately, determining which underlying factors are most important is more difficult than it appears due to differences in the outcomes under study and measures used. For example, a study using 1980 data found tobacco, hypertension, and overnutrition responsible for about three-fourths of deaths before age 65 and injury risks, alcohol, tobacco, and gaps in primary prevention accountable for about three-fourths of all YPLL before age 65.[8] Further complicating these analyses is the finding that individual risk factors may result in several different health outcomes. For example, alcohol use is linked with motor vehicle injuries, other injuries, cancer, and cirrhosis; tobacco use can result in heart disease, stroke, ulcers, fire and burn injuries, and low birth weight, as well as cancer.[6,8]

Despite problems with their measurement, the identification of antecedent causes is important for public health policy and interventions. Table 2–4 provides a frequently cited comparison of 1990 deaths by their listed causes of death, as given by the National Center for Health Statistics (NCHS), and their actual causes (major risk factors).[9] The two lists provide contrasting views as to the major health problems and needs of the U.S. population. Although this debate has continued since the days of Chadwick and Farr (see Chapter 1), it is by no means settled.

Coroners and medical examiners view immediate and underlying causes of death somewhat differently from the perspective offered in Table 2–4. Death certificates have two parts, one for entering the immediate and underlying conditions that caused the death and a second for identifying conditions or injuries that contributed to death but did not cause death. For example, a death attributed to cardiovascular disease might list cardiac tamponade as the immediate cause, due to or a consequence of a ruptured myocardial infarction, which itself was due to or a consequence of coronary arteriosclerosis. For this death, hypertensive cardiovascular disease might be listed as a significant condition contributing to, but not causing, the immediate and underlying causes.

Table 2–4 Listed and Actual Causes of Death, United States, 1990

10 Leading Causes of Death	Number	Actual Causes of Death	Number
Heart disease	720,058	Tobacco	400,000
Cancer	505,322	Diet/activity patterns	300,000
Cerebrovascular disease	144,088	Alcohol	100,000
Unintentional injuries	91,983	Certain infections	90,000
Chronic lung disease	86,679	Toxic agents	60,000
Pneumonia and influenza	79,513	Firearms	35,000
Diabetes	47,664	Sexual behavior	30,000
Suicide	30,906	Motor vehicles	25,000
Chronic liver disease	28,815	Drug use	20,000
HIV infection	25,188		
Total	1,760,216	Total	1,060,000

Source: Data from the National Center for Health Statistics and J.M. McGinnis and W. Foege, Actual Causes of Death in the United States, *Journal of the American Medical Association,* Vol. 270, pp. 2207–2212, © 1993, American Medical Association.

So where do smoking, obesity, diet, and physical inactivity get identified as the real causes of such deaths? Perhaps the Chadwick-Farr debate continues into the twenty-first century in terms of whether deaths in the year 2000 should be attributed to tobacco use, just as many of those in England in 1839 should have been attributed to starvation.

Social and Cultural Influences

Understanding the health effects of biologic, behavioral, and environmental risk factors is straightforward in comparison with understanding the effects of social, economic, and cultural factors on the health of populations. This is due in part to a lack of agreement as to what is being measured. Socioeconomic status and poverty are two factors that generally reflect position in society. There is considerable evidence that social position is an overarching determinant of health status, even though the indicators used to measure social standing are imprecise, at best.

Social class affects lifestyle, environment, and the utilization of services; it remains an important predictor of good and poor health in our society. Social class differences in mortality have long been recognized around the world. In 1842 Chadwick reported that the average ages at death for occupationally stratified groups in England were as follows: "gentlemen and persons engaged in the professions, 45 years; tradesmen and their families, 26 years; mechanics, servants and laborers, and their families, 16 years."[10] Life expectancies and other health indicators have improved considerably in England and elsewhere since 1842, but differences in mortality rates among the various social classes persist to the present day.

Some countries (such as Great Britain and the United States) have identifiable social strata that permit comparisons of health status by social class. Britain conducts ongoing analyses of socioeconomic differences according to

Table 2–5 Selected Outcomes and Relative Risk for Low-Income Families, as Compared with High-Income Families

Outcome	Relative Risk
Child neglect	9
Child abuse	4.5
Iron-deficiency anemia	3–4
Childhood mortality	>3
Fair or poor health	3
Fatal injuries	2–3
Growth retardation	2.5
Severe asthma	2
Pneumonia	1.6
Infant mortality	1.3–1.5
Low birth weight	1.2–2.2
Extreme behavioral problems	1.3

Source: Data from P. L. Geltman et al., Welfare Reform and Children's Health, *Health Policy and Child Health*, Vol. 3, No. 2, pp. 1–5, © 1996.

official categorizations based on general social standing within the community. For the United States, educational status, race, and family income are often used as indirect or proxy measures of social class. Despite the differences in approaches and indicators, there is little evidence of any real difference between Britain and the United States in terms of what is being measured. In both countries, explanations for the differences in mortality appear to relate primarily to inequalities in social position and material resources.[11,12] This effect operates all up and down the hierarchy of social standing; at each step improvements in social status are linked with improvements in measures of health status. For example, a study based on 1971 British census follow-up data found that a relatively affluent, home-owning group with two cars had a lower mortality risk than did a similar relatively privileged group with only one car.[11]

In the United States, epidemiologists have studied socioeconomic differences in mortality risk since the early 1900s. Infant mortality has been the subject of many studies that have consistently documented the effects of poverty. Findings from the 1988 National Maternal and Infant Health Survey, for example, demonstrated that the effects of poverty were greater for infants born to mothers with no other risk factors than for infants born to high-risk mothers.[13] Poverty status was associated with a 60 percent higher rate of neonatal mortality and a 200 percent higher rate for postneonatal mortality than for those infants of higher-income mothers.

Poverty affects many health outcomes, as illustrated in Figure 2–6 and Table 2–5. Low-income families in the United States have an increased likelihood (or relative risk) for a variety of adverse health outcomes, often two to five times greater than that of higher income families. The percentage of persons reporting fair or poor health is about four times as high for persons living below the poverty level as for those with family income at least twice the poverty level (22.2 percent and 5.5 percent, age adjusted).[1]

The implications of the consistent relationship between measures of social status and health outcomes suggest that studies need to consider how and how well social class is categorized and measured. Imprecise measures may under state the actual differences that are due to socioeconomic position in society. Importantly, if racial or ethnic differences are simply attributed to social class differences, factors that operate through race and ethnicity, such as racism or ethnism, will be overlooked. These additional factors also affect the difference between the social position one has and the position one would have attained, were it not for one's race or ethnicity. Race in the United States, independent of socioeconomic status, is linked to mortality, although these effects vary across age and disease categories.[14]

Studies of the effect of social factors on health status across nations add some interesting insights. In general, health appears to be closely associated with income differentials within countries, but there is only a weak link between national mortality rates and average income among the developed countries.[15] This pattern suggests that health is affected less by changes in absolute material standards across affluent populations than by relative income differences and the resulting disadvantage in each country. It is not the richest countries that have the greatest life expectancy. Rather, it is those developed nations with the narrowest income differentials between rich and poor, as illustrated in Figure 2–3. This finding argues that health in the developed world is less a matter of a population's absolute material wealth than of how their circumstances compare with those of other members of their society. A similar perspective views income to be related to health through two pathways: a direct effect on the material conditions necessary for survival, and an effect on social participation and the opportunity to control one's own life circumstances.[16] In settings or societies that provide little in the way of material conditions (clean water, sanitation services, ample food, adequate housing, etc.), income is more important for health. Where material conditions are conducive to good health, income acts through social participation.

The effects of culture on health and illness are also becoming better understood. To medical anthropologists, diseases are not purely independent phenomena. Rather, they are to be viewed and understood in relation to ecology and culture. Certainly, the type and severity of disease varies by age, sex, social class, and ethnic group. The different distributions and social patterns of diseases reveal differences in culture-mediated behaviors. Such insights are essential to developing successful prevention and control programs. Culture serves to shape health-related behaviors, as well as human responses to diseases including changes in the environment, which, in turn, affect health. As an adaptive mechanism to the environment, culture has great potential for both positively and negatively affecting health.

There is evidence that different societies shape the ways in which diseases are experienced and that social patterns of disease persist, even after risk factors are identified and effective interventions become available.[17-19] For example the link between poverty and various outcomes has been well established; yet even after advances in medicine and public health and significant improvement in general living and working conditions, the association persists. One explanation is that as some risks were addressed, others developed, such as health-related behaviors, including violent behavior and alcohol, tobacco, and drug use. In this way societies create and shape the diseases that they experience. This makes sense, especially if we view the social context in which health and disease reside—the setting and social networks. For problems such as HIV/AIDS, sexually transmitted diseases, and illicit drug use, spread is heavily influenced by the links between those at risk.[20] This also helps to explain why people in disorganized social structures are more likely to report their own health as poor than are similar persons with more social capital.[21,22]

Societal responses to diseases are also socially constructed. Efforts to prevent the spread of typhoid fever by limiting the rights of carriers (such as Typhoid Mary) differed greatly from those to reduce transmission risks from diphtheria carriers. Because many otherwise normal citizens would have been subjected to extreme measures in order to avoid the risk of transmission, it was not socially acceptable to invoke similar measures for these similar risks.

If these themes of social and cultural influences are on target, they place the study of health disparities at the top of the public health agenda. They also argue that health should be viewed as a social phenomenon. Rather than attempting to identify each and every risk factor that contributes only marginally to disparate health outcomes of the lower social classes, a more effective approach would be to directly address the broader social policies (distribution of wealth, education, employment, and the like) that foster the social disparities that cause the observed differences in health outcomes.[19] This broad view of health and its determinants is critical to understanding and improving health status in the United States, as well as internationally.

Global Health Influences

Considerable variation exists among the world's nations on virtually every measure of health and illness currently in use. The principal factors responsible for observed trends and obvious inequities across the globe fall into the general categories of the social and physical environment, personal behavior, and health services. Given the considerable variation in social, economic, and health status among the developed, developing, and underdeveloped nations, it is naive to make broad generalizations. Countries with favorable health status indicators, however, generally have a well-developed health infrastructure, ample opportunities for education and training, relatively high status for women, and economic development that counterbalances population growth. Nonetheless, countries at all levels of development share some problems, including the escalating costs involved in providing a broad range of health, social, and economic development services to disadvantaged subgroups within the population. Social and cultural upheaval associated with urbanization is another problem common to countries at all levels of development. Over the course of the twentieth century, the proportion of the world's population living in urban areas tripled—to about 40 percent; that trend is expected to continue into the new century.

The principal environmental hazards in the world today appear to be those associated with poverty. This is true for developed as well as developing and underdeveloped countries. Some international epidemiologists predict that, in the twenty-first century, the effects of overpopulation and production of greenhouse gases will join poverty as major threats to global health. These factors represent human effects on the world's climate and resources and are easily remembered as the "3 Ps" of global health (pollution, population, and poverty):

- pollution of the atmosphere by greenhouse gases, which will result in significant global warming, affecting both climate and the occurrence of disease
- worldwide population growth, which will result in a population of 10–12 billion people within the next century
- poverty, which is always associated with ill health and disease [23,24]

It surprises many Americans that population is a major global health concern. Birth rates vary inversely with the level of economic development and the status of women among the nations of the world. Continuing high birth rates and declining death rates will mean even more rapid growth in population in developing countries. It has taken all of history to reach the world's current population level, but it will take less than half a century to double that. Many factors have influenced this growth, including public health, which has increased the chances of conception by improving the health status of adults, increasing infant and child survival, preventing premature deaths of adults in the most fertile age groups, and reducing the number of marriages dissolved by one partner's death.

In general, public health approaches to dealing with world health problems must overcome formidable obstacles, including the unequal and inefficient distribution of health services, lack of appropriate technology, poor management, poverty, and inadequate or inappropriate government programs to finance needed services. Much of the preventable disease in the world is concentrated in the developing and underdeveloped countries, where the most profound differences exist in terms of social and economic influences. Table 2–6 provides estimates of the preventable toll caused by water-related diseases worldwide.

Although many of these factors appear to stem from low levels of national wealth, the link between national health status and national wealth is not firm, and comparisons across nations are seldom straightforward. Changes in standards of living; advances in literacy, education, and welfare policies; and advances in the politics of human relations generally have more to do with improved health status, as measured by current indicators, than with specific preventive interventions. The complexities involved in identifying and understanding these forces and their interrelationships often confound comparisons of health status between the United States and other nations.

Table 2–6 World Health Organization (WHO) Estimates of Morbidity and Mortality of Water-Related Diseases, Worldwide, 1995

Disease	Morbidity (Episodes per Year)	Mortality (Deaths per Year)	Relationship to Water Supply, Sanitation
Diarrheal (drinking)	1 billion	3.3 million	Unsanitary excreta disposal, poor personal and domestic hygiene, unsafe water
Infection with intestinal helminths	1.5 billion*	100,000	Unsanitary excreta disposal, poor personal and domestic hygiene
Schistosomiasis	200 million*	200,000	Unsanitary excreta disposal and absence of nearby sources of safe water
Dracunuliasis	100,000*†	—	Unsafe drinking water
Trachoma	150 million‡	—	Lack of face washing, often due to absence of nearby sources of safe water
Malaria	400 million	1.5 million	Poor water management and storage, poor operation of water points and drainage
Dengue fever	1.75 million	20,000	Poor solid wastes management, water storage, and operation of water points and drainage
Poliomyelitis (drinking)	114,000	—	Unsanitary excreta disposal, poor personal and domestic hygiene, unsafe water
Trypanosomiasis	275,000	130,000	Absence of nearby sources of safe water
Bancroftian filariasis	72.8 million*	—	Poor water management and storage, poor operation of water points and drainage
Onchocerciasis	17.7 million*§	40,000	Poor water management and large-scale projects

* People currently infected.
† Excluding Sudan.
‡ Case of active disease. Approximately 5.9 million cases of blindness or severe complications of trachoma occur annually.
§ Includes an estimated 270,000 blind.

Source: Reprinted from WHO Warns of Inadequate Communicable Disease Prevention, *Prevention Health Reports*, Vol. 111, pp. 296–297, 1996, U.S. Public Health Service.

ANALYZING HEALTH PROBLEMS FOR CAUSATIVE FACTORS

The ability to identify risk factors and pathways for causation is essential for rational public health decisions and actions to address important health problems in a population. First, however, it is necessary to define what is meant by *health problem*. Here, health problem means a condition of humans that can be represented in terms of measurable health status or quality-of-life indicators. In later chapters, additional dimensions will be added to this basic definition for the purposes of community problem solving and the development of interventions. This characterization of a health problem as something measured only in terms of outcomes is difficult for some to accept. They point to important factors, such as access to care or poverty itself, and feel that these should rightfully be considered as health problems. Important problems they may be, but if truly important in the causation of some unacceptable health outcome, they can be dealt with as related factors rather than health problems.

The factors linked with specific health problems are often generically termed *risk factors* and can exist at one of three levels. Those risk factors most closely associated with the health outcome in question are often termed *determinants*. Risk factors that play a role further back in the chain of causation are called *direct and indirect contributing factors*. Risk factors can be described at either an individual or a population level. For example, tobacco use for an individual increases the chances of developing heart disease or lung cancer, and an increased prevalence of tobacco use in a population increases that population's incidence of (and mortality rates from) these conditions.

Determinants are scientifically established factors that relate directly to the level of a health problem. As the level of the determinant changes, the level of the health outcome changes. Determinants are the most proximal risk factors through which other levels of risk factors act. The link between the determinant and the health outcome should be well established through scientific or epidemiologic studies. For example, for neonatal mortality rates, two well-established determinants are the low birth weight rate (the number of infants born weighing less than 2,500 grams, or about 5.5 pounds, per 100 live births) and weight-specific mortality rates. Improvement in the neonatal mortality rate cannot occur unless one of these determinants improves. Health outcomes can have one or many determinants.

Direct contributing factors are scientifically established factors that directly affect the level of a determinant. Again, there should be solid evidence that the level of the direct contributing factor affects the level of the determinant. For the neonatal mortality rate example, the prevalence of tobacco use among pregnant women has been associated with the risk of low birth weight. A determinant can have many direct contributing factors. For low birth weight, other direct contributing factors include low maternal weight gain and inadequate prenatal care.

Indirect contributing factors affect the level of the direct contributing factors. Although several steps distant from the health outcome in question, these factors are often proximal enough to be modified. The indirect contributing factor affects the level of the direct contributing factor, which, in

Table 2–7 Risk Factors

Determinant	Scientifically established factor that relates directly to the level of the health problem. A health problem may have any number of determinants identified for it.	Example: Low birth weight is a prime determinant for the health problem of neonatal mortality.
Direct contributing factor	Scientifically established factor that directly affects the level of the determinant.	Example: Use of prenatal care is one factor that affects the low-birth-weight rate.
Indirect contributing factor	Community-specific factor that affects the level of a direct contributing factor. Such factors can vary considerably from one community to another.	Example: Availability of day care or transportation services within the community may affect the use of prenatal care services.

Source: Data from Centers for Disease Control and Prevention Public Health Practice Program Office.

turn, affects the level of the determinant. The level of the determinant then affects the level of the health outcome. Many indirect contributing factors can exist for each direct contributing factor. For prevalence of tobacco use among pregnant women, indirect contributing factors might include easy access to tobacco products for young women, lack of health education, and lack of smoking cessation programs.

The health problem analysis framework begins with the identification of a health problem (defined in terms of health status indicators) and proceeds to establish one or more determinants; for each determinant, one or more direct contributing factors; and for each direct contributing factor, one or more indirect contributing factors. Intervention strategies at the community level generally involve addressing these indirect contributing factors. When completed, an analysis identifies as many of the causal pathways as possible to determine which contributing factors exist in the setting in which an intervention strategy is planned. The framework for this approach is presented in Table 2–7 and Figure 2–10. This framework forms the basis for developing meaningful interventions; it is used in several of the processes and instruments to assess community health needs that are currently in wide use at the local level. Community health improvement processes and tools will be further described in Chapter 5.

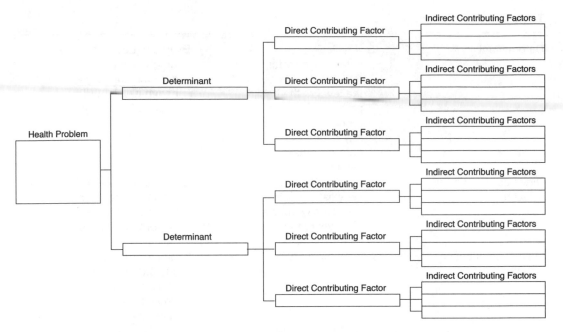

Figure 2–10 Health Problem Analysis Worksheet. *Source:* Reprinted from CDC Public Health Practice Program Office, 1991.

Although this framework is useful, it does not fully account for the relationships among the various levels of risk factors. Some direct contributing factors may affect more than one determinant, and some indirect contributing factors may influence more than one direct contributing factor. For example, illicit drug use during pregnancy influences both the likelihood of low birth weight and birth weight-specific survival rates. To account fully for these interactions, some direct and indirect contributing factors may need to be included in several different locations on the worksheet. Despite the advancement of epidemiologic methods, many studies ignore the contributing factors that affect the level of these major risk factors, leading to simplistic formulations of multiple risk factors for health problems that exist at the community level.[25]

ECONOMIC DIMENSIONS OF HEALTH OUTCOMES

The ability to measure and quantify outcomes and risks is essential for rational decisions and actions. Specific indicators, as well as methods of economic analysis, are available to provide both objective and subjective valuations. Several health indicators attempt to value differentially health status, outcomes, including age-adjusted rates, span of healthy life, and YPLL. For example, YPLL represents a method of weighting or valuing health outcomes by placing a higher value on deaths that occur at earlier ages. Years of life lost thus become a common denominator or, in one sense, a common currency. Health outcomes can be translated into this currency or into an actual currency, such as dollars. This translation allows for comparisons to be made among outcomes in terms of which costs more per person, per episode, or per another reference point. Cost comparisons of health outcomes and health events have become common in public health. Approaches include cost-benefit, cost-effectiveness, and cost-utility studies.

Cost-benefit analyses provide comprehensive information on both the costs and the benefits of an intervention. All health outcomes and other relevant impacts are included in the determination of benefits. The results are expressed in terms of net costs, net benefits, and time required to recoup an initial investment. If the benefits are expressed in health outcome terms, years of life gained or quality-adjusted life years (QALYs) may be calculated. This provides a framework for comparing disparate interventions. QALYs are calculated from a particular perspective that determines which costs and consequences are included in the analysis. For public health analyses, societal perspectives are necessary. When comprehensively performed, cost benefit analyses are considered the gold standard of economic evaluations.

Cost-effectiveness analyses focus on one outcome to determine the most cost-effective intervention when several options are possible. Cost-effectiveness examines a specific option's costs to achieve a particular outcome. Results are often specified as the cost per case prevented or cost per life saved. For example, screening an entire town for a specific disease might identify cases at a cost of $150 per new case, whereas a screening program directed only at high-risk groups within that town might identify cases at a cost of $50 per new case. Although useful for evaluating different strategies for achieving the same result, cost-effectiveness approaches are not very helpful in evaluating interventions intended for different health conditions.

Cost-utility analyses are similar to cost-effectiveness studies, except that the results are characterized as cost per quality-adjusted life years. These are most useful when the intervention affects both morbidity and mortality, and there is a variety of possible outcomes that include quality of life.

These approaches are especially important for interventions based on preventive strategies. The argument is frequently made that "an ounce of prevention is worth a pound of cure." If this wisdom is true, preventive interventions should result in savings equal to 16 times their actual cost. Not all preventive interventions measure up to this standard, but even crude information on the costs of many health outcomes suggests that prevention has economic as well as human savings. Table 2–8 presents information from Healthy People 2000[26] (HP2000) regarding the economics of prevention for a number of common diseases and conditions; for each, the potential savings represents an enormous sum. Figure 2–11 illustrates that the impacts of disease and injuries can be many in terms of medical care costs for treatment in outpatient, emergency department, and hospital settings.[27] The U.S. Public Health Service has estimated that as much as 11 percent of projected health expenditures for the year 2000 could have been averted through investments in public health for six conditions: motor vehicle injuries, occupationally related injuries, stroke, coronary heart disease, firearms-related injuries, and low-birth-weight infants.[28]

Table 2-8 The Economics of Prevention

Condition	Overall Magnitude	Avoidable Intervention*	Cost/Patient[†]
Heart disease	7 million with coronary artery disease 500,000 deaths/year 284,000 bypass procedures/year	Coronary bypass surgery	$30,000
Cancer	1 million new cases/year 510,000 deaths/year	Lung cancer treatment Cervical cancer treatment	$29,000 $28,000
Stroke	600,000 strokes/year 150,000 deaths/year	Hemiplegia treatment and rehabilitation	$22,000
Injuries	2.3 million hospitalizations per year 142,500 deaths/year 177,000 persons with spinal cord injuries in the United States	Quadriplegia treatment and rehabilitation Hip fracture treatment and rehabilitation Severe head injury treatment and rehabilitation	$570,000 (lifetime) $40,000 $310,000
HIV infection	1–1.5 million infected 118,000 AIDS cases (as of Jan. 1990)	AIDS treatment	$75,000 (lifetime)
Alcoholism	18.5 million abuse alcohol 105,000 alcohol-related deaths/year	Liver transplant	$250,000
Drug abuse	Regular users: 1–3 million, cocaine 900,000, IV drugs 500,000, heroin Drug-exposed infants: 375,000	Treatment of cocaine-exposed infant	$66,000 (5 years)
LBW infants	260,000 LBW infants/year 23,000 deaths/year	Neonatal intensive care for LBW infant	$10,000
Inadequate immunization	Lacking basic immunization series: 20–30% aged 2 and younger 3% aged 6 and older	Congenital rubella syndrome treatment	$354,000 (lifetime)

LBW, low birth weight.

*Interventions represent examples (other interventions may apply).

[†]Representative first-year costs, except as noted. Not indicated are nonmedical costs, such as lost productivity to society.

Source: Reprinted from *Healthy People 2000*, 1990, U.S. Public Health Service, Washington, DC.

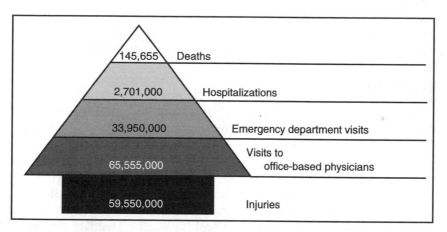

Figure 2–11 Health Impacts of Injuries. *Source:* Reprinted from C. W. Burt, Injury-Related Visits to Hospital Emergency Departments, *Advance Data 1995*, No. 261, 1992, NCHS.

Beyond the direct medical effects, there are often non-medical costs related to lost wages, taxes, and productivity.

Economists assert that the future costs for care and services that result from prevention of mortality must be considered a negative benefit of prevention. For example, the costs of preventing a death due to motor vehicle injuries should include all subsequent medical care costs for that individual over his or her lifetime, because these costs would not have occurred otherwise. They also argue that it is unfair to compare future savings to the costs of current prevention programs and that those savings must be discounted to their current value. If a preventive program will save $10 million 20 years from now, that $10 million must be translated into its current value in computing cost benefits, cost-effectiveness, or cost utility. It may be that the value of $10 million 20 years from now is only $4 million now. If the program costs $1 million, its benefit/cost ratio would be 4:1 instead of 10:1 before we even added any additional costs associated with medical care for the lives that were saved. These economic considerations contribute to the difficulty of marketing preventive interventions.

Two additional economic considerations are important for public health policy and practice. The first of these is what economists term *opportunity costs*. These represent the costs involved in choosing one course of action over another. Resources spent for one purpose are not available to be spent for another. As a result, there is a need to consider the costs of not realizing the benefits or gains from paths not chosen. A second economic consideration important for public health is related to the heavy emphasis of public health on preventive strategies. The savings or gains from successful prevention efforts are generally not reinvested in public health or even other health purposes. These savings or gains from investments in prevention are lost. Maybe this is proper because the overall benefits accrue more broadly to society, and public health remains, above all else, a social enterprise. However, imagine the situation for

American industry and businesses if they could not reinvest their gains to grow their businesses. This is often the situation faced by public health, further exacerbating the difficulty of arguing for and securing needed resources.

HEALTHY PEOPLE 2010

The data and discussion in this chapter only broadly describe health status measures in the United States in the early years of the new century. Several common themes emerge, however, that form the basis for national health objectives focusing on the year 2010.[29] Figure 2–12 (similar to the model illustrated in Figure 2–9) presents a *Healthy People 2010* (HP2010) process grounded in a broad view of the many factors influencing health. The year 2010 objectives build on the nation's experience with panels of health objectives established for the years 1990 and 2000. The Healthy People 1990 effort was initiated in the late 1970s through the efforts of Surgeon General Julius Richmond and coordinated by the Office of Disease Prevention and Health Promotion within the Office of the Assistant Secretary for Health.

Progress toward achievement of the year 2000 national health objectives was assessed in 1998. The status of each of the 319 objectives was reviewed and classified as moving in the right direction, moving in the wrong direction, showing no change, or unable to be tracked. The midcourse review found that 15 percent had been accomplished, another 44 percent were moving in the right direction, 18 percent were moving in the wrong direction, 3 percent showed no change, 6 percent showed mixed results, and 14 percent could not be tracked.[29] A substantially higher proportion of the objectives targeting special populations, especially blacks and American Indians, was found to be moving in the wrong direction. These findings raise concerns that disparities are persisting, if not increasing, in the United States. Progress toward some of the broader goals of the HP2000 effort was somewhat more positive; age-adjusted mortality targets for all age groups under age 70 were achieved.[29]

The year 2010 national health objectives include 467 specific objectives addressing health status measures, risk factor prevalence, and use of preventive health services. These objectives fall into 28 priority categories (Exhibit 2–1) and focus on two overarching goals: (1) to increase quality and years of healthy life and (2) to eliminate health disparities. Overall success will be gauged in relation to several age-adjusted summary measures for both the general population and racial and ethnic minorities: YPLL before age 75, hospital days per 100,000 population, and reported disability. Figure 2–13 presents data on several HP2010 objectives related to tobacco use. Because tracking 467 national targets is not practical, a list of leading indicators was developed (Exhibit 2–2); these focus on 10 important health issues by incorporating 21 of the HP2010 objectives.

Although the overall goals appear appropriate, they are only arguably linked. From one perspective, they represent two very different approaches to improving outcomes for the population as a whole. If we view the health status of the entire population as a Gaussian curve, one approach would be to shift the entire curve further toward better outcomes, and a second approach would be to change the shape of the curve, reducing the difference between

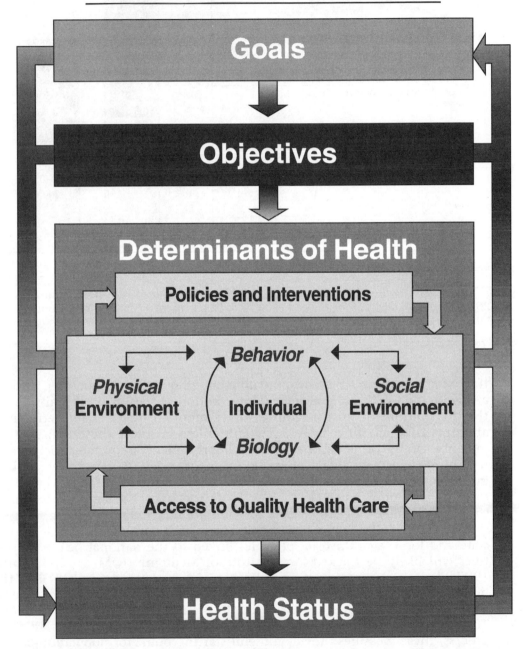

Figure 2–12 The Healthy People 2010 Model. *Source:* Reprinted from *Healthy People 2010: Understanding and Improving Health,* U.S. Department of Health and Human Services, Public Health Service, 2000.

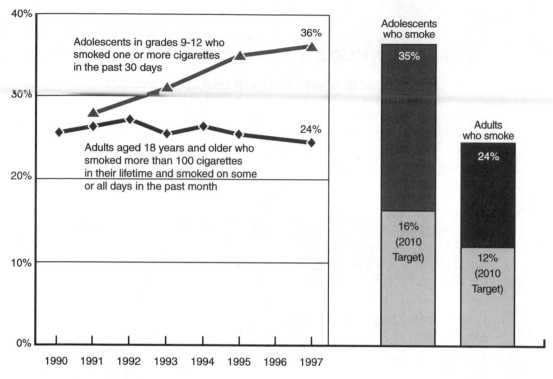

Figure 2–13 Cigarette Smoking, United States, 1990–1997. *Source:* Reprinted from *Healthy People 2010: Understanding and Improving Health,* U.S. Department of Health and Human Services, Public Health Service, 2000.

the extremes. These represent quite different strategies that would be associated with quite different policies and interventions. Focusing on the tail end of the distribution of health requires investment in questionably effective attempts that benefit relatively few and fail to promote the health of the majority. On the other hand, even small improvements in overall society-wide health measures have provided greater gains for society than very perceptible improvements in the health of a few.[30] The choice is one that can be viewed as focusing on "epiphenomena," such as risk factors or on the larger context and social environment. Healthy People 2010 ambitiously seeks to do both.

Monitoring all national health objectives is not considered feasible at the state and local level. Instead, priorities linked to the national health objectives will likely be tracked. An Institute of Medicine (IOM) committee in 1997 identified a basic set of indicators for use in community health improvement processes (Exhibit 2–3). This panel is notably more comprehensive than one promoted for use with the HP2000 activities of the 1990s. Together with the catalog of leading health indicators from the HP2010 process, these measures provide a useful starting point for population-based health improvement initiatives.

Exhibit 2–1 Healthy People 2010 Goals and Focus Areas

Goals
1. Increase Quality and Years of Healthy Life
2. Eliminate Health Disparities

Focus Areas
1. Access to Quality Health Services
2. Arthritis, Osteoporosis, and Chronic Back Conditions
3. Cancer
4. Chronic Kidney Disease
5. Diabetes
6. Disability and Secondary Conditions
7. Educational and Community-Based Programs
8. Environmental Health
9. Family Planning
10. Food Safety
11. Health Communication
12. Heart Disease and Stroke
13. HIV
14. Immunization and Infectious Disease
15. Injury and Violence Prevention
16. Maternal, Infant, and Child Health
17. Medical Product Safety
18. Mental Health and Mental Disorders
19. Nutrition and Overweight
20. Occupational Safety and Health
21. Oral Health
22. Physical Activity and Fitness
23. Public Health Infrastructure
24. Respiratory Diseases
25. Sexually Transmitted Diseases
26. Substance Abuse
27. Tobacco Use
28. Vision and Hearing

Source: Reprinted from *Healthy People 2010: Understanding and Improving Health,* U.S. Department of Health and Human Services, Public Health Service, 2000.

Exhibit 2–2 Healthy People 2010 Leading Indicators

Physical Activity
- Proportion of adolescents who engage in vigorous physical activity that promotes cardiorespiratory fitness 3 or more days per week for 20 or more minutes per occasion
- Proportion of adults who engage regularly, preferably daily, in moderate physical activity for at least 30 minutes a day

Overweight and obesity
- Proportion of children and adolescents who are overweight or obese
- Proportion of adults who are obese

Tobacco Use
- Proportion of adolescents who smoke
- Proportion of adults who smoke

Substance Abuse
- Proportion of adolescents not using alcohol or any illicit drugs during the past 30 days
- Proportion of adults using any illicit drug during the past 30 days
- Proportion of adults engaging in binge drinking of alcoholic beverages during the past month

Responsible Sexual Behavior
- Proportion of adolescents who abstain from sexual intercourse or use condoms if sexually active
- Proportion of sexually active persons who use condoms

Mental Health
- Proportion of adults with recognized depression who receive treatment

Injury and Violence
- Death rates due to motor vehicle crashes
- Death rates due to homicides

Environmental Quality
- Proportion of persons exposed to air that does not meet the U.S. Environmental Protection Agency's health-based standards for ozone
- Proportion of nonsmokers exposed to environmental tobacco smoke

Immunization
- Proportion of young children who receive all vaccines that have been recommended for universal administration for at least 5 years
- Proportion of noninstitutionalized adults who are vaccinated annually against influenza and ever vaccinated against pneumococcal disease

Access to Health Care
- Proportion of persons with health insurance
- Proportion of persons who have a specific source of ongoing care
- Proportion of pregnant women who begin prenatal care in the first trimester of pregnancy

Source: Reprinted from *Healthy People 2010: Understanding and Improving Health,* U.S. Department of Health and Human Services, Public Service, 2000.

Exhibit 2–3 Proposed Indicators for a Community Health Profile

Sociodemographic Characteristics

1. Distribution of the population by age and race/ethnicity.
2. Number and proportion of persons in groups such as migrants, homeless, or the non-English speaking for whom access to community services and resources may be a concern.
3. Number and proportion of persons aged 25 and older with less then a high school education.
4. Ratio of the number of students graduating from high school to the number of students who entered ninth grade three years previously.
5. Median household income.
6. Proportion of children less than 15 years of age living in families at or below the poverty level.
7. Unemployment rate.
8. Number and proportion of single-parent families.
9. Number and proportion of persons without health insurance.

Health Status

10. Infant mortality rate by race/ethnicity.
11. Numbers of deaths or age-adjusted death rates for motor vehicle crashes, work-related injuries, suicide, homicide, lung cancer, breast cancer, cardiovascular diseases, and all causes, by age, race, and gender, as appropriate.
12. Reported incidence of AIDS, measles, tuberculosis, and primary and secondary syphilis, by age, race, and gender, as appropriate.
13. Births to adolescents (ages 10–17) as proportion of total live births.
14. Number and rate of confirmed abuse and neglect cases among children.

Health Risk Factors

15. Proportion of two-year old children who have received all age appropriate vaccines, as recommended by the Advisory Committee on Immunization Practices.
16. Proportion of adults aged 65 and older who have ever been immunized for pneumococcal pneumonia; proportion who have been immunized in the past 12 months for influenza.
17. Proportion of the population who smoke, by age, race, and gender, as appropriate.
18. Proportion of the population aged 18 or older who are obese.
19. Number and type of U.S. Environmental Protection Agency air quality standards not met.
20. Proportion of assessed rivers, lakes, and estuaries that support beneficial uses (e.g., fishing-and swimming-approved).

Health Care Resource Consumption

21. Per-capita health care spending for Medicare beneficiaries (the Medicaid adjusted average per-capita cost [AAPCC]).

Functional Status

22. Proportion of adults reporting that their general health is good to excellent.
23. During the past 30 days, average number of days for which adults report that their physical or mental health was not good.

Quality of Life

24. Proportion of adults satisfied with the health care system in the community.
25. Proportion of persons satisfied with the quality of life in the community.

Source: Reprinted with permission from the Institute of Medicine. *Using Performance Monitoring to Improve Community Health: A Role for Performance Monitoring,* © 1997, National Academy Press.

CONCLUSION

From an ecological perspective, the health status of a population is influenced by many factors drawn from biology, behavior, the environment, and the use of health services. Social and cultural factors also play an important role in the disease patterns experienced by different populations, as well as in the responses of these populations to disease and illness. Globally, risks associated with population growth, pollution, and poverty result in mortality and morbidity that are still associated with infectious disease processes. In the United States, behaviorally mediated risks, including tobacco, diet, alcohol, and injury risks, rather than infectious disease processes, are the major contributors to health status, and the considerable gap between low-income minority populations and other Americans continues to widen. Reduction of the disparities in health status among population groups has emerged as the most critical national health goal for the year 2010. With the increasing availability of data on health status, as well as on determinants and contributing factors, the potential for more rational policies and interventions has increased. Over the long term, public policies that narrow income disparities and increase access to education, jobs, and housing do far more to improve the health status of populations than do efforts to provide more health care services. Health improvement efforts require more than data on health problems and contributing factors, which view health from a negative perspective. Also needed is information from a positive perspective, in terms of community capacities, assets, and willingness. More important still, there must be recognition and acceptance that the right to health is a basic human right and one inextricably linked to all other human rights, lest quality of life be seriously compromised.[31] It is this right to health that enables the practice of public health and challenges public health workers to measure health and quality of life in ways that promote its improvement.

DISCUSSION QUESTIONS AND EXERCISES

1. Is poverty a cause of poor health in a community, or is poor health a cause of poverty? How would different views of this question influence public health policy?
2. You have been asked to review and improve the consensus list of important health status indicators (see Exhibit 2–3). Identify and justify five indicators you would add to this list.
3. Visit the Internet website of one of the national print media and use the search features to identify articles on public health for a recent month. Catalog the health problems (both conditions and risks) from that search and compare this with the listing of health problems and issues on Table 2–4. Are the types of conditions and risks you encountered in the print media similar to those on Table 2–4? Were some conditions and risks either over- or underrepresented in the media, in comparison with their relative importance as sug-

gested by Table 2–4? What are the implications for the role of the media in informing and educating the public regarding public health issues?

4. Examine each of these websites. Which ones are most useful for the major topics examined in this part of the course? Why?

   - Healthfinder <http://www .healthfinder.gov>, a DHHS-sponsored gateway site that provides links to more than 550 websites (including more than 200 federal sites and 350 state, local, not-for-profit, university, and other consumer health sources), nearly 500 selected online documents, frequently asked questions on health issues, and databases and web search engines by topic and agency

   - Fedstats <http://www.fedstats.gov>, a gateway to a variety of federal agency data and information, including health statistics

   - National Center for Health Statistics (NCHS) <http://www.cdc.gov/nchswww>, an invaluable resource for data and information, especially "Health, United States," which can be downloaded from this site

   - CDC Mortality and Morbidity Weekly Reports <http://www2.cdc.gov/mmwr> and MMWR morbidity and mortality data by time and place <http://www2.cdc.gov/mmwr/distrnds.html>

   - U.S. Census data <http://www.census.gov>, the best general denominator data anywhere

5. Compare the "Public Health Achievements in Twentieth-Century America," presented in Chapter 1 (control of infectious diseases) and Chapter 2 (tobacco use). Which of these accomplishments, in your opinion, has had the greatest impact on the health status and quality of life of Americans living in the early twenty-first century? Justify your selection.

6. After reviewing "Public Health Achievements in Twentieth-Century America: Tobacco Use," select a health outcome related to tobacco use and analyze that problem for its determinants and contributing factors, using the method described in the text. Identify at least two major determinants for the problem that you select. For each determinant, identify at least two direct contributing factors, and for each direct contributing factor, identify at least two indirect contributing factors. At what level of your analysis does tobacco use appear as a risk factor?

7. Figure 2–13 presents data on several HP2010 objectives related to tobacco use. What are some important factors that must be addressed to achieve these targets in view of trends since 1990?

8. Population, poverty, and pollution are sometimes cited as the three most important factors influencing global health status today. After examining the WHO website <http://www.who.ch>, cite reasons for agreeing or disagreeing with this assertion.

9. Great Debate: There are three propositions to be considered. Proposition A: Disease entities should be listed as official causes of death. Proposition B: Underlying factors that result in these diseases should be listed as official causes of death. Proposition C: No causes of death should be listed on death certificates. Select one of these positions and develop a position statement with your rationale.

10. Projections call for a continuing increase in life expectancy through the first half of the twenty-first century. What effect will increased life expectancy have on the major goals of HP2010, increasing the quality and years of healthy life and eliminating health disparities?

REFERENCES

1. National Center for Health Statistics (NCHS). *Health United States 2002*. Hyattsville, MD: U.S. Public Health Service (PHS); 2002.

2. Allaire SH, LaValley MP, Evans SR et al. Evidence for decline in disability and improved health among persons aged 55 to 70 years: The Framingham heart study. *Am J Public Health*. 1999;89: 1678–1683.

3. Constitution of World Health Organization. In: *Chronicle of World Health Organization*. Geneva, Switzerland: World Health Organization (WHO); 1947;1:29–43.

4. Whaley RF, Hashim TJ. *A Textbook of World Health*. New York: Parthenon; 1995.

5. Centers for Disease Control and Prevention (CDC). First reportable underlying cause of death. *Morb Mortal Wkly Rep*. 1996;45:537.

6. Brownson RC, Remington PL, Davis JR, eds. *Chronic Disease Epidemiology and Control, 2nd ed*. Washington, DC: American Public Health Association; 1998.

7. Seitz F, Plepys C. Monitoring air quality in Healthy People 2000. *Healthy People 2000 Statistical Notes*. Hyattsville, MD: NCHS; 1995:No. 9.

8. Amler RW, Eddins DL. Cross-sectional analysis: Precursors of premature death in the U.S. In: Amler RW, Dull DL, eds. *Closing the Gap*. Atlanta, GA: Carter Center; 1985:181–187.

9. McGinnis JM, Foege W. Actual causes of death in the United States. *JAMA*. 1993;270: 2207–2212.

10. Chadwick E. *Report on the Sanitary Conditions of the Labouring Population of Great Britain 1842*. Edinburgh, Scotland: Edinburgh University Press; 1965.

11. Smith GD, Egger M. Socioeconomic differences in mortality in Britain and the United States. *Am J Public Health*. 1992;82:1079–1081.

12. Schrijvers CTMN, Stronks K, van de Mheen HD, Mackenbach JP. Explaining educational differences in mortality: The role of behavioral and material factors. *Am J Public Health*. 1999; 89:535–540.

13. CDC. Poverty and infant mortality: United States, 1988. *Morb Mortal Wkly Rep*. 1996;44:922–927.

14. Ng-Mak DS, Dohrenwend BP, Abraido-Lanza AF, Turner JB. A further analysis of race differences in the national longitudinal mortality study. *Am J Public Health*. 1999;89:1748–1751.

15. Wilkenson RG. National mortality rates: The impact of inequality. *Am J Public Health*. 1992;82:1082–1084.

16. Marmot M. The influence of income on health: views of an epidemiologist. *Health Affairs* 2002:21(2):31–46.

17. Sargent CF, Johnson TM, eds. *Medical Anthropology: Contemporary Theory and Method. Rev ed.* Westport, CT: Praeger Publishers; 1996.

18. Susser M, Watson W, Hopper K. *Sociology in Medicine.* New York: Oxford University Press; 1985.

19. Link BG, Phelan JC. Understanding sociodemographic differences in health: The role of fundamental social causes. *Am J Public Health.* 1996;86:471–473.

20. Friedman SR, Curtis R, Neaigus A, Jose B, Des Jarlais DC. *Social Networks, Drug Injectors' Lives and HIV/AIDS.* New York: Kluwer Academic Publishers; 1999.

21. Kawachi I, Kennedy BP, Glass R. Social capital and self-rated health: A contextual analysis. *Am J Public Health.* 1999;89:1187–1193.

22. Malmstom M, Sundquist J, Johansson SE. Neighborhood environment and self-reported health status: A multilevel analysis. *Am J Public Health.* 1999;89:1181–1186.

23. Doll R. Health and the environment in the 1990s. *Am J Public Health.* 1992;82:933–941.

24. Winkelstein W. Determinants of worldwide health. *Am J Public Health.* 1992;82:931–932.

25. Fielding JE. Public health in the twentieth century: Advances and challenges. *Ann Rev Public Health.* 1999;20:xiii–xxx.

26. U.S. Department of Health and Human Services (DHHS). *Healthy People 2000.* Washington, DC: DHHS-PHS; 1990.

27. Burt CW. *Injury-Related Visits to Hospital Emergency Departments, U.S., 1992.* Hyattsville, MD: PHS; 1995:261.

28. *For a Healthy Nation: Return on Investments in Public Health.* Washington, DC: PHS; 1994.

29. National Center for Health Statistics. *Healthy People 2000 Final Review.* Hyattsville MD: PHS; 2001.

30. McKinlay JB, Marceau LD. A tale of 3 tails. *Am J Public Health.* 1999;89:295–298.

31. Universal Declaration of Human Rights. *GA res* 217 A(iii), UN Doc A/810, art 25(1);1948.

Public Health
and the Health System

This chapter picks up where Chapter 2 left off—with influences on health. The influences to be examined in Chapter 3, however, are the interventions and services available through the health system.

The relationship between public health and other health-related activities has never been clear, but in recent years, it has become even less well defined. Some of the lack of clarity may be due to the several different images of public health described in Chapter 1, but certainly not all. In addition to the U.S. health system remaining poorly understood by the public, there are different views among health professionals and policymakers as to whether public health is part of the health system or the health system is part of the public health enterprise. Most agree that these components serve the same ends but disagree as to the balance between the two and the locus for strategic deci sions and actions. The issue of ownership—which component's leadership and strategies will predominate—underlies these different perspectives. In this text, the term health system will refer to all aspects of the organization, financing, and provision of programs and services for the prevention and treatment of illness and injury. The public health system is a component of this larger health system. This view conflicts with the image that most people have of our health system; the public commonly perceives the health system to include only the medical care and treatment aspects of the overall system. Both public health and the overall health sector will be referred to as *systems*, with the understanding that public health activities are part of a larger set of activities that focus on health, well-being, disease, and illness.

Although the relationships may not be clear, there is ample cause for public health interest in the health system. Perhaps most compelling is the sheer size and scope of the U.S. health system, characteristics that have made the health system an ethical issue. Nearly 12 million workers and $1.5 trillion in resources are devoted to health-related purposes.[1] However, this huge investment in fiscal and human resources may not be accomplishing what it can and should in terms of health outcomes. Lack of access to needed health services for an increasing number of Americans and inconsistent quality contribute to less than optimal health outcomes. Although access and quality have long been public health concerns, the excess capacity of the health system is a relatively new issue for public health.

This chapter examines the U.S. health system from several perspectives that consider the public health implications of costs and affordability, as well as several other important public policy and public health questions:

- Does the United States have a rational strategy for investing its resources to maintain and improve people's health?
- Is the current strategy excessive in ways that inequitably limit access to and benefit from needed services?
- Is the health system accountable to its end-users and ultimate payers for the quality and results of its services?

It is these issues of health, excess, access, accountability, and quality that make the health system a public health concern.

Complementary, even synergistic, efforts involving medicine and public health are apparent in many of the important gains in health outcomes achieved during the twentieth century. Progress since 1900 in improving pregnancy outcomes and promoting the health of mothers and infants (see "Public Health Achievements in Twentieth-Century America: Improved Maternal and Infant Health" following) tell this story from one perspective. Another perspective will be drawn from a framework for linking various health strategies and activities to their strategic intent, level of prevention, relationship to medical and public health practice, and community or individual focus. Key economic, demographic, and resource trends will then be briefly presented as a prelude to understanding important themes and emerging paradigm shifts. New opportunities afforded by sweeping changes in the health system, many of which relate to managed care strategies, will be apparent in the review of these issues.

Example

Public Health Achievements in Twentieth-Century America: Improved Maternal and Infant Health

Both medical and public health strategies have contributed to the impressive improvement in maternal and infant health measures achieved over the twentieth century. Reducing infant mortality, for example, calls for either decreasing the proportion of infants born at low birth weight (prevention) or by improving the chances of those infants to survive through more effective medical care. Prevention and treatment should not be considered mutually exclusive strategies.

Improved Pregnancy Outcomes

At the beginning of the twentieth century, for every 1,000 live births, 6–9 women in the United States died of pregnancy-related complications, and approximately 100 infants died before the age of 1 year.

Table 3–1 Percentage Reduction in Infant, Neonatal, and Postneonatal Mortality, by Year—United States, 1915–1997*

| | Percentage Reduction in Mortality | | |
Year	Infant (aged 0–364 days)	Neonatal (aged 0–27 days)	Postneonatal (aged 28–364 days)
1915–1919	13%	7%	19%
1920–1929	21%	11%	31%
1930–1939	26%	18%	35%
1940–1949	33%	26%	46%
1950–1959	10%	7%	15%
1960–1969	20%	17%	27%
1970–1979	35%	41%	14%
1980–1989	22%	27%	12%
1990–1997	22%	17%	29%
1915–1997	93%	89%	96%

*Percentage reduction is calculated as the reduction from the first year of the time period to the last year of the time period.
Source: Reprinted from Achievements in Public Health, United States, 1900–1999: Healthier Mothers and Babies. *Morbidity and Mortality Weekly Report*, Vol. 48, No. 38, pp. 849–858, the Centers for Disease Control and Prevention, 1999.

From 1915 through 1997, the infant mortality rate declined greater than 90 percent to 7.2 per 1,000 live births; and, from 1900 through 1997, the maternal mortality rate declined almost 99 percent to less than 0.1 reported death per 1,000 live births (7.7 deaths per 100,000 live births in 1997) (Table 3–1 and Figure 3–1). Environmental interventions, improvements in nutrition, advances in clinical medicine, improvements in access to health care, improvements in surveillance and monitoring of disease, increases in education levels, and improvements in standards of living contributed to this remarkable decline. Despite these improvements in maternal and infant mortality rates, significant disparities by race and ethnicity persist.

The decline in infant mortality is unparalleled by other mortality reduction this century. If turn-of-the-century infant death rates had continued, an estimated 500,000 live-born infants during 1997 would have died before age 1 year; instead, 28,045 infants died.

In 1900 in some U.S. cities, up to 30 percent of infants died before reaching their first birthdays. Efforts to reduce infant mortality focused on improving environmental and living conditions in urban areas. Urban environmental interventions (e.g., sewage and refuse disposal and safe drinking water) played key roles in reducing infant mortality. Rising standards of living, including improvements in economic and education levels of families, helped to promote health. Declining fertility rates also contributed to reductions in infant mortality through longer spacing of children, smaller family size, and better nutritional

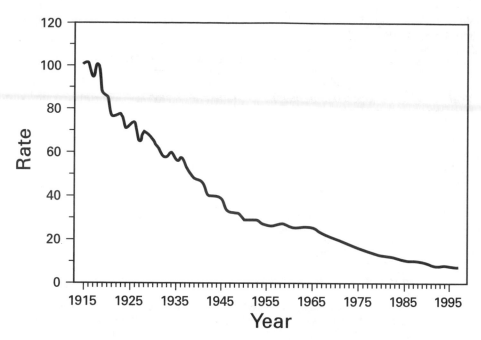

Figure 3–1 Infant Mortality Rate (per 1,000 live births) by Year—United States, 1915–1997. *Source:* Reprinted from Achievements in Public Health, United States, 1900–1999: Healthier Mothers and Babies, *Morbidity and Mortality Weekly Report,* Vol. 48, No. 38, pp. 849–858, the Centers for Disease Control and Prevention, 1999.

status of mothers and infants. Milk pasteurization, first adopted in Chicago in 1908, contributed to the control of milk-borne diseases (e.g., gastrointestinal infections) from contaminated milk supplies.

During the first three decades of the century, public health, social welfare, and clinical medicine (pediatrics and obstetrics) collaborated to combat infant mortality. This partnership began with milk hygiene but later included other public health issues. In 1912 the Children's Bureau was formed and became the primary government agency to work toward improving maternal and infant welfare until 1946, when its role in maternal and child health diminished; the Bureau was eliminated in 1969. The Children's Bureau defined the problem of infant mortality and shaped the debate over programs to ameliorate the problem. The Bureau also advocated comprehensive maternal and infant welfare services, including prenatal, natal, and postpartum home visits by health-care providers. By the 1920s the integration of these services changed the approach to infant mortality from one that addressed infant health problems to an approach that included infant and mother and prenatal care programs to educate, monitor, and care for pregnant women.

The discovery and widespread use of antimicrobial agents (e.g., sulfonamide in 1937 and penicillin in the 1940s) and the development of fluid and electrolyte replacement therapy and safe blood transfusions accelerated the declines in infant mortality; from 1930 through 1949, mortality rates declined 52 percent.

The percentage decline in postneonatal (age 28–364 days) mortality (66 percent) was greater than the decline in neonatal (age 0–27 days) mortality (40 percent). From 1950 through 1964, infant mortality declined more slowly. An increasing proportion of infant deaths was attributed to perinatal causes and occurred among high-risk neonates, especially low-birth-weight (LBW) and preterm babies. Although no reliable data exist, the rapid decline in infant mortality during earlier decades probably was not influenced by decreases in LBW rates because the decrease in mortality was primarily in postneonatal deaths that are less influenced by birth weight. Inadequate programs during the 1950s and 1960s to reduce deaths among high-risk neonates led to renewed efforts to improve access to prenatal care—especially for the poor—and to a concentrated effort to establish neonatal intensive-care units and to promote research in maternal and infant health, including research into technologies to improve the survival of LBW and preterm babies.

During the late 1960s, after Medicaid and other federal programs were implemented, infant mortality (primarily postneonatal mortality) declined substantially. From 1970 to 1979, neonatal mortality plummeted 41 percent (Table 3–1) because of technologic advances in neonatal medicine and in the regionalization of perinatal services; postneonatal mortality declined 14 percent. During the early to mid-1980s, the downward trend in U.S. infant mortality slowed. However, during 1989–1991, infant mortality declined slightly faster, probably because of the use of artificial pulmonary surfactant to prevent and treat respiratory distress syndrome in premature infants. During 1991–1997, infant mortality continued to decline primarily because of decreases in sudden infant death syndrome (SIDS) and other causes.

Although improvements in medical care were the main force for declines in infant mortality during the second half of the century, public health actions played a role. During the 1990s, a greater than 50 percent decline in sudden infant death syndrome (SIDS) rates (attributed to the recommendation that infants be placed to sleep on their backs) has helped to reduce the overall infant mortality rate. The reduction in vaccine-preventable diseases (e.g., diphtheria, tetanus, measles, poliomyelitis, and *Haemophilus influenzae* type b meningitis) has reduced infant morbidity and has had a modest effect on infant mortality. Advances in prenatal diagnosis of severe central nervous system defects, selective termination of affected pregnancies, and improved surgical treatment and management of other structural anomalies have helped to reduce infant mortality attributed to these birth defects. National efforts to encourage reproductive-aged women to consume foods or supplements containing folic acid could reduce the incidence of neural tube defects by half.

Family Planning

During the twentieth century, the hallmark of family planning in the United States has been the ability to achieve desired birth spacing and family size (Figure 3–2). Fertility decreased as couples chose to have fewer children; concurrently, child mortality declined, people moved from farms to cities, and the age at marriage increased. Smaller families and longer birth intervals have contributed to the better health of infants, children, and women, and have improved the social and economic role of women. Despite high failure rates, traditional methods of fertility control contributed to the decline in family size. Modern contraception and reproductive health-care systems that became available later in the century further improved couples' ability to plan their families. Publicly supported family planning services prevent an estimated 1.3 million unintended pregnancies annually.

Family size declined between 1800 and 1900 from 7.0 to 3.5 children. In 1900, 6 to 9 of every 1,000 women died in childbirth, and 1 in 5 children died during the first 5 years of life. Distributing information and counseling patients about contraception and contraceptive devices was illegal under federal and state laws; the timing of ovulation, the length of the fertile period, and other reproductive facts were unknown.

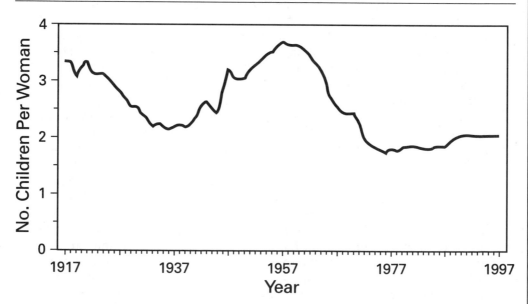

Figure 3–2 Fertility Rates, United States, 1917–1997. *Source:* Reprinted from Achievements in Public Health, United States, 1900–1999: Family Planning, *Morbidity and Mortality Weekly Report,* Vol. 48, No. 47, pp. 1073–1080, the Centers for Disease Control and Prevention, 1999.

Maternal Mortality

Maternal mortality rates were highest in this century during 1900–1930 (Figure 3–3). Poor obstetric education and delivery practices were mainly responsible for the high numbers of maternal deaths, most of which were preventable. Obstetrics as a specialty was shunned by many physicians, and obstetric care was provided by poorly trained or untrained medical practitioners. Most births occurred at home with the assistance of midwives or general practitioners. Inappropriate and excessive surgical and obstetric interventions (e.g., induction of labor, use of forceps, episiotomy, and Caesarean deliveries) were common and increased during the 1920s. Deliveries, including some surgical interventions, were performed without following the principles of asepsis. As a result, 40 percent of maternal deaths were caused by sepsis (half following delivery and half associated with illegally induced abortion), with the remaining deaths primarily attributed to hemorrhage and toxemia.

The 1933 White House Conference on Child Health Protection, Fetal, Newborn, and Maternal Mortality and Morbidity report demonstrated the link between poor aseptic practice, excessive operative deliveries, and high maternal mortality. This and earlier reports focused attention on the state of maternal health and led to calls for action by state medical associations. During the 1930s and 1940s, hospital and

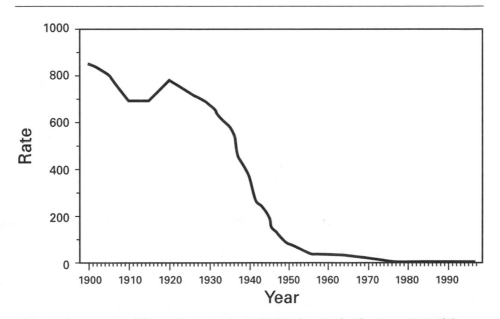

Figure 3–3 Maternal Mortality Rates (per 100,000 live births) by Year, United States, 1900–1997. *Source:* Reprinted from Achievements in Public Health, United States, 1900–1999: Healthier Mothers and Babies, *Morbidity and Mortality Weekly Report,* Vol. 48, No. 38, pp. 849–858, the Centers for Disease Control and Prevention, 1999.

state maternal mortality review committees were established. During the ensuing years, institutional practice guidelines and guidelines defining physician qualifications needed for hospital delivery privileges were developed. At the same time, a shift from home to hospital deliveries was occurring throughout the country; during 1938–1948, the proportion of infants born in hospitals increased from 55 percent to 90 percent. However, this shift was slow in rural areas and southern states. Safer deliveries in hospitals under aseptic conditions and improved provision of maternal care for the poor by states or voluntary organizations led to decreases in maternal mortality after 1930. Medical advances (including the use of antibiotics, oxytocin to induce labor, and safe blood transfusion and better management of hypertensive conditions during pregnancy) accelerated declines in maternal mortality. During 1939–1948, maternal mortality decreased by 71 percent. The legalization of induced abortion, beginning in the 1960s, contributed to an 89 percent decline in deaths from septic illegal abortions during 1950–1973.

Since 1982, maternal mortality has not declined. However, more than half of maternal deaths can be prevented with existing interventions. In 1997, 327 maternal deaths were reported based on information on death certificates; however, death certificate data underestimate these deaths, and the actual numbers are 2–3 times greater. The leading causes of maternal death are hemorrhage, including hemorrhage associated with ectopic pregnancy, pregnancy-induced hypertension (toxemia), and embolism.

Sources: Adapted from Achievements in Public Health, United States, 1900–1999: Healthier Mothers and Babies, *Morbidity and Mortality Weekly Report*, Vol. 48, No. 38, pp. 849–858, the Centers for Disease Control and Prevention, 1999; and Public Health Achievements, United States, 1900–1999: Family Planning, *Morbidity and Mortality Weekly Report*, Vol. 48, No. 47, pp. 1073–1080, the Centers for Disease Control and Prevention, 1999.

PREVENTION AND HEALTH SERVICES

As evidenced in improvements in pregnancy outcome and the health of mothers and children, the health system influences health status through a variety of intervention strategies and services.[2] Key relationships among health, illness, and various interventions intended to maintain or restore health are summarily presented in Table 3–2. As discussed in Chapter 2, health and illness are dynamic states that are influenced by a wide variety of biologic, environmental, behavioral, social, and health service factors. The complex interaction of these factors results in the occurrence or absence of disease or injury, which, in turn, contributes to the health status of individuals and populations. Several different intervention points are possible, including two general strategies that seek to maintain health by intervening prior to the development of disease or injury.[2] These are health promotion and specific protection strategies. Both involve activities that alter the interaction of

Table 3–2 Health Strategies, Prevention Levels, Practice Domains, and Targets

Strategy	State Addressed	Prevention Level	Practice Domain	Target
Health promotion	Health	Primary	Public health	Community
Specific protection	Health	Primary	Public health	Community or risk group
Early case finding and prompt treatment	Illness	Secondary	Public health and primary medical care	Individual
Disability limitation	Illness	Tertiary	Secondary/tertiary medical care	Individual
Rehabilitation	Illness	Tertiary	Long-term care	Individual and group

Source: Data from H. R. Leavell and E. G. Clark, *Preventive Medicine for the Doctor in His Community, Third Edition* © 1965, McGraw-Hill.

the various health-influencing factors in ways that contribute to either averting or altering the likelihood of occurrence of disease or injury.

Health Promotion and Specific Protection

Health promotion activities attempt to modify human behaviors to reduce those known to affect adversely the ability to resist disease or injury-inducing factors, thereby eliminating exposures to harmful factors. Examples of health promotion activities include interventions such as nutrition counseling, genetic counseling, family counseling, and the myriad activities that constitute health education. However, health promotion also properly includes the provision of adequate housing, employment, and recreational conditions, as well as other forms of community development activities. What is clear from these examples is that many fall outside the common public understanding of what constitutes health care. Several of these are viewed as the duty or responsibility of other societal institutions, including public safety, housing, education, and even industry. It is somewhat ironic that activities that focus on the state of health and that seek to maintain and promote health are not commonly perceived to be "health services." To some extent, this is also true for the other category of health-maintaining strategies—specific protection activities.

Specific protection activities provide individuals with resistance to factors (such as microorganisms like viruses and bacteria) or modify environments to decrease potentially harmful interactions of health-influencing factors (such as toxic exposures in the workplace). Examples of specific protection include activities directed toward specific risks (e.g., the use of protective equipment for asbestos removal), immunizations, occupational and environmental engineering, and regulatory controls and activities to protect individuals from environmental carcinogens (such as exposure to second-hand or side-stream smoke) and toxins. Several of these are often identified with settings other than traditional health care settings. Many are implemented and enforced through governmental agencies. Exhibit 3–1 presents a catalog of health-related prevention organizations, agencies, and institutions.

Exhibit 3–1 Example of Health-Related Prevention Organizations, Agencies, and Institutions

---

Federal Agencies

Department of Agriculture
Department of Transportation
Department of Energy
Department of Health and Human Services
Department of Homeland Security
Department of Labor
Department of Education
Department of Justice
Department of the Interior
Department of Veterans Administration
Department of Commerce
Department of Treasury
Department of Housing and Urban Development
Environmental Protection Agency
Consumer Product Safety Commission
Federal Mine Safety and Health Review Commission
National Transportation Safety Board
Nuclear Regulatory Commission
Occupational Safety and Health Review Commission
Federal Emergency Management Agency

State Agencies (different agency names in different states)

Aging
Agriculture
Alcoholism and Substance Abuse
Children and Family Services
Council on Health and Fitness
Emergency Services and Disaster Agency
Energy and Natural Resources
Environmental Protection Agency
Guardianship and Advocacy Commission
Health Care Cost Containment Agency
Health Facilities Planning Board and Agency
Mental Health and Developmental Disabilities
Nuclear Safety
Pollution Control Board
Professional Regulation Agency
Public Health
Rehabilitation Services
State Fire Marshall
State Board of Education
State Board of Higher Education
Veterans Affairs

Miscellaneous Organizations and Sites

Foundations
Corporations
Voluntary Health Associations
United Way of America
Physician Office Visits
HMO visits
Dental Visits

Early Case Finding and Prompt Treatment, Disability Limitation, and Rehabilitation

Although health promotion and specific protection both focus on the healthy state and seek to prevent disease, a different set of strategies and activities is necessary if the interaction of factors results in disease or injury. When disease occurs, the strategies that become necessary are those facilitating early detection, rapid control, or rehabilitation, depending on the stage of development of the disease.

In general, early detection and prompt treatment reduce individual pain and suffering and are less costly to both the individual and society than treatment initiated only after a condition has reached a more advanced state. Interventions to achieve early detection and prompt treatment include screening tests, case-finding efforts, and periodic physical exams. Screening tests are increasingly available to detect illnesses before they become symptomatic. Case-finding efforts for both infectious and noninfectious conditions are directed at populations at greater risk for the condition on the basis of criteria appropriate for that condition. Periodic physical exams, such as those mentioned in the age-specific recommendations of the U.S. Preventive Health Services Task Force,[3] incorporate these practices and are best provided through an effective primary medical care system. Primary care providers who are sensitive to disease patterns and predisposing factors can play substantial roles in the early identification and management of most medical conditions.

Another strategy targeting disease is disability limitation through effective and complete treatment. It is this set of activities that most Americans equate with the term *health care,* largely because this strategy constitutes the lion's share of the U.S. health system in terms of resource deployment. Quite appropriately, these efforts largely aim to arrest or eradicate disease or to limit disability and prevent death. The final intervention strategy focusing on disease—rehabilitation—is designed to return individuals who have experienced a condition to the maximum level of function consistent with their capacities.

Links with Prevention

There are several useful aspects of this framework. It emphasizes the potential for prevention inherent in each of the five health service strategies. Prevention can be categorized in several ways. The best known approach classifies prevention in relation to the stage of the disease or condition.

Preventive intervention strategies are considered primary, secondary, or tertiary. Primary prevention involves prevention of the disease or injury itself, generally through reducing exposure or risk factor levels. Secondary prevention attempts to identify and control disease processes in their early stages, often before signs and symptoms become apparent. In this case, prevention is akin to preemptive treatment. Tertiary prevention seeks to prevent disability through restoring individuals to their optimal level of functioning after damage is done. The selection of an intervention point at the primary, secondary, or tertiary level is a function of knowledge, resources, acceptability, effectiveness, and efficiency, among other considerations.

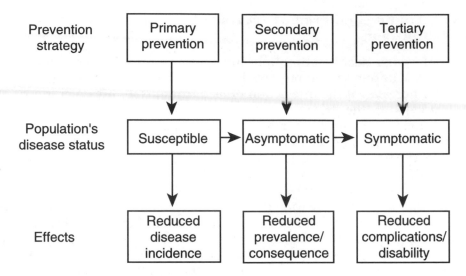

Figure 3–4 Levels of Prevention with Effects. *Source:* Reprinted from RC Brownson, PL Remington, and JR Davis, *Chronic Disease Epidemiology and Control,* 2nd Edition, © 1998, American Public Health Association.

The relationship of health promotion and specific protection to these levels of prevention is also presented in Table 3–2. Health promotion and specific protection are primary prevention strategies seeking to prevent the development of disease. Early case finding and prompt treatment represent secondary prevention because they seek to interrupt the disease process before it becomes symptomatic. Both disability limitation and rehabilitation are considered tertiary-level prevention in that they seek to prevent or reduce disability associated with disease or injury. Although these are considered tertiary prevention, they receive primary attention under current policy and resource deployment.

Figure 3–4 illustrates each of the three levels of prevention strategies in relation to population disease status and effect on disease incidence and prevalence. The various potential benefits from the three intervention levels derive from the basic epidemiologic concepts of incidence and prevalence. Prevalence (the number of existing cases of illness, injury, or a health event) is a function of both incidence (the number of new cases) and duration. Reducing either component can reduce prevalence. Primary prevention aims to reduce the incidence of conditions, whereas secondary and tertiary prevention seek to reduce prevalence by shortening duration and minimizing the effects of disease or injury. It should be apparent that there is a finite limit to how much a condition's duration can be reduced. As a result, approaches emphasizing primary prevention have greater potential benefit than do approaches emphasizing other levels of prevention. This basis for understanding the differential impact of prevention and treatment approaches to a particular health problem or condition cannot be overstated.

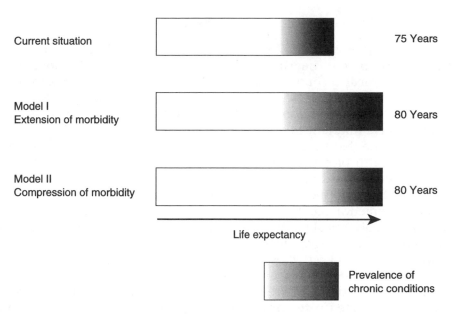

Figure 3–5 Alternative Models of Extension or Compression of Morbidity as Life Expectancy Is Extended. *Source:* Reprinted from RC Brownson, PL Remington, and JR Davis, *Chronic Disease Epidemiology and Control,* 2nd Edition, © 1998, American Public Health Association.

These same considerations are pertinent to the idea of postponement of morbidity as a prevention strategy, as illustrated in Figure 3–5. As demonstrated in Model I, increased life expectancy without postponement of morbidity may actually increase the burden of illness within a population, as measured by prevalence. However, postponement may result in the development of a condition so late in life that it results in either no or less disability in functioning.

Another approach to classifying prevention efforts groups interventions by the nature of the intervention into clinical, behavioral, or environmental categories. Clinical interventions are provided to individuals, whereas environmental interventions are organized for populations or groups. Behavioral interventions can be provided either for individuals or for populations, including subgroups identified as being at higher risk for a particular condition.

Within this framework for considering intervention strategies aimed at health or illness, the potential for prevention as an element of all strategies is clear. There are substantial opportunities to use primary and secondary prevention strategies to improve health in general and reduce the burden of illness for individuals and for society. As noted in Chapter 2, reducing the burden of illness carries the potential for substantial cost savings. These concepts serve to promote a more rational intervention and investment strategy for the U.S. health system.

Links with Public Health and Medical Practice

Another useful aspect of this framework is in its allocation of responsibilities for carrying out the various interventions. Three practice domains can be roughly delineated: public health practice, medical practice, and long-term care practice.[2] The framework assigns public health practice primary responsibility for health promotion, specific protection, and a good share of early case finding. It is important to note that the concept of public health practice here is a broad one that accommodates the activities carried out by many different types of health professionals and workers, not only those working in public health agencies. Although many of these activities are carried out in public health agencies of the federal, state, or local government, many are not. Public health practice occurs in voluntary health agencies, as well as in settings such as schools, social service agencies, industry, and even traditional medical care settings. In terms of prevention, public health practice embraces all of the primary prevention activities in the model, as well as some of the activities for early diagnosis and prompt treatment.

The demarcations between public health and medical practice are neither clear nor absolute. In recent decades, public health practice has been extensively involved in screening and has become an important source of primary medical care for populations with diminished access to care. At the same time, medical practice has also been extensively involved with early case finding while traditionally providing the major share of primary care services to most segments of the population.

Medical practice, meaning those services usually provided by or under the supervision of a physician or other traditional health care provider, can be viewed as including three levels (Exhibit 3–2). Primary medical care has been variously defined but generally focuses on the basic health needs of individuals and families. It is first-contact health care in the view of the patient; provides at least 80 percent of necessary care; includes a comprehensive array of services, on site or through referral, including health promotion and disease prevention, as well as curative services; and is accessible and acceptable to the patient population. This comprehensive description of primary care differs substantially from what is commonly encountered as primary care in the U.S. health system. Often lacking from current so-called primary care services are those relating to health promotion and disease prevention.

The concept of *disease management* has evolved from efforts to provide a more integrated approach to healthcare delivery in order to improve health outcomes and reduce costs, often for defined populations such as Medicaid enrollees. Disease management focuses on identifying and proactively monitoring high-risk populations, assisting patients and providers to adhere to treatment plans that are based on proven interventions, promoting provider coordination, increasing patient education, and preventing avoidable medical complications.

Beyond primary medical care are two more specialized types of care that are often termed *secondary care* and *tertiary care*. Secondary care is specialized care serving the major share of the remaining 20 percent of the need that lies beyond the scope of primary care. Physicians or hospitals generally provide

Exhibit 3–2 Health Care Pyramid Levels

- Tertiary Medical Care
  Subspecialty referral care requiring highly specialized personnel and facilities
- Secondary Medical Care
  Specialized attention and ongoing management for common and less frequently encountered medical conditions, including support services for people with special challenges due to chronic or long-term conditions
- Primary Medical Care
  Clinical preventive services, first-contact treatment services, and ongoing care for commonly encountered medical conditions
- Population-Based Public Health Services
  Interventions aimed at disease prevention and health promotion that shape a community's overall health profile

Source: Reprinted from *For a Healthy Nation: Return on Investments in Public Health,* U.S. Public Health Service, 1994.

secondary care, ideally upon referral from a primary care source. Tertiary medical care is even more highly specialized and technologically sophisticated medical and surgical care for those with unusual or complex conditions (generally no more than a few percent of the need in any service category). Tertiary care is frequently provided in large medical centers or academic health centers.

Long-term care is appropriately classified separately because of the special needs of the population requiring such services and the specialized settings where many of these services are offered. This, too, is changing as specialized long-term care services increasingly move out of long-term care facilities and into home settings.

Within the health services pyramid presented in Figure 3–6, primary prevention activities are largely associated with population-based public health services at the base of the pyramid, although some primary prevention in the form of clinical preventative services is also associated with primary medical care services. Secondary prevention activities are split somewhat more evenly between the population-based public health services and primary medical care. Tertiary prevention activities fall largely in the secondary and tertiary medical care components of the pyramid. The use of a pyramid to represent health services implies that each level serves a different proportion of the total population. Everyone should be served by population-wide public health services, and nearly everyone should be served by primary medical care. However, increasingly smaller proportions of the total population require secondary- and tertiary-level medical care services. In any event, the system should be built from the bottom up. It would not be rational to build such a system from the top down; there might not be enough resources to address the lower levels that served as the foundation for the system. Nonetheless, there is evidence in later sections of this chapter that this is exactly what has occurred with the U.S. health system.

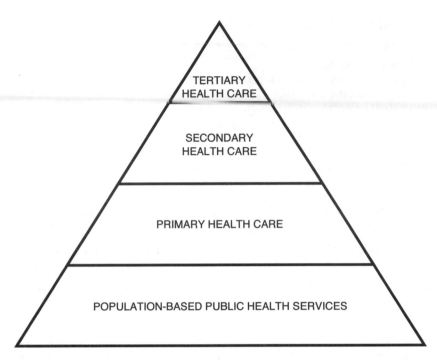

Figure 3–6 Health Services Pyramid. *Source:* Reprinted from *For a Healthy Nation: Return on Investments in Public Health,* 1994, Public Health Service, Washington, DC.

Targets of Health Service Strategies

A final facet of this model characterizes the targets for the strategies and activities. Generally, primary preventive services are community-based and are targeted toward populations or groups rather than individuals. Early case-finding activities can be directed toward groups or toward individuals. For example, many screening activities target groups at higher risk when these are provided through public health agencies. The same screening activities can also be provided for individuals through physicians' offices and hospital outpatient departments. Much of primary and virtually all of secondary and tertiary medical care is appropriately individually-oriented. It should be noted that there is a concept, termed *community-oriented primary care,* in which primary care providers assume responsibility for all of the individuals in a community, rather than only those who seek out care from the provider. Even in this model, however, care is provided on an individual basis. Long-term care involves elements of both community-based service and individually-oriented service. These services are tailored for individuals but often in a group setting or as part of a package of services for a defined number of recipients, as in a long-term care facility.

Public Health and Medical Practice Interfaces

This framework also sheds light on the potential conflicts between public health and medical practice. Although the two are presented as separate domains of practice, there are many interfaces that provide a template for either collaboration or conflict. Both paths have been taken over the past century. Public health practitioners have traditionally deferred to medical practitioners for providing the broad spectrum of services for disease and injuries in individuals. Medical practitioners have generally acknowledged the need for public health practice for health promotion and specific protection strategies. The interfaces raise difficult issues. For example, for one specific protection activity—childhood immunizations—it can be argued that the extensive role of public health practice has served to fragment health services for children. It would be logical to provide these services within a well-functioning primary care system, where they could be better integrated with other services for this population. Despite occasional differences as to roles, in most circumstances, medical practice has supported the role of public health to serve as the provider of last resort in ensuring medical care for persons who lack financial access to private health care. This, too, has varied over time and from place to place.

Advances in bacteriologic diagnoses in public health laboratories, for example, fostered friction between medical practitioners and public health professionals for diseases such as tuberculosis and diphtheria that were often difficult to identify from other common but less serious maladies. Clinicians feared that laboratory diagnoses would replace clinical diagnoses and that, in highly competitive medical markets, paying patients would abandon private physicians for public health agencies. Issues of turf and scope of practice persist in many communities.

Some of the most serious conflicts have come in the area of primary care services, including early case-finding activities. Because of the increased yield of screening tests when these are applied to groups at higher risk, public health practice has sought to deploy more widely risk group or community case-finding methods (including outreach and linkage activities). This has, at times, been perceived by medical practitioners as encroachment on their practice domain for certain primary care services, such as prenatal care. Although there has been no rule that public health practice could not be provided within the medical practice domain and vice versa, the perception that these are separate, but perhaps unequal, territories has been widely held by both groups.

It is important to note that this territoriality is not based only on turf issues. There are significant differences in the world views and approaches of these two domains. Medical practice quite properly seeks to produce the best possible outcome through the development and execution of individualized treatment plans. Seeking the best possible outcome for an individual suggests that decisions are made primarily for the benefit of that individual. Costs and resource availability are secondary considerations. Public health practice, on the other hand, seeks to deploy its limited resources to avoid the worst outcomes (at the level of the group). Some level of risk is tolerated at the collective level to prevent an unacceptable level of adverse outcomes from occurring. These are quite different approaches to practice: maximizing individual positive outcomes, as opposed to minimizing adverse collective outcomes. As a result, differences in perspective and philosophy often underlie differences in approaches that initially appear to be concerns over territoriality.

An example that illustrates these differences is apparent in approaches to widespread use of human immunodeficiency virus (HIV) antibody testing in the mid and late 1980s. Medical practitioners perceived that HIV antibody testing would be very useful in clinical practice and that its widespread use would enhance case finding. As a result, medical practitioners generally opposed restrictions on use of these tests, such as specific written informed consent and additional confidentiality provisions. Public health practitioners perceived that widespread use of the test without safeguards and protections would actually result in fewer persons at risk being tested and decreased case-finding in the community. With both groups focusing on the same science in terms of the accuracy of the specific testing regimen, these differences in practice approaches may be difficult to understand. However, in view of their ultimate aims and concerns as to individual versus collective outcomes, the conflict is more understandable.

Perspectives and roles may differ for public health and medical practice, but both are important and necessary. The real question is what blending of these approaches will be most successful in improving health status throughout the population. There is sufficient cause to question current policy and investment strategies. Table 3–3 examines the potential contributions of various strategies (personal responsibility, health care services, community action, and social policies) toward reducing the impact of the actual causes of death identified in Chapter 2. This table suggests that more medical care services are not as likely to reduce the toll from these causes as are public health approaches (community action and social policies). Yet, there are opportunities available through the current system and perhaps even greater opportunities in the near term as the system seeks to address the serious problems that have brought it to the brink of major reform.

Medicine and Public Health Collaborations

The need for a renewed partnership between medicine and public health generated several promising initiatives in the final years of the twentieth century. Just as bacteriology brought together public health professionals and practicing physicians at the turn of the twentieth century to battle diphtheria and other infectious diseases, technology and economics may become the driving forces for a renewed partnership at the dawn of the twenty-first century. In pursuit of this vision, the American Medical Association and the American Public Health Association established the Medicine/Public Health Initiative in 1994 to provide an ongoing forum to define mutual interests and promote models for successful collaborations. Regional and state meetings followed a National Congress in 1996. A variety of collaborative structures were identified

Table 3–3 Actual Causes of Death in the United States and Potential Contribution to Reduction

Causes	Deaths		Potential Contribution to Reduction*			
	Estimated No.	%	Personal	Health Care System	Community Action	Social Policy
Tobacco	400,000	19	++++	+	+	++
Diet/activity patterns	300,000	14	+++	+	+	++
Alcohol	100,000	5	+++	+	+	+
Microbial agents	90,000	4	+	++	++	++
Toxic agents	60,000	3	+	+	++	++++
Firearms	35,000	2	++	+	+++	+++
Sexual behavior	30,000	1	++++	+	+	+
Motor vehicles	25,000	1	++	+	+	++
Illicit use of drugs	20,000	<1	+++	+	++	++

*Plus sign indicates relative magnitude (∠+ scale).
Source: Reprinted from Fielding and Halfon, *Journal of the American Medical Association,* Vol. 272, pp. 1292–1296, © 1995, American Medical Association. All rights reserved.

and promoted through the widely circulated monograph, *Medicine and Public Health: The Power of Collaboration*.[4] More than 400 examples of collaborations are highlighted in the monograph. General categories of collaboration include coalitions, contracts, administrative/management systems, advisory bodies, and intra-organizational platforms. This initiative represents a major breakthrough for public health interests, one long overdue and welcome; in fact, it represents the first time that these two major professional organizations have met around mutual interests.

Collaborations between public health and hospitals have also gained momentum. Increasingly, hospitals and managed care organizations have begun to pursue community health goals, at times in concert with public health organizations and at other times filling voids that exist at the community level. In many parts of the United States, hospitals have taken the lead in organizing community health planning activities. More frequently, however, they participate as major community stakeholders in health planning efforts organized through the local public health agency. A variety of positive interfaces with managed care organizations has been documented.[5] Hospital boards and executives now commonly include community benefit objectives in their annual performance evaluations. Examples of community health strategies include:

- Establishing "boundary spanner" positions that report to the chief executive officer, but focus on community-wide, rather than institutional, interests
- Changing reward systems in terms of salaries and bonuses that executives and board members linked to the achievement of community health goals
- Educating staff on the mission, vision, and values of the institution, and linking these with community health outcomes
- Exposing board to the work of community partners
- Engaging board members with the staff and community
- Reporting on community health performance (report cards)[6]

THE HEALTH SYSTEM IN THE UNITED STATES

There are many sources of more complete information on the health system in the United States than will be provided in this chapter. Here, the intent is to examine those aspects of the health industry and health system that interface with public health or raise issues of public health significance. There is no shortage of either. This section will examine some of the issues facing the health system in the United States, with a special focus on the problems of the system that are fueling reform and change. Interfaces with public health will be identified and discussed, as will possible effects of these changes on the various images of public health. Throughout these sections, data from the Health United States series, published annually by the National Center for Health Statistics, will be used to describe the economic, demographic, and resources aspects of the American health system.

Economic Dimensions

The health system in the United States is immense and growing rapidly, as shown in Figure 3–7. Total national health expenditures in the United States nearly doubled during the 1990s to $1.3 trillion by 2000, more than four times the sum expended in 1980 and nearly 50 times more than in 1960. It is naive to consider the possible public health interfaces with the health system in the United States without understanding the context in which they take place—the health sector of modern America. In the early years of the new century, economic growth and employment in the United States weakened after nearly two decades of prosperity and improved productivity. The health care sector is now a powerful component in the overall U.S. economy. By the year 2000, the health care sector represented nearly one-seventh of the total national gross domestic product (GDP).[1] Figure 3–8 traces the growth in health expenditures as a proportion of GDP.

The United States spends a greater share of the national gross domestic product (GDP) on health care services than any other industrialized nation. Health expenditures in the United Kingdom and Japan are about half and Germany and Canada about three-fourths the U.S. figure (13.2 percent). Per

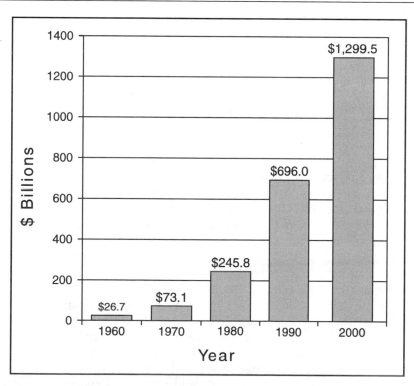

Figure 3–7 National Health Expenditures, United States, 1960–2000. *Source:* Adapted from National Center for Health Statistics. *Health United States 2002.* PHS, 2002.

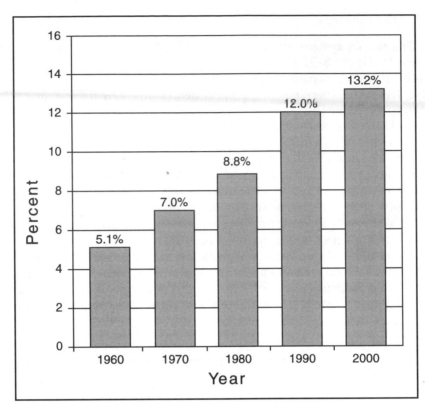

Figure 3–8 Percent of National Gross Domestic Expenditures Spent for Health-Related Purposes, U.S. 1960–2000. *Source:* Adapted from National Center for Health Statistics. *Health United States 2002.* PHS, 2002.

capita expenditures on health show the same pattern, with more than $4,600 per capita spent on health in the United States in 2000, compared with about $2,500 per capita in Germany and Canada, and only $1,600–1,800 per capita in Japan and the United Kingdom.[1] Several factors suggest that this is too much: the current system is reaching the point of no longer being affordable; the U.S. population is no healthier than other nations that spend far less; and the opportunity costs are considerable.

Expenditures for personal health care services comprise 87 percent of all health expenditures. Administrative costs in both the public and private sector account for 6.4 percent and investments (research and construction) comprise another 3.4 percent. The remaining 3.4 percent is devoted to government public health activities (about $8.3 billion in 2000), including personal health care services provided directly by government.[1] Chapters 4 and 6 examine governmental health and public health expenditure trends for the various levels of government in the United States.

There are three general sources for the $1.1 trillion in personal health care expenditures: government at all levels pays 43 percent; private health insurance covers 35 percent; individuals pay about 17 percent out of pocket; and the remaining 5 percent is covered by other private funds.[1] The rapidly increasing costs for health services have hit all these sources in their pocket-books, and each is reaching the point where further increases may not be affordable. The largest single purchaser of health care in the United States remains the federal government, but the ultimate payers are individuals. Even those individuals covered by health insurance plans are experiencing a steady increase in the triple burden of higher premiums, increased cost-sharing, and reduced benefits.

Only limited information is available on expenditures for prevention and population-based public health services. A study using 1988 data estimated that total national expenditures for all forms of health-related prevention (including clinical preventive services provided to individuals and population-based public health programs, such as communicable disease control and environmental protection) amounted to $33 billion.[7] The analysis sought to include all activities directed toward health promotion, health protection, disease screening, and counseling. As a result, the $33 billion figure approximates expenditures for primary and secondary prevention efforts. Included in this total, however, was $14 billion for activities not included in the calculation of national health expenditures (such as sewage systems, water purification, and air traffic safety). The remaining $18 billion in prevention-related health expenditures were included in the calculation of total national health expenditures, but represented only 3.4 percent of all national health expenditures for that year.

Nearly one-half (48 percent) of the health-related prevention resources identified in this analysis came from the federal government; another 31 percent represented expenditures for clinical preventive services, often paid out of pocket by individuals.[7] Preventive health services were the largest category of health-related prevention expenditures (36 percent), although health protection (30 percent)and health promotion services (23 percent) were also significant targets of prevention-related expenditures. The share of these expenditures that represents population-based preventive services cannot be directly determined from this study. However, it appears that population-based services constituted about $6–7 billion in 1988, in view of the prominence of health protection and health promotion services.

As part of the development of a national health reform proposal in 1994, federal officials developed an estimate of national health expenditures for population-based services.[8] On the basis of expenditures in 1993, this analysis concluded that about 1 percent of all national health expenditures ($8.4 billion) supported population-based programs and services. Based on data available, this analysis found that the proportion of all health expenditures attributed to population-based services declined slightly during the 1980s from 1.2 percent in 1980 to 0.9 percent a decade later. U.S. Public Health Service (PHS) agencies spent $4.3 billion for population-based services in 1993, and state and local health agencies expended another $4.1 billion. PHS officials estimated that achieving an "essential" level of population-based services nationwide would require doubling 1993 expenditure levels and that achieving a "fully effective" level would require tripling the 1993 levels.

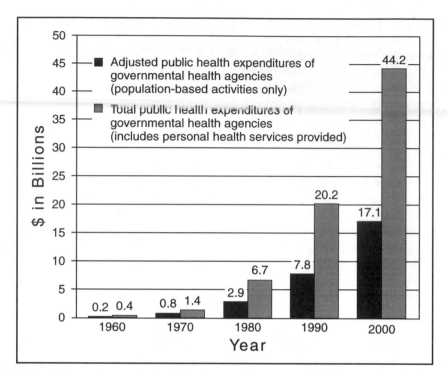

Figure 3–9 Total Expenditures (in $ Billions) of Governmental Health Agencies (Including Personal Health Services) and Adjusted Total Governmental Public Health Spending (Population-Based Services Only), United States, 1960–2000. *Sources and Notes:* Data compiled from National Centers for Health Statistics, *Health United States 2002*, PHS, 2002 and Centers for Medicare and Medicaid Services, National Health Accounts (NHA) 1960–2000. The NHA breaks down health spending by source of funding and by activity and type of service provided. Adjusted total public health expenditures include expenditures at both the federal and state/local level. State/local public health expenditures are adjusted in an attempt to include only funding for essential (that is, population-based) public health services and to exclude personal health care services.

Consistent with these earlier analyses, data from the National Health Accounts identify levels of population-based health expenditures by federal, state, and local governments to have been $7.8 billion in 1990, $12.3 billion in 1995, and $17.1 billion in 2000 (see Figure 3–9). [9,10] On a per capita basis, governmental expenditures for population-based public health activities increased more than 1200 percent between 1960 and 2000 (Figure 3–10), but governmental public health agencies continue to spend more of their resources on providing personal health care series than on population-based public health activities, as Figure 3–9 illustrates.

The implications of these expenditure patterns will be discussed in Chapter 4, and non-governmental expenditures for public health activities will be examined in Chapter 6. Here, however, these gross figures are presented in

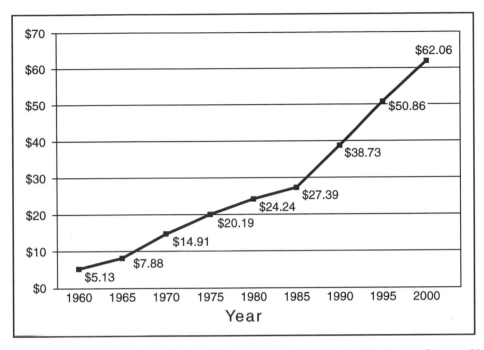

Figure 3–10 Per Capita Adjusted Total Governmental Public Health Expenditures, United States, 1960–2000. *Sources and Notes:* Data compiled from National Centers for Health Statistics, *Health United States 2002,* PHS, 2002 and Centers for Medicare and Medicaid Services, National Health Accounts (NHA) 1960–2000. The NHA breaks down health spending by source of funding and by activity and type of service provided. Adjusted total public health expenditures include expenditures at both the federal and state/local level. State/local public health expenditures are adjusted in an attempt to include only funding for essential (that is, population-based) public health services and to exclude personal health care services.

order to demonstrate the very small slice of the national health expenditure pie devoted to population-based preventive services and the public health system. As shown in Figure 3–11, governmental public health spending as a percent of total national health expenditures grew from 1960 through 1975, then declined from 1975 to 1985, and has been increasing steadily since 1985. The availability of resources from the 1998 settlement between states and the major tobacco companies, together with bioterrorism preparedness funding from Congress beginning in 2002, presented an opportunity to achieve the doubling of expenditures for population-based prevention deemed necessary to achieve an essential level of services by the PHS in 1994. Although such a doubling would require only a small shift in resource allocation strategies within a $1.5 trillion dollar enterprise, there was little hope for increased resources for population-based public health activities until the tobacco settlement and bioterrorism preparedness funds appeared. Subsequent chapters will provide additional information as to the effect these additional resources are having on the public health system.

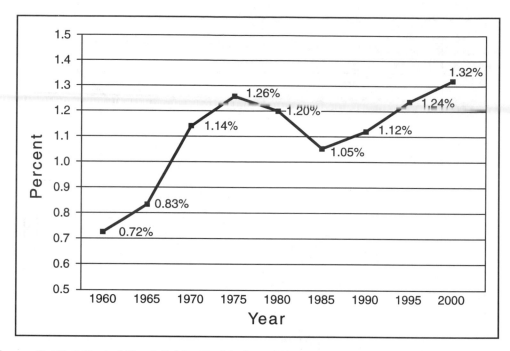

Figure 3–11 Adjusted Total Public Health Spending as a Percent of Total Health Spending, United States, 1960–2000. *Sources and Notes:* Data compiled from National Centers for Health Statistics, *Health United States 2002*, PHS, 2002 and Centers for Medicare and Medicaid Services, National Health Accounts (NHA) 1960–2000. The NHA breaks down health spending by source of funding and by activity and type of service provided. Adjusted total public health expenditures include expenditures at both the federal and state/local level. State/local public health expenditures are adjusted in an attempt to include only funding for essential (that is, population-based) public health services and to exclude personal health care services.

But macro-economic trends tell only part of the story. The disparities between rich and poor in the United States are also growing, leaving an increasing number of Americans without financial access to many health care services. These and other important aspects will be examined as we review the demands on and resources of the U.S. health system.

Demographic and Utilization Trends

Several important demographic trends affect the U.S. health care system. These include the slowing population growth rate, the shift toward an older population, the increasing diversity of the population, changes in family structure, and persistent lack of access to needed health services for too many Americans. The relative prevalence of particular diseases is another demographic phenomenon but will not be addressed here, although recent history with diseases such as HIV infections illustrates how specific conditions can place increasing demands on fragile health care systems.

Census studies document that the growth of the U.S. population has been slowing, a trend that would be expected to restrain future growth in demand for health care services. However, this must be viewed in light of projected changes in the age distribution of the U.S. population. Between 2000 and 2030, the population over age 65 will double, whereas the younger age groups will grow little, if at all.

Utilization of health care services, in general, is closely correlated with the age distribution of the population. For example, adults 75 years and older visit physicians 3–4 times as frequently as do children under the age of 17. Because older persons utilize more health care services than do younger people, their expenditures are higher. Obvious reasons for the higher utilization of health care resources by the elderly include the high prevalence of chronic conditions, such as arteriosclerosis, cerebrovascular disease, diabetes, senility, arthritis, and mental disorders. As the population ages, it is expected that the prevalence of chronic disorders and the treatment costs associated with them will also increase. This could be minimized through prevention efforts that either avert or postpone the onset of these chronic diseases. Nonetheless, these important demographic shifts portend greater use of health care services in the future.

Another important demographic trend is the increasing diversity of the population. The nonwhite population is growing three times faster than the white population, and the Hispanic population is increasing at five times the rate for the entire U.S. population. Between 1980 and 2000, Hispanics increased from 6.4 percent to 12.5 percent of the U.S. population. African Americans increased from 11.5 to 14.5 percent of the total population while Asian/Pacific Islanders grew more than doubled from 1.6 to 3.7 percent. The white population declined from 79.7 to 69.1 percent of the total population over these two decades. Figure 3–12 projects these trends through the years 2025 and 2050. These trends reflect differences in fertility and immigration patterns and disproportionately affect the younger age groups, suggesting that services for mothers and children will face considerable challenges in their ability to provide culturally sensitive and acceptable services. At the same time, the considerably less diverse baby boom generation will be increasing its ability to affect public policy decisions and resource allocations into the next century. These trends also underscore the importance of cultural competence for health professionals. Cultural competence is a set of behaviors and attitudes, as well as a culture within an institution or system, that respects and takes into account the cultural background, cultural beliefs, and values of those served and incorporates this into the way services are delivered.

Changes in family structure also represent a significant demographic trend in the United States. There is only a 50 percent chance that married partners will reach their 25th anniversary. One in three children live part of their lives in a one-parent household; for black children, the chances are two in three. Labor force participation for women more than doubled from under 25 percent in 1950 to 54 percent by 1985. Even more indicative of gender changes in the labor market, the proportion of married women in the work force with children under age five grew from 44 percent in 1975 to 64 percent in 1987. Many American households have maintained their economic status

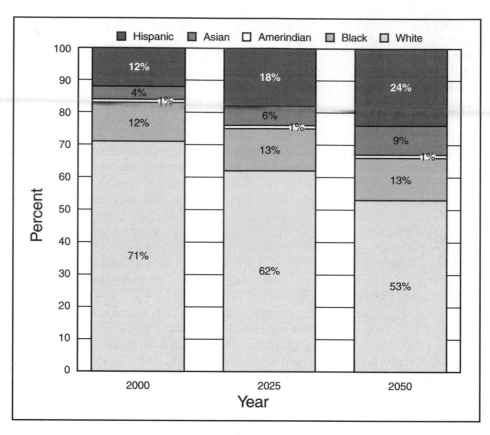

Figure 3–12 Current and Projected Racial and Ethnic Composition of U.S. Population, 2000, 2025, 2050. *Source:* U.S. Census Bureau, 2001.

over the past two decades with the second paychecks from women in the work force. As the nature of families changes, so do their needs for access, availability, and even types of services (such as substance abuse, family violence, and child welfare services).

Intermingled with many of these trends are the persistent inequalities in access to services for low-income populations, including blacks and Hispanics. For example, despite higher rates of self-reported fair or poor health and greater utilization of hospital inpatient services, low-income persons are 50 percent more likely to report no physician contacts within the past two years than are persons in high-income households. Utilization rates for prenatal care and childhood immunizations are also lower for low-income populations.

Despite outspending other developed countries on health services, the United States leads other industrialized nations by a wide margin in the rate of its citizens who lack health insurance coverage. Various studies since 1998 place the figure at approximately 45 million Americans and rising. Health insurance coverage of the population has been declining since 1980 for all age groups except those under age five, whose access was improved through Med-

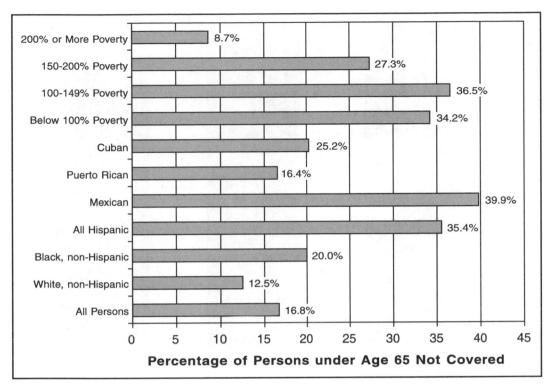

Figure 3–13 Persons Under Age 65 Not Covered by Health Insurance by Selected Characteristics, United States, 2000. *Source:* Adapted from National Center for Health Statistics. *Health United States 2002.* Hyattsville MD; PHS; 2002.

icaid eligibility changes. The age-adjusted percentage of persons who were not covered by health insurance increased from 14 percent in 1984 to almost 17 percent in 2000. Young adults 18–24 years of age were most likely (30 percent) to be uninsured in 2000.[1]

Blacks were two-thirds more likely than whites, and Hispanics were almost three times as likely as whites to be uninsured in 2000. Individuals in households at 150 percent or less of the poverty level were more than four times more likely to be uninsured than were persons living in households at 200 percent or more of the poverty level (Figure 3–13). Still, of the 41 million uninsured people under the age of 65, about two-thirds are 15–44 years of age, three-fourths are white, and one-third live in families earning $25,000 or more. Lack of insurance coverage may disproportionately affect minority low-income individuals, but its growth in recent years has affected individuals in almost all groups. About two-thirds of uninsured individuals in the United States are either employed or are dependents of an employed family member. Part-time workers and the self-employed are as likely as the unemployed to be uninsured. Access to health services is one of the ten leading indicators of the health status of the United States; Figure 3–14 illustrates targets set for the nation as part of the Healthy People 2010 initiative.

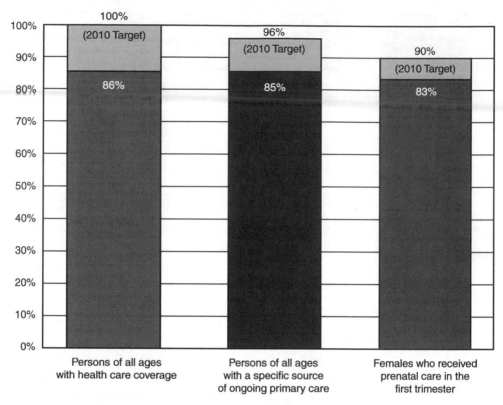

Figure 3–14 Access to Health Care, United States, 1997, and Year-2010 Targets. *Source:* Reprinted from *Healthy People 2010: Understanding and Improving Health,* U.S. Department of Health and Human Services, Public Health Service, 2000.

Health Care Resources

The supply of health care resources is another key dimension of the health care system. During the past quarter-century, the number of active U.S. physicians increased by more than two-thirds, with even greater increases among women physicians and international medical graduates. The specialty composition of the physician population also changed during this period, as a result of many factors, including changing employment opportunities, advances in medical technology, and the availability of residency positions. Suffice it to say that medical and surgical subspecialties grew more rapidly than did the primary care specialties. Recent projections suggest that the early twenty-first century will see a substantial surplus of physicians, primarily those trained in the surgical and medical specialties.

Health care delivery models have also experienced major changes in recent years. For example, hospital-based resources have changed dramatically. Since the mid-1970s, the number of community hospitals has decreased, and the numbers of admissions, days of care, average occupancy rates, and average

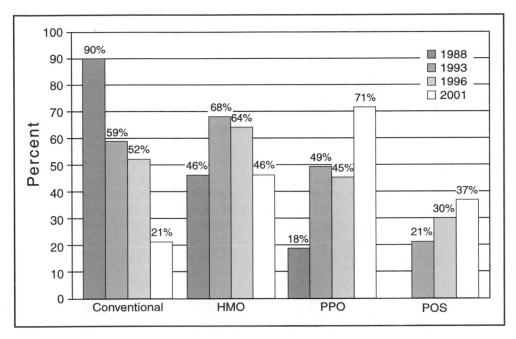

Figure 3–15 Percent of Covered Workers with a Choice of Conventional, HMO, PPO, or POS Plans, 1988–2001 *Sources:* Data from Kaiser Family Foundation/Health Research and Education Trust Survey of Employer-Sponsored Health Benefits: 2001; KPMG Survey of Employer-Sponsored Health Benefits: 1988, 1993, 1996. Information was not obtained for POS plans in 1988. HMO refers to health maintenance organizations; PPO refers to preferred provider organizations; and POS refers to point-of-service plans

length of stay have all declined, as well. On the other hand, the number of hospital employees per 100 average daily patients has continued to increase. Hospital outpatient visits have also been increasing since the mid-1970s.

The growth in the number and types of health care delivery systems in recent years is another reflection of a rapidly changing health care environment. Figure 3–15 traces changes in the types of health plan options available to workers with health insurance coverage between 1988 and 2001. Increasing competition, combined with cost containment initiatives, has led to the proliferation of group medical practices, health maintenance organizations (HMOs), preferred provider organizations, ambulatory surgery centers, and emergency centers. Common to many of these delivery systems since the early 1990s have been managed care strategies and methods that seek to control the utilization of services. Managed care represents a system of administrative controls intended to reduce costs through managing the utilization of services. Elements of managed care strategies generally include some combination of the following:

- Risk sharing with providers to discourage the provision of unnecessary diagnostic and treatment services and, to some degree, to encourage preventive measures

- To attract specific groups, designing of tailored benefit packages that include the most important (but not necessarily all) services for that group; cost sharing for some services through deductibles and co-payments can be built into these packages
- Case management, especially for high-cost conditions, to encourage seeking out of less expensive treatments or settings
- Primary care gatekeepers, generally the enrollee's primary care physician, who control referrals to specialists
- Second opinions as to the need for expensive diagnostic or elective invasive procedures
- Review and certification for hospitalizations, in general, and hospital admissions through the emergency department, in particular
- Continued-stay review for hospitalized patients as they reach the expected number of days for their illness (as determined by diagnostic related groupings)
- Discharge planning to move patients out of hospitals to less expensive care settings as quickly as possible

The growth and expansion of these delivery systems has significant implications for the cost of, access to, and quality of health services. These, in turn, have substantial impact on public health organizations and their programs and services.[5] By the year 2000, more than half of the U.S. population was served through a managed care organization. Within the next decade, managed care will capture 80–90 percent of the market. The growth of managed care also has significant implications for both the population-based services of governmental public health agencies and the clinical services that have been provided in the public sector. Appendix 3–A examines some of these emerging and future issues as public health and managed care seek to coexist peacefully with each other in a rapidly changing health sector.

The dramatic growth in the number of HMOs during the early and mid-1980s was followed by a period of slower growth and consolidations and mergers. Rapid growth resumed in the 1990s with more than one-third of the population, about 80 million Americans, enrolled in HMOs in 2001, up from only 4 percent in 1980. Considerable variation is apparent across regions of the country, ranging from 35–40 percent in the west and northeast to 21–22 percent in the midwest and south. The structure of HMOs varies, as well, with about 80 percent of enrollees found in independent practice and mixed-model HMOs; only about 20 percent are served by group model HMOs. Recent growth has come largely in the form of the mixed-model HMOs, which include aspects of both the staff and independent models. In general, cost-control measures are more effectively implemented through group model HMOs.

CHANGING ROLES, THEMES, AND PARADIGMS IN THE HEALTH SYSTEM

Even a cursory review of the health sector requires an examination of the key participants or key players in the health industry. The list of major stake holders has been expanding as the system has grown and now includes government, business, third-party payers, health care providers, drug companies, and labor, as well as consumers. The federal government has grown to become the largest purchaser of health care and, along with business, has attempted to become a more prudent buyer by exerting more control over payments for services. Government seeks to reduce rising costs by altering the economic performance of the health sector through stimulation of a more competitive health care market. Still, budget problems at all levels make it increasingly difficult for government to fulfill commitments to provide health care services to the poor, the disadvantaged, and the elderly. Over recent years, new and expensive medical technology, inflation, and unexpected increases in utilization forced third parties to pay out more for health care than they anticipated when premiums were determined. As a result, insurers have joined government in becoming more aggressive in efforts to contain health care costs. Many commercial carriers are exploring methods to anticipate utilization more accurately and to control outlays through managed care strategies. Business, labor, patients, hospitals, and professional organizations are all trying to restrain costs while maintaining access to health services.

Reducing the national deficit and balancing the federal budget will look in part to proposals that will control costs within Medicare and Medicaid, as well as in discretionary federal health programs. Except for Medicare, these recommendations are likely to be politically popular, even though the public has little understanding of the federal budget. For example, a 1994 poll[11] found that Americans believe health care costs constitute 5 percent of the federal budget, although these costs actually constitute 16 percent. At the same time, Americans believe that foreign aid and welfare constitute 27 and 19 percent, respectively, of the federal budget when, in fact, they constitute only 2 and 3 percent, respectively. When the time comes to balance the federal budget and reduce the national deficit, the American public will face difficult choices as to which programs can be reduced. Public health programs, largely discretionary spending, may not fare well in this scenario.

As these stakeholders search for methods to reduce costs and as competition intensifies, efforts to preserve the quality of health care will become increasingly important. An Institute of Medicine study concluded that medical errors account for as many deaths each year as motor vehicle crashes and breast cancer (Figure 3–16).[12] Public debate will continue to focus on how to define and measure quality. Despite the difficulty in measuring quality of medical care, it is likely that quality measurement systems will increase substantially. Dialogue and debate among the major stakeholders in the health system will be influenced by the tension between cost containment and regulation; the interdependence of access, quality, and costs; the call for greater accountability; and the slow but steady acceptance of the need for health reform.

Almost certainly, health policy issues will become increasingly politicized. The debate on health care issues will continue to expand beyond the health care community. Many health policy issues may no longer be determined by sound science and practice considerations, but rather by political factors. Changes in the health sector may lead to unexpected divisions and alliances on health policy issues. The intensity of economic competition in the health sector is likely to continue to increase because of the increasing supply of health care personnel and because of the changes in the financing of care.

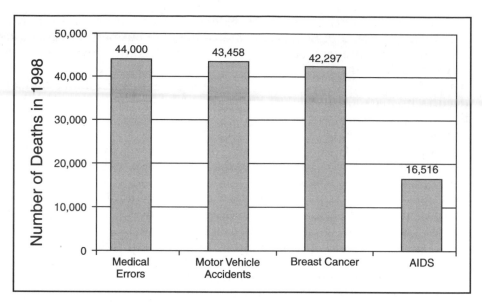

Figure 3–16 Selected Causes of Death in the United States, 1998 *Source:* Institute of Medicine. *To Err is Human.* Washington, DC: National Academy of Sciences, 1999.

Increased competition is likely to cause realignments among key participants in the health care sector, often depending on the particular issue involved.

The failure of health reform at the national policy level in 1994 did not preclude the implementation of significant improvements in either the public or the private components of the health sector. With or without changes in national health policies, the health system in the United States is clearly reforming itself. With the persistence of cost and access as the system's twin critical problems, new approaches and models were both needed and expected. The federal, as well as state, governments have moved to control the costs of Medicaid services, primarily through attempts to enroll non-disabled Medicaid populations (largely, mothers and children) into capitated managed care programs. The rapid conversion of Medicaid services to managed care operations and the growth of private managed care organizations pose new issues for the delivery of clinical preventive and public health services.[5] Although it is anticipated that these changes will result in fewer clinical preventive and treatment services being provided through public health agencies, both the extent and impact of these shifts remain unclear. Appendix 3–A explores these issues in greater depth.

In any event, the underlying investment strategy of the U.S. health system appears to remain unchanged, with 97 percent of the available resources allocated for treatment services, approximately 2 percent for clinical preventive services, and 1 percent for population-based public health services. Without at least some additional investment in prevention and public health approaches, the long-term prospects for controlling costs within the U.S. health system are bleak. In the meantime, some 40–45 million Americans remain outside the system and will continue to incur excessive costs when they inappropriately access needed services. Universal access is a prerequisite for eventual control of costs. However, it is not clear how true reform can be effected without reform of both our medical care and public health subsystems.

Although progress along this road has been painfully slow, there is evidence that a paradigm shift is already under way. The Pew Health Professions Commission argues that the American health care system of the twenty-first century will be quite different from its 1990s counterpart.[13] The health system of the twenty-first century will be

- More managed, with better integration of services and financing
- More accountable to those who purchase and use health services
- More aware of and responsive to the needs of enrolled populations
- More able to use fewer resources more effectively
- More innovative and diverse in how it provides for health
- More inclusive in how it defines health
- Less focused on treatment and more concerned with education, prevention, and care management
- More oriented to improving the health of the entire population
- More reliant on outcomes data and evidence

These gains, however, are likely to be accompanied by pain. The number of hospitals may decline by as much as 50 percent and the number of hospital beds by even more than that. There will be continued expansion of primary care in community and other ambulatory settings; this will foster replication of services in different settings, a development likely to confuse consumers. These forces also suggest major traumas for the health professions, with projected deficits of some professions, such as nurses and dentists, and surpluses of others, such as physicians and pharmacists.[13] An estimated 100,000–150,000 excess physicians, mainly specialists, could be joined by 200,000–300,000 excess nurses as the hospital sector consolidates and as many as 40,000 excess pharmacists as drug dispensing is automated and centralized. The massive fragmentation among 200 or more allied health fields will cause consolidation into multi-skilled professions to meet the changing needs of hospitals and other care settings. One of the few professions likely to flourish in this environment will be public health, with its focus on populations, information-driven planning, collaborative responses, and broad definition of health and health services.

Where these forces will move the health system is not yet known. To blend better the contributions of preventive and treatment-based approaches, several important changes are needed. There must be a new and more rational understanding of what is meant by "health services." This understanding must include a broad view of health promotion and health protection strategies, and must provide these equal standing with treatment-based strategies. Once and for all, health services must be seen to include services that focus on health, as well as those that focus on ill health. This should result in support for a more comprehensive approach to defining a basic benefit package that would be provided to all Americans. A second and companion change needed is to finance this enhanced basic benefit package from the same source, rather than funding public health and most prevention from one source (government resources) and treatment and the remaining prevention activities from private sources (business, individuals, insurance). With these changes, a gradual reallocation of resources can move the system toward a more rational and effective investment strategy.

The sheer size and scope of the American health system make it a force to be reckoned with, engendering comparisons with a similar force that existed in the United States in the 1950s and 1960s. At that time, and as he left office, President Eisenhower warned the nation of the potentially dangerous influence of the nation's "military industrial complex." His observations were both ominous and insightful as he decried a powerful industry whose self-interest was coloring the nation's view of other countries and their people. The plight of the American health system raises the specter of a modern analogue in a "medical industrial complex." One danger posed by these complexes is their ability to influence the way we address (or even think about) a major public policy problem or issue. This occurs through interpreting and recasting the issues involved, sometimes even to the extent of altering public perceptions as to what is occurring and why.

Public understanding of the meaning of the terms *health reform* and *health care* is a case in point. Although, as a society, we have come to substitute the term health care for what is really medical or treatment care, these are simply not the same. The health status of a population is largely determined by a different set of considerations, as discussed in Chapter 2. Those considerations are very much the focus of the public health system. If the ultimate goal is a healthier population and, more specifically, the prevention of disease and disability, the national health system must aggressively balance treatment with population- and community-based prevention strategies.

There is a term for when an organization finds that it is unable to achieve its primary objectives and outcomes (bottom line), then justifies its existence in terms of how well it does the things it is doing. *Outcome displacement* is that term; it means that the original outcome (here, improved health status) has been displaced by a focus on how well the means to that end (the organization, provision, and financing of services) are being addressed. These, then, become the new purpose or mission for that system. Instead of "doing the right things" to affect health status, the system focuses on "doing things right" (regardless of whether they maximally affect health). It is possible to have the best medical care services in the world but still have an inadequate health system.

CONCLUSION

Every day in America, decisions are made that influence the health status of individuals and groups of individuals. The aggregate of these decisions and the activities necessary to carry them out constitute our health system. It is important to view interventions as linked with health and illness states, as well as with the dynamic processes and multiple factors that move an individual from one state to another. Preventive interventions act at various points and through various means to prevent the development of a disease state or, if it occurs, to minimize its effects to the extent possible. These interventions differ in their linkages with public health practice, medical practice, and long-term care, as well as in their focus on individuals or groups. The framework represents a rational one, reflecting known facts concerning each of its aspects and their relationships with each other.

As this chapter has described, current health policy in the United States reflects a different view of the factors incorporated in the model. Current policy focuses unduly on disease states and strategies for restoring, as opposed to promoting or protecting, health. It directs the vast majority of human, physical, and financial resources to tertiary prevention, particularly to acute treatment. It focuses disproportionately on individually-oriented secondary and tertiary medical care. In so doing, it raises questions as to whether these policies are effective and ethical.

Characterized in the past largely by federalism, pluralism, and incrementalism, the health sector in the United States is undergoing fundamental change, primarily in response to economic realities that have invested a trillion dollars in a model that equates medical care with health care. We are now realizing that this investment strategy is not producing results commensurate with its resource consumption. Health indicators, including those characterizing large disparities in outcomes and access among important minority groups, are not responding to more resources being deployed in the usual ways. The major problems have been widely characterized as cost and access, with the former being considered a cause of the latter. How to fix the cost question without aggravating the access issue has yet to be addressed, although managed care approaches are serving to place some controls on the utilization of specific services. A better representation of the twin problems facing the U.S. health sector might be excess and access, suggesting a return to the strategic drawing boards for approaches that reduce and redeploy resources, rather than only reducing them. Within this reexamination of purpose and strategies for the health sector, the need to address health, as well as disease and prevention, as well as treatment, should be apparent. To accomplish these aims, there must be consensus that basic health services include population-based public health services and clinical preventive services, as well as diagnostic and treatment services. To facilitate rational policy making and investment decisions, these services should be funded from a common source. This may require that health insurance premiums replace governmental appropriations as the source of funding for public sector activities. It is to be hoped that these realizations will take place before the health sector reaches its meltdown point.

DISCUSSION QUESTIONS AND EXERCISES

1. What are the most critical issues facing the health care system in the U.S. today? Before answering this question, see what insights you can find at the websites of these major health organizations: American Medical Association <http://www.ama-assn.org>,

American Hospital Association <http://www.aha.org>, American Nurses Association <http://www.ana.org>, and the American Association of Medical Colleges <http://www.aamc.org>.

2. What forces are most likely to fuel further movement toward major health care reform in America?

3. Why is there less concern over national policy solutions (or "health reform") today than there was in 1994?

4. Select an important health problem (disease or condition) related to maternal and infant health (see "Public Health Achievements in Twentieth-Century America: Improved Maternal and Infant Health") and describe interventions for this problem across the five strategies of health- and illness-related interventions (health promotion, specific protection, early detection, disability limitation, rehabilitation) presented in Chapter 3.

5. For the same health problem related to maternal and infant health (see "Public Health Achievements in Twentieth-Century America: Improved Maternal and Infant Health") selected in Question 4, describe interventions for this problem across the three levels of preventive interventions (primary, secondary, tertiary) presented in Chapter 3.

6. Exhibit 3–1 lists organizations, agencies and institutions that might be considered part of an overall national prevention effort. Identify those elements that should be included in a compilation of health-related prevention efforts. On the basis of what you know of these agencies, which of their programs or services should be included? Explain why in terms of categories of preventive activities (e.g., health promotion, health protection, clinical preventive services). Identify those that you would include if you had the task of quantifying the scope and cost of all health-related prevention activities and expenditures in the United States. Which would you choose to leave off this list? Why?

7. Examine the data on the health system in a city or county of interest that is available through a state or local health agency. What elements from this site are most useful?

8. Great Debate: This debate examines contributors to improvement in health status in the United States since 1900. There are two propositions to be considered. Proposition A: Public health interventions are responsible for these improvements. Proposition B: Medical care interventions are responsible for these improvements. Select one of these positions to argue and submit a summary of arguments.

9. Is an ounce of prevention still worth a pound of cure in the United States? If not, what is the relative value of prevention, in comparison with treatment?

10. Review Appendix 3–A. Has the recent growth of managed care strategies within the health sector had a positive or a negative impact on the public's health? How? Why?

REFERENCES

1. National Center for Health Statistics. *Health United States, 2002.* Hyattsville, MD: U.S. Public Health Service (PHS); 2002.

2. Leavell HR, Clark EG. *Preventive Medicine for the Doctor in His Community, 3rd ed.* New York: McGraw-Hill; 1965.

3. U.S. Preventive Services Task Force. *Guide to Clinical Preventive Services, 2nd ed.* Washington, DC: U.S. Department of Health and Human Services (DHHS); 1995.

4. Lasker RD. *Medicine & Public Health: The Power of Collaboration.* New York: New York Academy of Medicine; 1997.

5. Halverson PK, Kaluzny AD, McLaughlin CP. *Managed Care & Public Health.* Gaithersburg, MD: Aspen Publishers; 1998.

6. Weil PA, Bogue RJ. Motivating community health improvement: Leading practices you can use. *Healthcare Executive.* 1999:Nov/Dec:18–24.

7. Brown RE, Elixhauser A, Corea J, Luce BR, Sheingold S. *National Expenditures for Health Promotion and Disease Prevention Activities in the United States.* Washington, DC: Medical Technology Assessment and Policy Research Center; 1991.

8. Core Functions Project, PHS, Office of Disease Prevention and Health Promotion. *Health Care Reform and Public Health: A Paper Based on Population-Based Core Functions.* Washington, DC: PHS; 1993.

9. Centers for Medicare and Medicaid Services, National Health Accounts, 1960–2000.

10. Frist B. Public Health and National Security: The Critical Role of Increased Federal Support. *Health Affairs* 2002;21(6):117–130.

11. Blendon RJ. *Kaiser/Harvard/KRC National Election Night Survey.* Menlo Park, CA: Henry J. Kaiser Family Foundation; 1994.

12. Institute of Medicine. *To Err is Human.* Washington DC: National Academy of Sciences, 1999.

13. Pew Health Professions Commission. *Critical Challenges: Revitalizing the Health Professions for the Twenty-First Century.* San Francisco: University of California Center for Health Professions; 1995.

Managed Care and Public Health: Strange Bedfellows?

The forces of reform buffeted the U.S. health system during much of the 1990s, resulting in significant change in the organization, provision, and financing of health services. These changes certainly constitute reform, although this type of reform takes decades, rather than months or years. Central to these changes are managed care plans and the competitive purchase of health services from large health systems. The links with public health have not always been clear, but what is clear is that public health practitioners need a better understanding of managed care and how it works. The most important reason is that effective partnerships with managed care will be critical to solving many public health problems. In addition, public health surveillance will depend, in part, on the nature and quality of information available from managed care plans. Finally, the mix and match of public health programs and services will depend on what the medical-care system does and does not do. For these reasons, the basic concepts and practices of managed care organizations are presented here.

Managed Care at the Turn of Century

Managed care organizations exist for two related purposes, to insure plan members and to furnish and manage the care that they receive. There are many different variations on this theme, but definitions of managed care characterize a system that is under the management of a single entity that insures its members, then furnishes benefits to those members through a defined network of participating providers. Services may be furnished either directly or through intermediaries. In any event, the system strives to manage the health care practices of its participating providers. Still, it is the providers who manage the patients. Because it is provider decisions, more than the decisions of patients that influence service utilization and costs, modern managed care organizations must manage providers.

In the United States, managed care organizations function as corporations. Insurance companies established some, although many are now investor-owned. Generally, the largest investors are health care providers themselves; the principal stakeholders are hospitals, physicians, and specialized entities that offer a single-service product line, such as behavioral health benefits. The common denominator among managed care organizations is their assumption of risk on a complete or partial basis. Profits are derived from the difference between premium payments and costs of providing services to patients.

Health maintenance organizations and other forms of managed care grew rapidly in the 1990s. By the end of the decade, more than 80 million privately insured individuals were covered by managed care plans. Managed care has also begun to penetrate governmentally financed health services, with more than one-half of all Medicaid beneficiaries and nearly 1 in 10 Medicare recipients receiving services through managed care operations. These numbers will grow rapidly over the next decade.

Many forces are at work to promote the growth of managed care arrangements in the United States. First and foremost are rising costs associated with health care. As costs escalated, and because the majority of Americans are covered through employers, businesses moved to control costs. Many businesses had already acted to self-insure their workers and dependents, in an effort to control decisions affecting costs better. They soon began to treat health services as they would other costs of doing business and looked for insurance products that would allow them to control costs through controlling providers. Managed care was an attractive strategy. Managed care also afforded an opportunity for government to control its costs in a manner that would overcome at least some of the obstacles that had traditionally discouraged providers from serving Medicaid recipients (such as delayed payments and extensive paper work). With predictable reimbursement levels and lower utilization of services, at least in comparison with the greater risk and need, the opportunity for profit margins has attracted interest from managed care organizations in virtually every state. Managed care for Medicare beneficiaries has advanced less rapidly than for the private sector and Medicaid. Official predictions of inadequate resources to serve baby boomers when they reach senior citizenship, however, suggest that managed care will eventually penetrate the Medicare program.

The jargon and terminology of modern managed care confuses even the most knowledgeable individuals. More important than familiarity with the jargon, however, is understanding how these plans work. In general, there are both open and closed variations of managed care plans. *Open* and *closed* refer to the relationship between the managed care plan and its patients in terms of freedom to choose providers other than those controlled by the managed care organization. Closed plans have tighter control over providers, and enrolled plan members have little ability to secure covered services outside of these panels of providers. Many traditional staff-model HMOs are examples of closed plans. Open panels are looser arrangements that allow members to obtain services from a wider (and less tightly controlled) network of providers. Preferred provider organizations and physician/hospital networks are examples of open panels. In this form of managed care, enrolled members can obtain services at very little additional cost out of-pocket, unless that service is received outside the plan. When that occurs, members pay more, although they generally remain partially covered by the plan.

A hybrid arrangement is the point-of-service model. Here, services provided by plan providers are tightly controlled, but services can also be obtained outside of the plan through a looser network of providers, for an added fee. This allows for greater consumer choice as to providers, but still provides for some control of costs for basic benefits.

Naturally, the more interested the purchaser is in controlling costs, the less open the plan will be. Medicaid managed care plans and even private plans less concerned over patient freedom to choose among providers find the closed panels more conducive to aggressive cost-control strategies. Decisions to go the closed-panel route require that assessments have been made of the capacity of the managed care organization to provide covered services, including both primary and specialized care services. Unfortunately, methods and tools for such assessments are seldom afforded the same priority as controlling costs.

Methods for controlling costs are straightforward, with utilization control serving as a primary approach. Services and procedures that cannot be quickly and cheaply provided during a provider visit are reviewed for appropriateness in terms of whether such services are actually needed and, if needed, from whom and in what settings they will be provided. In short, the plan determines whether the service is covered and where the member can get it. Denial of approval can be tantamount to denial of care for those who lack the ability to secure the services using their own resources. Until recently, there has been little opportunity for insured individuals to challenge these decisions in the courts.

Sharing of costs between the plan and the enrollee is another approach for controlling costs. When costs are shared, the plan ends up paying less. Such cost sharing also serves to discourage the member from actually receiving the service, another savings for the managed care plan. Other cost-control measures relate to member selection. Marketing to potential members from healthier age groups and populations also serves to control costs down the road. Some marketing efforts are even more explicit in terms of more actively enrolling (even door-to-door) the healthier members of an eligible group—a practice that has been identified especially with the development of Medicaid managed care programs.

In addition to risk-profiling potential members, similar profiles can be assembled on providers to identify those whose practice patterns and decisions result in "unnecessary" costs for the plan. Patterns for use of screening tests, performance of office procedures, return visits, and hospital admissions are examined to identify providers whose practice patterns might be modified or even whose participation might be excluded. There is some scientific merit to these reviews in the face of numerous studies describing greatly varying rates of medical procedures across the United States, often with no apparent differences in health outcomes.

These approaches to economic credentialing often do not consider differences in the risk mix of populations served. Asthma management of a white teenage male in the suburbs may not be the same as for an inner-city, African American teenager. Identification and consideration of different risk mixes and contributing factors is a public health skill that is not widely available in managed care operations.

Opportunities for Improving Public Health

Despite the tensions and conflicts that have emerged between managed care organizations and both providers and consumers, aspects of managed care offer opportunities for improving public health. Fragmentation and lack of coordination of health services have long been a hallmark of the American health system. Managed care imposes some semblance of a structure on this pluralistic "non-system" and establishes a framework for effective health services that can reach more individuals. In the past, this could only be done on a provider-by-provider basis. There are now access and leverage points for networks of providers to provide clinical preventive services more extensively and to integrate their activities with community prevention efforts. There are even financial incentives for these to occur. Diseases and conditions prevented today will mean lower expenditures and greater profits tomorrow. Although managed care organizations with a long-term view and a stable base of enrollees recognize this opportunity, many newly established managed care operations focus on shorter-term financial viability concerns, such as expanding enrollment and rapid generation of profits.

However, profit orientations cut both ways, and public health agencies may find themselves cut out of the picture for many services they have been providing in recent decades. Some services, such as primary and even treatment care services, may shift to managed care organizations for individuals covered by Medicaid or other third-party insurers. Other services are specialized public health services, such as treatment services for tuberculosis, HIV infections, and sexually transmitted diseases. The future for these services is very much an open question. Managed care plans would prefer not to enroll individuals who need specialized, often high-cost services. Providers of specialized services are also worrisome to managed care plans because these might serve to attract more individuals with high-cost needs. Yet these needs will exist, and it is unclear how and by whom they will be addressed.

One approach is to require that managed care plans include specialized public health providers in their networks. Needless to say, this approach is not very popular among managed care organizations. Another option is to tax a portion of the revenues of managed care plans to support specialized public health providers through grants or contracts. The public health agencies would not be formally part of the managed care networks, but they would share information on individuals as referrals were made back and forth. Another approach is to carve out certain services from the managed care plans and let individuals seek out these services on an as-needed basis. This approach, however, fosters fragmentation and lack of continuity of care. The advantages of defining and carving out specific services as public health rather than components of a comprehensive benefit package have not been well established to date.

Another opportunity is afforded by the information systems necessary to manage networks of providers and services. Traditionally, public health surveillance has been not been able to access and utilize information on health status and health conditions of living persons captured in the ambulatory care system. Combining this information with other data sources can greatly bene-fit public health surveillance efforts, as well as inform the needs of managed care plans and providers. However, public health interests are not the only ones likely to be seeking access to health plan data and information. The very same stakeholders whose priorities promoted the expansion of managed care will be looking for information that proves that their resources are being used effectively and efficiently. Businesses and the government will be demanding information that demonstrates the value that their health dollars are realizing and that allows them and their employees to evaluate and compare health plan performance. Ideally, health outcome concerns should drive these devel-opments, but financial concerns are more likely to dictate what information is collected and how it is used.

The managed care industry has developed a data set for use in evaluating and comparing health plan performance, the Health Plan Employer Data and Information Set (HEDIS). Revisions of HEDIS have sought to incorporate com-munity and public health performance measures; the public health commu-nity is actively seeking to build on HEDIS so that public health data needs might be better addressed. At least three categories of data may have applica-tions for public health purposes:

1. administrative data sets, such as provider names and payments
2. enrollment data, such as basic demographic information that can be useful in identifying high-risk individuals and communities
3. encounter data profiling what their providers order and the frequency of hospital admissions

Encounter data, however, tend to be limited because these are the most expensive form of data to obtain, especially if on-site inspection and abstract-ing information from medical records are required. Also, managed care plans do not rely on encounter data for reimbursement, as is common with fee-for-service systems.

There has been little agreement to date as to which information from encounter data would be both useful for public health purposes and appropri-ate for managed care plans to provide. The many issues surrounding data questions are only beginning to be explored. It is likely that additional oppor-tunities will surface as they are discussed and developed. For example, school health may represent another opportunity for forging closer working relation-ships between managed care plans and public health organizations. In many parts of the country, school health programs are being dismantled because of financial pressures on state and local government. School health nurses have long been the linchpins of school health programs. These, too, are declining in numbers, even while new mandates and expectations are being established in areas such as compliance with immunization requirements, vision and hearing screenings, medical assessments for special education students, med-ication administration, and crisis intervention services. With these duties, their involvement in health curriculum issues is greatly diluted. However, as Medicaid managed care conversions develop and as managed care penetrates further into the private sector, school health may represent an opportunity to integrate managed care plans with public health objectives. For example, children at a single school may be served by 10–20 managed care plans currently, and in the future, perhaps by only 5–10. These plans could contribute proportionately to the funding of school nurses and support staff to carry out the duties described above in ways that would be less expensive than either providing them at plan provider sites or not providing them and dealing with preventable disease outbreaks or asthma attacks requiring hospitalization.

The many opportunities afforded by the expansion of managed care call for new thinking and new roles, such as those suggested in Exhibit 3–A1. Both managed care plans and public health agencies must approach these challenges with common objectives.

Still, there remains one role that is likely to be aggravated by the expansion of managed care plans—the role of providing medical services for those who have no coverage. This number has been estimated to include 40–45 million Americans at any one time. The expansion of managed care, with its heavy emphasis on price competition and financial bottom lines, will serve to reduce the amount of so-called charity care previously furnished by private sector providers. This is already apparent in communities where managed care has captured large segments of the market, and it is likely to occur in many, if not most, U.S. communities. These circumstances suggest once again that reform of the medical care system must be accompanied by reform within the public health system.

Exhibit 3–A1 Managed Care and Public Health Issues for the Future

Public health goals and Medicaid services	How these can be merged • to increase the focus on health • to simplify and increase access for Medicaid recipients • to incorporate health services (broadly defined) essential for good health outcomes
Case management and enabling services	How to ensure • inclusion of these services in view of evidence that they improve access and yield better health outcomes for enrollees than systems that only coordinate medical treatment
System capacity and the roles of providers	How these can be clearly articulated • to clarify the sometimes conflicting case management roles of both patient advocates and cost-containment agents
Fluctuations in enrollment	How these will • complicate efforts to supply case management to Medicaid Populations • affect provider accountability for continuity of care • increase the likelihood that public health agencies will maintain a significant role in delivering services as "providers of last resort"

continues

Exhibit 3–A1 continued

Assurance of quality	How to deal with issues of quality so that • quality will not be compromised • quality will be monitored by government • there is a public health focus on access and clinical care, as well as a financial focus on solvency and enrollment composition • there is a careful analysis of broad outcome data • encounter data will facilitate consumer choice and identify problems in the shift from fee-for-service care delivery to managed care with capitated payments • the appropriate roles of government, employers, and consumers are identified
Data	How to address • the need for data essential for a successful "outcome-oriented" approach to continuing quality processes within managed-care systems • integration in systems that collect, make meaningful, and disseminate data to facilitate decision making
Provider and consumer acceptance	How to resolve • dependence on the degree to which provider concerns regarding practice autonomy and consumer perceptions of diminished choice are addressed • the need for a consumer-oriented approach to quality, requiring consumer support, and independent access to medical advice, such as second opinions

Source: Adapted from *Challenge and Opportunity: Public Health in an Era of Change,* 1996, Illinois Department of Public Health.

Chapter 4

Law, Government, and Public Health

Public health is not limited to what governmental public health agencies do, although this is a widely held misperception among those inside and outside the field. Still, particular aspects of public health rely on government. For example, the enforcement of laws remains one of those governmental responsibilities important to the public's health and public health practice. Yet, law and the legal system are important for public health purposes above and beyond the enforcement of laws and regulations. Laws at all levels of government bestow the basic powers of government and distribute these powers among various agencies, including public health agencies. Law represents governmental decisions and their underlying collective social values; it provides the basis for actions that influence the health of the public.

Decisions and actions that take place outside the sphere of government also influence the health of the public, perhaps even more than those made by our elected officials and administrative agencies. Private sector and voluntary organizations play key roles in identifying factors important for health and advancing actions to promote and protect health for individuals and groups. Public health involves collective decisions and actions, rather than purely personal ones; however, it is often governmental forums that raise issues, make decisions, and establish priorities for action. Many governmental actions reflect the dual roles of government often portrayed on official governmental seals and vehicles of local public safety agencies—to protect and to serve. As they relate to health, the genesis of these two roles lies in separate, often conflicting, philosophies and legacies of government. This chapter will examine how these roles are organized in the United States. This examination particularly emphasizes the relationships among law, government, and public health, seeking answers to the following questions:

- What are the various roles for government in serving the public's health?
- What is the legal basis for public health in the United States?
- How are public health responsibilities and roles structured at the federal, state, and local levels?

To review the organization and structure of governmental public health, this chapter, unlike the history briefly traced in Chapter 1, will begin with federal public health roles and activities, to be followed, in turn, by those at the state and local levels. The focus is primarily on form and structure, rather than function, which will be addressed in Chapter 5. In most circumstances, it is logical for form to follow function. Here, however, it is necessary to understand the legal and organizational framework of governmental public health as part of the context for public health practice. The framework established through law and governmental agencies is a key element of the public health's infrastructure and one of the basic building blocks of the public health system. Other important building blocks, including human, informational, fiscal, and other aspects of organizational resources, will be examined in Chapter 6. The topics in this chapter have been separated from other public health system structures somewhat arbitrarily. However, the legal basis of public health and the governmental agencies that have been created to serve the public health are basic and important concepts in their own right. This structure is a product of our uniquely American approach to government.

AMERICAN GOVERNMENT AND PUBLIC HEALTH

Former Speaker of the U.S. House of Representatives, Tip O'Neil, frequently observed, "all politics is local." If this is so, public health must be considered primarily a local phenomenon, as well, because politics are embedded in public health processes. After all, public health represents collective decisions as to which health outcomes are unacceptable, which factors contribute to those outcomes, which unacceptable problems will be addressed in view of resource limitations, and which participants need to be involved in addressing the problems. These are political processes, with different viewpoints and values being brought together to determine which collective decisions will be made. All too often, the term *politics* carries a very different connotation, one frequently associated with overtones of partisan politics. However, political processes are necessary and productive, and perhaps the best means devised by humans to meet our collective needs.

The public health system in the United States is a product of many forces that have shaped governmental roles in health. The framers of the U.S. Constitution did not plan for the federal government to deal directly with health or, for that matter, many other important issues. The word *health* does not even appear in that famous document, relegating health to the group of powers reserved to the states or the people. The Constitution explicitly authorized the federal government to promote and provide for the general welfare (in the Preamble and Article I, Section 8) and to regulate commerce (also in Article I, Section 8). Federal powers evolved slowly in the area of health on the basis of these explicit powers and subsequent U.S. Supreme Court decisions that broadened federal authority by determining that additional powers are implied in the explicit language of the Constitution.

The initial duties to regulate international affairs and interstate commerce led the federal government to concentrate its efforts on preventing the importation of epidemics and assisting states and localities, upon request, with their episodic needs for communicable disease control. The earliest federal health unit, the Marine Hospital Service, was established in 1798, partly to serve merchant seamen and partly to prevent importation of epidemic diseases; it evolved over time into what is now the U.S. Public Health Service.

However, the power to promote health and welfare did not always translate into the ability to act. The federal government acquired the ability to raise significant financial resources only with the authority to levy a federal tax on income, provided by the Sixteenth Amendment in the early twentieth century. The ability to raise vast sums generated the capacity to address health problems and needs through transferring resources to state and local governments in various forms of grants-in-aid. Despite its powers to provide for the general welfare and regulate commerce, the federal government could not act directly in health matters; it could act only through states as its primary delivery system. After 1935 the power and influence of the federal government grew rapidly through its financial influence over state and local programs, such as the Hospital Services and Construction (Hill-Burton) Act of 1946 and, after 1965, through its emergence as a major purchaser of health care through Medicare and Medicaid. As for a public health presence at the federal level, the best-known and most widely respected federal public health agency, now known as the Centers for Disease Control and Prevention (CDC), was not established until 1946.[1]

The emergence of the federal government as a major influence in the health system displaced states from a position they had held since before the birth of the American republic. States were sovereign powers before agreeing to share their powers with the newly established federal government; their sovereignty included powers over matters related to health emanating from two general sources. First, they derived from the so-called police powers of states, which provide the basis for government to limit the actions of individuals in order to control and abate hazards and nuisances. A second source for state health powers lay in the expectation for government to serve those individuals unable to provide for themselves. This expectation had its roots in the Elizabethan Poor Laws and carried over to states in the new American form of government. Despite this common heritage, states assumed these roles quite differently and at different points in time because the evolution of states themselves during the nineteenth century took place unevenly.

States developed structures and organizations needed to use their police powers to protect citizens from communicable diseases and environmental hazards, primarily from wastes, water, and food. State health agencies developed first in Massachusetts, then across the country, during the latter half of the nineteenth century. When federal grants became available, especially after 1935, states eagerly sought out federal funding for maternal and child health services, public health laboratories, and other basic public health programs. In so doing, states surrendered some of their autonomy over health issues. Priorities were increasingly dictated by federal grants tied to specific programs and services. It is fair to say that the grantor-grantee arrangement has never been fully satisfactory to either party, and the results in terms of health, welfare, education, and environmental policy suggest that better frameworks may be possible.

States possess the ultimate authority to create the political subunits that provide various services to the residents of a particular jurisdiction. In this manner, counties, cities, and other forms of municipalities, townships, boroughs, parishes, and the like are established. Special-purpose districts for every conceivable purpose—from library services and mosquito control to emergency medical services and education—have also abounded. The powers delegated to or authorized for all of these local jurisdictions are established by state legislatures for health and other purposes. Although many big-city health departments were established prior to the establishment of their respective state health agencies, states are free to use a variety of approaches to structuring public health roles at the local level. Because most states use the county form of subdividing the state, counties became the primary local governmental jurisdictions with health roles after 1900.

State constitutions and statutes impart the authority for local governments to influence health. This authority comes in two forms: those responsibilities of the state specifically delegated to local governments and additional authorities allowed through home rule powers. Home rule options permit local jurisdictions to enact a local constitution or charter and to take on additional authority and powers, such as the ability to levy taxes for local public health services and activities.

Counties generally carry out duties delegated by the state. More than two-thirds of U.S. counties have a county commission form of government, with anywhere from 2 to 50 elected county commissioners (supervisors, judges, and other titles are also used).[2] These commissions carry out both legislative and executive branch functions, although they share administrative authority with other local elected officials, such as county clerks, assessors, treasurers, prosecuting attorneys, sheriffs, and coroners. Some counties—generally, the more populous ones—have a county administrator accountable to elected commissioners, and a small number of counties (less than 5 percent) have an elected county executive. Elected county executives often have veto power over the county legislative body; home rule jurisdictions are more likely to have an elected county executive than are other counties.

Local governments in U.S. cities were first on the scene in terms of public health activities, as noted in Chapter 1. Big-city health agencies remain an important force in the public health system in the United States. However, after about 1875 when states became more extensively involved, the relative role of municipal governments began to erode. Both local and state governments were overwhelmed by the availability of federal funding in comparison with their own resources, finding it easier to take what they could get from the federal government rather than generating their own revenue to finance needed services.

Many forces have been at work to alter the initial relationships among the three levels of government for health roles, including:

- Gradual expansion and maturation of the federal government
- Staggered addition of new states and variability in the maturation of state governments
- Population growth and shifts over time

- Ability of the various levels of government to raise revenues commensurate with their expanding needs
- Growth of science and technology as tools for addressing public health and medical care needs
- Rapid growth of the U.S. economy
- Expectations and needs of American society for various services from their government[3,4]

The last of these factors is perhaps the most important. For the first 150 years of U.S. history, there was little expectation that the federal government should intervene in the health and welfare needs of its citizenry. The massive need and economic turmoil of the Great Depression years drastically altered this longstanding value as Americans began to turn to government to help deal with current needs and future uncertainties.

The complex public health network that exists today evolved slowly, with many different shifts in relative roles and influence. Economic considerations and societal expectations, both reaching a critical point in the 1930s, set the tone for the rest of the twentieth century. In general, power and influence were initially greatest at the local level, residing there until states began to develop their own machinery to carry out their police power and welfare roles. States then served as the primary locus for these health roles until the federal government began to use its vast resource potential to meet changing public expectations in the 1930s. Federal grant programs for public health and, eventually, personal health care service programs soon drove state actions, especially after the 1960s. It was then that several new federal health and social service programs were targeted directly to local governments, bypassing states. At the same time, a new federal-state partnership for the medically indigent (Medicaid) was established to address the national policy concern over the plight of the medically indigent.

Political and philosophical shifts since about 1980 are altering roles once again.[3] Debates over federal versus state roles continued throughout the 1980s and 1990s, although current indications suggest that some diminution of federal influence and enhancement of state influence is likely to persist for the near term. Still, the federal government has considerable ability to influence the health system through its fiscal muscle power, as well as its research, regulatory, technical assistance, and training roles.

PUBLIC HEALTH LAW

One of the chief organizing forces for public health lies in the system of law. Law has many purposes in the modern world, and many of these are evident in public health laws. Unfortunately, there is no one repository where the entire body of law, even the body of public health law, can be found. This has occurred because laws are products of the legal system, which, in the United States, includes a federal system and 50 separate state legal systems. These developed at different times in response to somewhat different circumstances and issues. Common to each is some form of a state constitution, a considerable amount of legislation, and a substantial body of judicial decisions. If there is any road map through this maze, it lies in the federal and state constitutions, which establish the basic framework dividing governmental powers among the various branches of government in ways that allow each to create its own laws.

As a result, four different types of law can be distinguished by virtue of their form or authority:

1. constitutionally based law,
2. legislatively based law,
3. administratively based law, and
4. judicially based law.

This framework still allows latitude for judicial interpretation and oversight. A brief description of each of these forms of law follows.

Types of Law

Constitutional law is ultimately derived from the U.S. Constitution, the legal foundation of the nation, in which the powers, duties, and limits of the federal government are established. States basically gave up certain powers (defense, foreign diplomacy, printing money, etc.), ceding these to the federal government while retaining all other powers and duties. Health is not one of those powers explicitly bestowed upon the federal government. The federal constitution also included a Bill of Rights intended to protect the rights of individuals from abuses by their government. States, in turn, have developed their own state constitutions, often patterned after the federal framework, although state constitutions tend to be more clear and specific in their language, leaving less room and need for judicial interpretation. State constitutions provide the broad framework from which states determine which activities will be undertaken and how those activities will be organized and funded. These decisions and actions come in the form of state statutes.

Statutory law includes all of the acts and statutes enacted by Congress and the various state and local legislative bodies. This collection of law represents a wide range of governmental policy choices, including:

- Simple expressions of preferences in favor of a particular policy or service (such as the value of home visits by public health nurses)
- Authorizations for specific programs (such as the authority for local governments to license restaurants)
- Mandates or requirements for an activity to occur or, alternatively, to be prohibited (such as requiring all newborns to be screened for specific metabolic diseases or prohibiting smoking in public places)
- Providing resources for specific purposes (such as the distribution of medications to patients with acquired immune deficiency syndrome [AIDS])

If the legislative intent is for something to occur, the most effective approaches are generally to require or prohibit an activity.

The basic requirement for statutory-based laws is that they must be consistent with the U.S. Constitution and, for state and local statutes, with state constitutions as well. State laws also establish the various subunits of the state and delineate their responsibilities for carrying out state mandates, as well as the limits of what they can do. At the local level, the legislative bodies of these subunits (e.g., city councils and county commissions) enact ordinances and statutes setting forth the duties and authorizations of local government and its agencies. Laws affecting public health are created at all levels in this hierarchy, but especially at the state and local levels. Among other purposes, these laws establish state and local boards of health and health departments, delineate the responsibilities of these agencies, including their programs and budgets, and establish health-related laws and requirements. Many of these laws are enforced by governmental agencies.

Administrative law is law promulgated by administrative agencies within the executive branch of government. Rather than enact statutes that include extensive details of a professional or technical nature and to allow greater flexibility in their design and subsequent revision, administrative agencies are provided with the authority to establish law through rule-making processes. These rules, administrative law, carry the force of law and represent a unique situation in which legislative, judicial, and executive powers are carried out by one agency. Administrative agencies include cabinet-level departments, as well as other boards, commissions, and the like that are granted this power through an enactment of the legislative body. Because of its importance and pervasiveness for public health actions, Appendix 4-A examines administrative law in more depth.

The fourth type of law is judicial law, also known as common law. This includes a wide range of tradition, legal custom, and previous decisions of federal and state courts. To ensure fairness and consistency, previous decisions are used to guide judgments on similar disputes. This form of law becomes especially important in areas in which laws have not been codified by legislative bodies. In public health, nuisances (unsanitary, noxious, or otherwise potentially dangerous circumstances) are one such area in which few legislative bodies have specified exactly what does and what does not constitute a public health nuisance. In this situation, the common law for nuisances is derived from previous judicial decisions. These determine under what circumstances and for what specific conditions a public health official can take action, as well as the actions that can be taken.

Purposes of Public Health Law

Two broad purposes for public health law can be described: protecting and promoting health and ensuring the protection of rights of individuals in the processes used to protect and promote health. Public health powers ultimately derive from the U.S. Constitution, which bestows the authority to regulate commerce and provide for the general welfare, and from the various state constitutions, which often provide clear but broad authorities, based largely on the police power of the state. States often have reasonably well-defined public health codes. However, there is considerable diversity in their content and scope, despite similarities in their basic sources of power and authority.

Many public health laws are enacted and enforced under what is known as the state's "police power." This is a broad concept that encompasses the functions historically undertaken by governments in protecting the health, safety, welfare, and general well-being of their citizens. A wide variety of laws derives from the police power of the state, a power that is considered one of the least limitable of all governmental powers. The police power of the state can be vested in an administrative agency, such as a state health agency, which becomes accountable for the manner in which these responsibilities are executed. In these circumstances, its use is a duty, rather than a matter of choice, although its form is left to the discretion of the user.

The courts have upheld laws that appear to limit severely or restrict the rights of individuals where these were found to be reasonable, rather than arbitrary and capricious attempts to accomplish government's ends. The state's police power is not unlimited, however. Interference with individual liberties and the taking of personal property are considerations that must be balanced on a case-by-case basis. At issue is whether the public interest in achieving a public health goal outweighs the public interest in protecting civil liberties. Public health laws requiring vaccinations or immunizations to protect the community have generally withstood legal challenges claiming that they infringed upon the rights of individuals to make their own health decisions. A precedent-setting judicial opinion upheld a Massachusetts ordinance authorizing local boards of health to require vaccinations for smallpox to be administered to residents if deemed necessary by the local boards.[5] Such decisions argue that laws that place the common good ahead of the competing rights of individuals should govern society. Similarly, courts have weighed the power of the state to appropriate an individual's property or limit the individual's use of it if the best interests of the community make such an action desirable. In some circumstances, equitable compensation must be provided. Issues of community interest and fair compensation are commonly encountered in dealing with public health nuisances in which an individual's private property can be found to be harmful to others.

The various forms of law and the changing nature of the relationships among the three levels of government have created a patchwork of public health laws. Despite its relatively limited constitutionally-based powers, the federal government can preempt state and local government action in key areas of public health regulation involving commerce and aspects of communicable disease control. States also have authority to preempt local government actions in virtually all areas of public health activity. Although this legal framework allows for a clear and rational delineation of authorities and responsibilities, a quite variable set of arrangements has arisen. Often, the higher level of government chooses not to exercise its full authority and shifts that authority to a lower level of government. This can be accomplished in some instances by delegating or requiring, and in other instances by authorizing (with incentives), the lower level of government to exercise authorities of the higher level. This has made for a complex set of relationships among the three levels of government and for 50 variations of the theme to be played in the 50 states. These relationships and their impact on the form and structure of governmental public health agencies will be evident in subsequent sections of this chapter.

There have been many critiques of the statutory basis of public health in the United States. A common one is that public health law, not unlike law affecting other areas of society, simply has not kept pace with the rapid and extensive changes in science and technology. Laws have been enacted at different points in time in response to different conditions and circumstances. These laws have often been enacted with little consideration as to their consistency with previous statutes and their overall impact on the body of public health law. For example, many states have different statutes and legal frameworks for similar risks, such as general communicable diseases, sexually transmitted diseases (STDs), and human immunodeficiency virus (HIV) infections. Confidentiality and privacy provisions, which trace their origins to the vow in the Hippocratic oath not to reveal patient's secrets, are often inconsistent from law-to-law, and enforcement provisions vary as well. Beyond these concerns, public health laws often lack clear statements of purpose or mission and are not linked to public health core functions and essential public health services.

In view of these criticisms, recommendations have been advanced calling for a complete overhaul and recodification of public health law. Recommendations for improvement of the public health codes often call for

- stronger links with the overall mission and core functions of public health.
- uniform structures for similar programs and services.
- confidentiality provisions to be reviewed and made more consistent.
- clarification of police power responsibilities to deal with unusual health risks and threats.
- greater emphasis on the least restrictive means necessary to achieve the law's intent through use of intermediate sanctions and compulsive measures, based on proven effectiveness.
- fairer and more consistent enforcement and administrative practices.

Although these recommendations have been advanced for several decades, little progress has been made at either the federal or state level. At times, states have sought to recodify public health statutes by relocating their placement in the statute books, rather than dealing with the more basic issues of reviewing the scope and allocation of their public health responsibilities so that these are clearly presented and assigned among the various levels of government. The intricacies of public health law often help drive the inner workings of federal, state, and local public health agencies. We will now turn to the form and structure of these agencies.

GOVERNMENTAL PUBLIC HEALTH: FEDERAL HEALTH AGENCIES

The U.S. Public Health Service (PHS) serves as the focal point for health concerns at the federal level. Although there have been frequent reorganizations affecting the structure of PHS and its placement within the massive Department of Health and Human Services (DHHS), the restructuring completed in 1996 was the most significant in recent decades. The changes were undertaken as part of the federal Reinvention of Government Initiative to bring expertise in public health and science closer to the Secretary of DHHS.

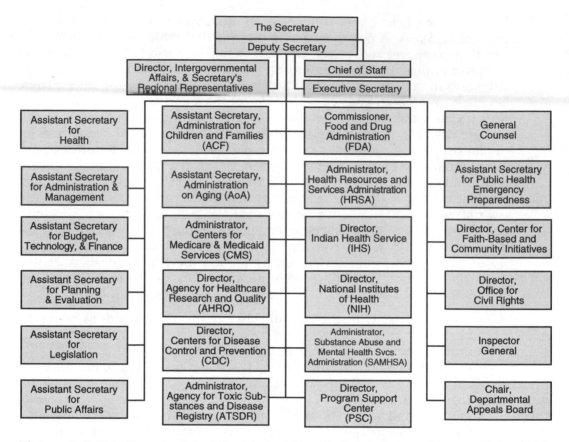

Figure 4–1 U.S. Department of Health and Human Services Organization Chart, 2003. *Source:* Reprinted from U.S. Department of Health and Human Services, 2003.

In the restructuring, the line authority of the Assistant Secretary for Health over the various agencies within PHS was abolished, with those agencies now reporting directly to the Secretary of Health and Human Services, as illustrated in Figure 4–1. The Assistant Secretary for Health became the head of the Office of Public Health and Science (OPHS), a new division reporting to the Secretary that also includes the Office of the Surgeon General. Each of the former PHS agencies became a full HHS operating division. These eight operating agencies, the OPHS, and the regional health administrators for the 10 federal regions of the country now constitute the PHS. In effect, PHS has become a functional rather than an organizational unit of DHHS. In 2003 several activities related to emergency preparedness and response were moved into the newly established Department of Homeland Security (see Chapter 8). An Office of Public Health Emergency Preparedness and Response remained at DHHS to coordinate bioterrorism and other public health emergency activities managed by various PHS agencies.

The PHS agencies address a wide range of public health activities, from research and training to primary care and health protection, as described in Exhibit 4–1. The key PHS agencies are:

- Health Resources and Services Administration (HRSA)
- Indian Health Service (IHS)
- Centers for Disease Control and Prevention (CDC)
- National Institutes of Health (NIH)
- Food and Drug Administration (FDA)
- Substance Abuse and Mental Health Services Administration (SAMHSA)
- Agency for Toxic Substances and Disease Registry (ATSDR)
- Agency for Health Care Research and Quality (AHRQ)

Exhibit 4–1 U.S. Public Health Service Agencies

Health Resources and Services Administration (HRSA)	HRSA helps provide health resources for medically under-served populations. The main operating units of HRSA are the Bureau of Primary Health Care, Bureau of Health Professions, Maternal and Child Bureau, and the HIV/AIDS Bureau. A nationwide network of 643 community and migrant health centers, plus 144 primary care programs for the homeless and residents of public housing, serve 8.1 million Americans each year. HRSA also works to build the health care workforce and maintains the National Health Service Corps. The agency provides services to people with AIDS through the Ryan White Care Act programs. It oversees the organ transplantation system and works to decrease infant mortality and improve maternal and child health. HRSA was established in 1982 by bringing together several existing programs. HRSA has more than 1300 employees at its headquarters in Rockville, MD and another 750 employees in 10 regional offices throughout the U.S.
Indian Health Service (IHS)	The Indian Health Service (IHS) is responsible for providing federal health services to American Indians and Alaska Natives. The provision of health services to members of federally-recognized tribes grew out of the special government-to-government relationship between the federal government and Indian tribes. This relationship, established in 1787, is based on Article I, Section 8 of the Constitution, and has been given form and substance by numerous treaties, laws, Supreme Court decisions, and Executive Orders. The IHS is the principal federal health care provider and health advocate for Indian people, and its goal is to raise their health status to the highest possible level. The IHS currently provides health services to approximately 1.5 million American Indians and Alaska Natives who belong to more than 557 federally recognized tribes in 35 states. IHS was established in 1924; its mission was transferred from the Interior Department in 1955. Agency headquarters are in Rockville, MD.

continues

Exhibit 4–1 continued

Centers for Disease Control and Prevention (CDC)	Working with states and other partners, CDC provides a system of health surveillance to monitor and prevent disease outbreaks, including bioterrorism events and threats, and maintains national health statistics. CDC also provides for immunization services, supports research into disease and injury prevention, and guards against international disease transmission, with personnel stationed in more than 25 foreign countries. CDC was established in 1946 (see Exhibit 4–2); its headquarters are in Atlanta, GA. CDC has 8,500 employees.
National Institutes of Health (NIH)	Begun as a one-room Laboratory of Hygiene in 1887, the National Institutes of Health (NIH) today is one of the world's foremost medical research centers and the federal focal point for health research. NIH is the steward of medical and behavioral research for the Nation. Its mission is science in pursuit of fundamental knowledge about the nature and behavior of living systems and the application of that knowledge to extend healthy life and reduce the burdens of illness and disability. In realizing its goals, the NIH provides leadership and direction to programs designed to improve the health of the nation by conducting and supporting research: in the causes, diagnosis, prevention, and cure of human diseases; in the processes of human growth and development; in the biological effects of environmental contaminants; in the understanding of mental, addictive, and physical disorders; in directing programs for the collection, dissemination, and exchange of information in medicine and health, including the development and support of medical libraries and the training of medical librarians and other health information specialists. Though the majority of NIH resources sponsor external research, there is also a large in-house research program. NIH includes 27 separate health institutes and centers; its headquarters are in Bethesda, MD. NIH has more than 16,000 employees.
Food and Drug Administration (FDA)	FDA ensures that the food we eat is safe and wholesome, that the cosmetics we use won't harm us, and that medicines, medical devices, and radiation-transmitting products such as microwave ovens are safe and effective. FDA also oversees feed and drugs for pets and farm animals. Authorized by Congress to enforce the Federal Food, Drug, and Cosmetic Act and several other public health laws, the agency monitors the manufacture, import, transport, storage, and sale of $1 trillion worth of goods annu-

continues

Exhibit 4–1 continued

	ally, at a cost to taxpayers of about $3 a person. FDA has over 9,000 employees, located in 167 U.S. cities. Among its staff, FDA has chemists, microbiologists, and other scientists, as well as investigators and inspectors who visit 16,000 facilities a year as part of their oversight of the businesses that FDA regulates. FDA, established in 1906, has its headquarters in Rockville, MD.
Substance Abuse and Mental Health Services Administration (SAMHSA)	The Substance Abuse and Mental Health Services Administration (SAMHSA) was established by Congress under Public Law 102-321 on October 1, 1992, to strengthen the Nation's health care capacity to provide prevention, diagnosis, and treatment services for substance abuse and mental illnesses. SAMHSA works in partnership with States, communities, and private organizations to address the needs of people with substance abuse and mental illnesses as well as the community risk factors that contribute to these illnesses. SAMHSA serves as the umbrella under which substance abuse and mental health service centers are housed, including the Center for Mental Health Services (CMHS), the Center for Substance Abuse Prevention (CSAP), and the Center for Substance Abuse Treatment (CSAT). SAMHSA also houses the Office of the Administrator, the Office of Applied Studies, and the Office of Program Services. In fiscal year 2000, SAMHSA's budget was approximately $2.6 billion. SAMHSA headquarters are in Rockville, MD; the agency has about 600 employees.
Agency for Toxic Substances and Disease Registry (ATSDR)	Working with states and other federal agencies, ATSDR seeks to prevent exposure to hazardous substances from waste sites. The agency conducts public health assessments, health studies, surveillance activities, and health education training in communities around waste sites on the U.S. Environmental Protection Agency's National Priorities List. ASTDR also has developed toxicological profiles of hazardous chemicals found at these sites. The agency is closely associated administratively with CDC; its headquarters are in Atlanta, GA. ASTDR has more than 400 employees.
Agency for Health Care Research and Quality (AHRQ)	AHRQ supports cross-cutting research on health care systems, health care quality and cost issues, and effectiveness of medial treatments. The agency has about 300 employees; its headquarters are in Rockville, MD. Formerly known as the Agency for Health Care Policy and Research, AHRQ was established in 1989, assuming broadened responsibilities of its predecessor agency, the National Center for Health Services Research and Health Care Technology Assessment.

PHS agencies actually represent only a small part of DHHS. Other important operating divisions within DHHS include the Administration for Children and Families, the Health Care Financing Administration, and the Office of the Assistant Secretary for Aging. In addition there are several administrative and support units within DHHS for management and the budget, intergovernmental affairs, legal counsel, civil rights, the inspector general, departmental appeals, public affairs, legislation, and planning and evaluation.

Beyond DHHS, health responsibilities have been assigned to several other federal agencies, including the federal Environmental Protection Agency (EPA) and the Departments of Homeland Security, Education, Agriculture, Defense, Transportation, and Veterans Affairs, just to name a few. The importance of some of these other federal agencies should not be underestimated in terms of the level and proportion of their resources devoted to health purposes. Health-specific agencies at the federal level are a relatively new phenomenon. PHS itself remained a unit of the Treasury Department until 1944, and the first cabinet-level federal human services agency of any kind was the Federal Security Agency in 1939. This historical trivia demonstrates that federal powers and authority in health and public health are a relatively recent phenomenon in U.S. history. The history of CDC in Exhibit 4–2 further documents this claim, describing the expansion of the federal presence in both traditional and emerging public health practice.

Exhibit 4–2 History of CDC

The Centers for Disease Control and Prevention (CDC), an institution synonymous around the world with public health, was 50 years old on July 1, 1996. The Communicable Disease Center was organized in Atlanta, Georgia, on July 1, 1946; its founder, Dr. Joseph W. Mountin, was a visionary public health leader who had high hopes for this small and comparatively insignificant branch of the Public Health Service (PHS). It occupied only one floor of the Volunteer Building on Peachtree Street and had fewer than 400 employees, most of whom were engineers and entomologists. Until the previous day, they had worked for Malaria Control in War Areas, the predecessor of CDC, which had successfully kept the southeastern states free of malaria during World War II and, for approximately 1 year, free from murine typhus fever. The new institution would expand its interests to include all communicable diseases and would be the servant of the states, providing practical help whenever called.

Distinguished scientists soon filled CDC's laboratories, and many states and foreign countries sent their public health staffs to Atlanta for training. Any tropical disease with an insect vector and all those of zoologic origin came within its purview. Dr. Mountin was not satisfied with this progress, and he impatiently pushed the staff to do more. He reminded them that, except for tuberculosis and venereal disease, which had separate units in Washington, DC, CDC was responsible for any communicable disease. To survive, it had to become a center for epidemiology.

Medical epidemiologists were scarce, and it was not until 1949 that Dr. Alexander Langmuir arrived to head the epidemiology branch. Within months, he launched the first-ever disease surveillance program, which confirmed his suspicion that malaria, on which CDC spent the largest portion of its budget, had long since disappeared. Subse-

---

continues

Exhibit 4–2 continued

quently, disease surveillance became the cornerstone on which CDC's mission of service to the states was built and, in time, changed the practice of public health.

The outbreak of the Korean War in 1950 was the impetus for creating CDC's Epidemiologic Intelligence Service (EIS). The threat of biologic warfare loomed, and Dr. Langmuir, the most knowledgeable person in PHS about this arcane subject, saw an opportunity to train epidemiologists who would guard against ordinary threats to public health while watching out for alien germs. The first-class EIS officers arrived in Atlanta for training in 1951 and pledged to go wherever they were called for the next 2 years. These "disease detectives" quickly gained fame for "shoe-leather epidemiology," through which they ferreted out the cause of disease outbreaks.

The survival of CDC as an institution was not at all certain in the 1950s. In 1947, Emory University gave land on Clifton Road for a headquarters, but construction did not begin for more than a decade. PHS was so intent on research and the rapid growth of the National Institutes of Health that it showed little interest in what happened in Atlanta. Congress, despite the long delay in appropriating money for new buildings, was much more receptive to CDC's pleas for support than either PHS or the Bureau of the Budget.

Two major health crises in the mid-1950s established CDC's credibility and ensured its survival. In 1955, when poliomyelitis appeared in children who had received the recently approved Salk vaccine, the national inoculation program was stopped. The cases were traced to contaminated vaccine from a laboratory in California; the problem was corrected, and the inoculation program, at least for first and second graders, was resumed. The resistance of these 6- and 7-year-olds to polio, compared with that of older children, proved the effectiveness of the vaccine. Two years later, surveillance was used again to trace the course of a massive influenza epidemic. From the data gathered in 1957 and subsequent years, the national guidelines for influenza vaccine were developed.

CDC grew by acquisition. The venereal disease program came to Atlanta in 1957 and with it the first Public Health Advisors, non-science college graduates destined to play an important role in making CDC's disease-control programs work. The tuberculosis program moved in 1960, immunization practices and the Morbidity and Mortality Weekly Report in 1961. The Foreign Quarantine Service, one of the oldest and most prestigious units of PHS, came in 1967; many of its positions were switched to other uses as better ways of doing the work of quarantine, primarily through overseas surveillance, were developed. The long-established nutrition program also moved to CDC, as well as the National Institute for Occupational Safety and Health, and work of already established units increased. Immunization tackled measles and rubella control; epidemiology added family planning and surveillance of chronic diseases. When CDC joined the international malaria-eradication program and accepted responsibility for protecting Earth from moon germs and vice versa, CDC's mission stretched overseas and into space.

CDC played a key role in one of the greatest triumphs of public health, the eradication of smallpox. In 1962, it established a smallpox surveillance unit, and a year later tested a newly developed jet gun and vaccine in the Pacific Island nation of Tonga. After refining vaccination techniques in Brazil, CDC began work in Central and West Africa in 1966. When millions of people there had been vaccinated, CDC used surveillance to speed the work along. The World Health Organization used this "eradication escalation" technique elsewhere with such success that global eradication of smallpox was achieved in 1977. The United States spent only $32 million on the project, about the cost of keeping smallpox at bay for 2.5 months.

continues

Exhibit 4–2 continued

CDC also achieved notable success at home, tracking new and mysterious disease outbreaks. In the mid-1970s and early 1980s, it found the cause of Legionnaires' disease and toxic shock syndrome. A fatal disease, subsequently named acquired immunodeficiency syndrome (AIDS), was first mentioned in the June 5, 1981, issue of MMWR. Since then, MMWR has published numerous follow-up articles about AIDS, and one of the largest portion of CDC's budget and staff is assigned to address this disease.

Although CDC succeeded more often than it failed, it did not escape criticism. For example, television and press reports about the Tuskegee study on long-term effects of untreated syphilis in black men created a storm of protest in 1972. This study had been initiated by PHS and other organizations in 1932 and was transferred to CDC in 1957. Although the effectiveness of penicillin as a therapy for syphilis had been established during the late 1940s, participants in this study remained untreated until the study was brought to public attention. CDC was also criticized because of the 1976 effort to vaccinate the U.S. population against swine flu, the infamous killer of 1918-19. When some vaccinees developed Guillain-Barre syndrome, the campaign was stopped immediately; the epidemic never occurred.

As the scope of CDC's activities expanded far beyond communicable diseases, its name had to be changed. In 1970 it became the Center for Disease Control, and in 1981, after extensive reorganization, Center became Centers. The words "and Prevention" were added in 1992, but, by law, the well-known three-letter acronym was retained. In health emergencies, CDC means an answer to SOS calls from anywhere in the world, such as the recent one from Zaire, where Ebola fever raged.

Fifty years ago, CDC's agenda was non-controversial (hardly anyone objected to the pursuit of germs), and Atlanta was a backwater. In 1996, CDC's programs are often tied to economic, political, and social issues, and Atlanta is as near to Washington as the tap of a keyboard.

Source: Reprinted from History of CDC, *Morbidity and Mortality Weekly Report,* Vol. 45, pp. 526–528, the Centers for Disease Control and Prevention, 1996.

The federal government is the largest purchaser of health-related services, although spending on health purposes represents only a fraction of the total federal budget. Figure 4–2 compares total national health expenditures with health expenditures attributed to the federal government and to state local governments. Health expenditures constituted about 23 percent of total federal expenditures in 2000, up from 12 percent in 1980, and only 3 percent in 1960 (Figure 4–3). Escalating costs for health care services seriously constrain efforts to reduce the federal budget deficit, and there is little public or political support for additional taxes for health purposes

It is no simple task to describe the federal budget development and approval process that determines funding levels for federal health programs. Although nearly one-fourth of the federal budget supports health activities, the major share is spent on Medicare and Medicaid. These and other entitlement programs constitute two-thirds of the federal budget; this spending is mandatory and cannot be easily controlled. The remaining one-third repre-

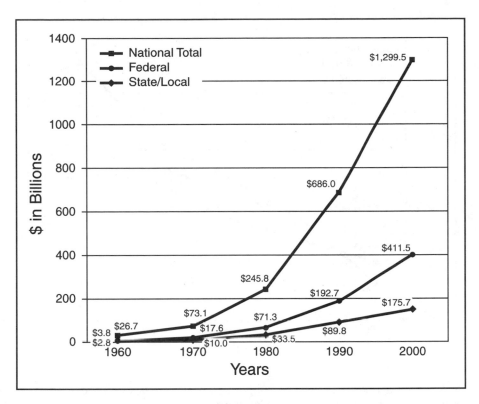

Figure 4–2 Total National Health Expenditures, and Federal and State/Local Government Expenditures Spent for Health-Related Purposes, United States, 1960–2000. *Source:* Adapted from National Center for Health Statistics. *Healthy United States 2002,* Public Health Service, 2002.

sents discretionary spending; half of this is related to national defense purposes. Spending for discretionary programs is more readily controlled. Non-defense discretionary spending for health purposes competes with a wide array of programs, including education, training, science, technology, housing, transportation, and foreign aid. Despite a small increase due to national terrorism preparedness initiatives, it has declined as a proportion of all federal spending, from 23 percent in 1966 to 19 percent in 2003.

Decisions authorizing and funding health programs are made in an annual budget approval process. The current process is a complex one that establishes ceilings for broad categories of expenditures and then reconciles individual programs and funding levels within those ceilings in omnibus budget reconciliation acts. For discretionary programs, Congress must act each year to provide spending authority. For mandatory programs, Congress may act to change the spending that current laws require. The result is a mixture of substantive decisions as to which programs will be authorized and what they will be authorized to do, together with budget decisions as to the level of resources to be made available through 13 annual appropriations bills. In recent years federal

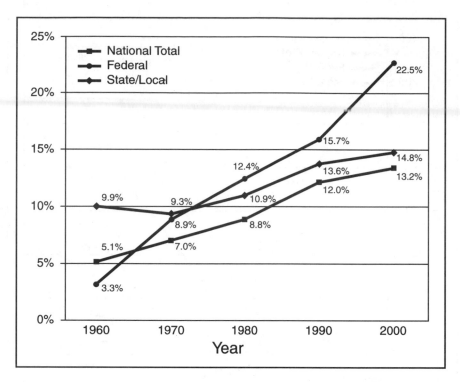

Figure 4–3 Percentage of National Gross Domestic Expenditures, and Federal and State/Local Government Expenditures Spent for Health-Related Purposes, United States, 1960–2000. *Source:* Adapted from National Center for Health Statistics. *Healthy United States 2002*, Public Health Service, 2002.

law has imposed a cap on total annual discretionary spending and requires that spending cuts must offset increased mandatory spending or new discretionary programs. This budgetary environment presents major challenges for new public health programs and, not infrequently, threatens continued funding for programs that have been operating for decades.

The organization of federal health responsibilities within DHHS is quite complex fiscally and operationally. In federal fiscal year 2004, the overall DHHS budget is about $500 billion.[6] DHHS has nearly 65,000 employees and is the largest grant-making agency in the federal government, with some 60,000 grants each year. DHHS manages more than 300 programs through its 11 operating divisions. The major share of the DHHS budget supports the Medicare and Medicaid programs within HCFA. PHS activities account for less than one-tenth of the fiscal year 2004 DHHS budget. In addition to HCFA and the PHS agencies, DHHS also includes the Administration for Children and Families and the Administration on Aging.

Budgets for PHS operating division budgets in federal fiscal year 2004 range from $28 billion for NIH to $300 million for AHRQ (Figure 4–4). Sixty percent of all PHS funds support NIH research activities, and another $18 billion sup-

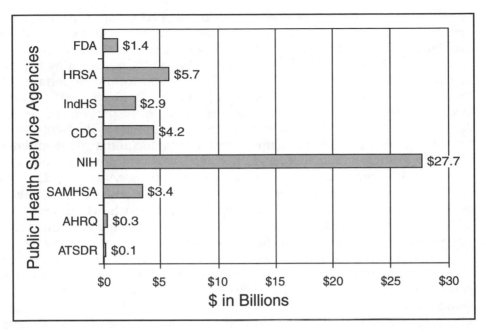

Figure 4–4 Fiscal Year 2004 U.S. Public Health Service Agency Budgets. *Source:* Adapted from the Fiscal Year 2004 Budget, U.S. Department of Health and Human Services, 2003.

port the remaining PHS agencies with HRSA and CDC together accounting for about $10 billion, which represents about 2 percent of total DHHS resources and about 0.5 percent of all federal spending.

Since the late 1970s, the Office of Health Promotion and Disease Prevention within the Office of the Assistant Secretary for Health has coordinated the development of the national agenda for public health and prevention efforts. Results of these efforts are apparent in the establishment of national health objectives that targeted the years 1990, 2000, and 2010 (see Chapter 2). Only one of more than 500 objectives from the 1990 and 2000 processes related to the public health system; that objective called for 90 percent of the population to be served by a local public health agency (LPHA) that was effectively carrying out public health's core functions by the year 2000.[7] Current estimates are that about 95 percent of the U.S. population is served by an LPHA functioning at some level of capability. Baseline data on how many local agencies were effectively carrying out the core functions were not available when this objective was established in 1990. Several studies of core function-related performance in the 1990s suggest that the nation fell far short of achieving its year 2000 target. Chapter 5 will describe core functions and performance measures used in these assessments and will identify some of the issues that impede progress toward this important national objective. Chapter 6 will describe an extensive panel of public health infrastructure objectives developed for Healthy People 2010.

PHS agencies have promoted greater use of performance measures in key federal health programs, including immunizations, tuberculosis control, STDs, substance abuse, and mental health services. As previously described, federal grants-in-aid have long been the prime strategy and mechanism by which the federal government generates state and local action toward important health problems. A variety of approaches to grant-making has been used over recent decades. These can be categorized by the extent of restrictions or flexibility imparted to grantees. The greatest flexibility and lack of requirements are associated with revenue-sharing grants. Block grants, including those initiated in the early 1980s, consolidate previously categorical grant programs into a block that generally comes with fewer restrictions than the previous collection of categorical grants. Formula grants are awarded on the basis of some predetermined formula, often based at least partly on need, which determines the level of funding for each grantee. Project grants are more limited in availability and are generally intended for a specific demonstration program or project.

In the 1990s DHHS proposed a series of federal partnership performance grants to address some of the shortcomings attributed to block grants implemented in the early 1980s. At that time restrictions were relaxed for the categorical programs folded into the block grants, including the Maternal and Child Health (MCH) Block Grant and the Prevention Block Grant. Lessons learned from the previous experience suggest the need for a cautious approach to new federal block grant proposals. In the 1980s the new block grants indeed came with fewer strings attached. However, they also came at funding levels that were reduced about 25 percent from the previous arrangement. The blocking of several categorical programs into one mega-grant also served to dissipate the constituencies for the categorical programs. Without active and visible constituencies advocating for programs, restoration or even maintenance of previous funding levels proved difficult. In addition, the reduction in reporting requirements made it more difficult to justify budget requests. Any new federal approaches to overcome these obstacles will be watched closely by advocates, as well as by state and local public health officials.

In addition to being a prime strategy to influence services at the state and local level, federal grants also serve to redistribute resources to compensate for differences in the ability of states to fund and operate basic health services. They have also served as a useful approach to promoting minimum standards for specific programs and services. For example, federal grants for maternal and child health promoted personnel standards in state and local agencies that fostered the growth of civil service systems across the country. Other effects on state and local health agencies will be apparent as these are examined in the following sections.

GOVERNMENTAL PUBLIC HEALTH: STATE HEALTH AGENCIES

Several factors place states at center stage when it comes to health. The U.S. Constitution gives states primacy in safeguarding the health of their citizens. From the mid-nineteenth century until the 1930s, states largely exercised that leadership role with little competition from the federal government and only occasional conflict with the larger cities. Federal funding turned the tables on states after 1935, reaching its peak influence in the 1960s and 1970s. At that time, numerous federal health and human service initiatives (such as model cities, community health centers, and community mental health services) were funded directly to local governments and even to community-based organizations. This practice greatly concerned state capitals and served to damage tenuous relationships among the three levels of government. The relative influence of states began to grow once again after 1980, with both increasing rhetoric and federal actions restoring some powers and resources to states and their state health agencies. Although states were finding it increasingly difficult to finance public health and medical service programs, they demanded more autonomy and control over the programs they managed, including those operated in partnership with the federal government. At the same time, local governments were making demands on state governments similar to those that states were making on the federal government. States have found themselves uncomfortably in the middle between the two other levels of government. At the same time, states are one step removed from both the resources needed to address the needs of their citizens and the demands and expectations of the local citizenry. For health issues, especially those affecting oversight and regulation of health services and providers, states often appear unduly influenced by large, politically active lobbies representing various aspects of the health system.

States carry out their health responsibilities through many different state agencies, although the overall constellation of health programs and services within all of state government is similar across states. Exhibit 4–3 outlines more than 20 state agencies that carry out health responsibilities or activities in a typical state. Somewhere in the maze of state agencies is an identifiable lead agency for health. These official health agencies are often free-standing departments reporting to the governor of the state. In about two-thirds of the states, the state health agency reports to a state board of health, although the prevalence of this reporting relationship is declining. Another approach to the organizational placement of state health agencies finds them within a multipurpose human service agency, often with the state's social services and substance abuse responsibilities. This approach has waxed and waned in popularity, although its popularity increased in the 1990s with the hopes of fostering better integration of community services across the spectrum of health and social services. State health agencies are freestanding agencies in about 30 states and are part of multipurpose health and/or human services agencies in the others.

The range of responsibilities for the official state health agency varies considerably in terms of specific programs and services. Staffing levels and patterns also show a wide range, reflecting the diversity in agency responsibilities. Comprehensive information on the resources and programs of state health agencies has not been available since the early 1990s, due to the demise of a national reporting system coordinated by the Association of State and Territorial Health Officials (ASTHO) and the Public Health Foundation. The data presented on state health agencies in this chapter are derived from the most recent compilation available;[8] this information was collected as part

Exhibit 4–3 Typical State Agencies with Health Roles (Names Vary from State to State)

- Official State Health Agency (Department of Health/Public Health)
- Department of Aging
- Department of Agriculture
- Department of Alcoholism and Substance Abuse
- Asbestos Abatement Authority
- Department of Children and Family Services
- Department of Emergency and Disaster Services
- Department of Energy and Natural Resources
- Environmental Protection Agencies
- Guardianship and Advocacy Commissions
- Health and Fitness Council
- Health Care Cost Containment Council
- Health Facilities Authority
- Health Facilities Planning Board
- Department of Mental Health and Developmental Disabilities
- Department of Mines and Minerals
- Department of Nuclear Safety
- Pollution Control Board
- Department of Professional Regulation
- Department of Public Aid
- Department of Rehabilitation Services
- Rural Affairs Council
- State Board of Education
- State Fire Marshall
- Department of Transportation
- State University System
- Department of Veterans Affairs

of a salary survey of state health officials in 2002. Figure 4–5 illustrates the variability in state health agencies' responsibilities for programs. In 2002, for example, 90 percent of the official state health agencies administered the Supplemental Food Program for Women, Infants and Children (WIC), vital statistics systems, public health laboratories, and tobacco prevention and control programs. Less than half of the state health agencies administered the state Medicaid Program, mental health and substance abuse services, and licensed health professionals. Most state health agencies administered programs for environmental health services, most frequently involving food and drinking water safety. However, only 25 percent of the state health agencies served as the environmental regulatory agency within their state, which often includes responsibility for clean air, resource conservation, clean water, superfund sites, toxic substance control, and hazardous substances.

As illustrated in Figure 4–2, state and local governments spent $176 billion on health-related purposes in 2000. Health expenditures have comprised 13–15 percent of state and local government expenditures since 1990 (Figure 4–3). Before the advent of Medicaid and Medicare in 1965, state and local governments actually spent more for health purposes than did the federal government.

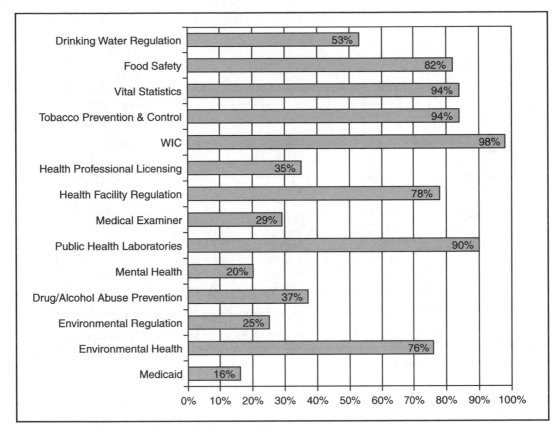

Figure 4–5 Selected Organizational Responsibilities of State Health Agencies, 2002. *Source:* Adapted from Association of State and Territorial Health Officials. *2002 Salary Survey of State and Territorial Health Officials.* Washington, DC: ASTHO; 2003.

With public health responsibilities allocated differently across the various states, data on state health agency expenditures are both difficult to interpret and incomplete in several important respects. These data do not allow for meaningful comparison across states because of the variation in responsibilities assigned to the official state health agency and those assigned to other state agencies. More importantly, these data do not differentiate between population-based public health activities and personal health services. Also lacking is a composite picture of resource allocations for important public health purposes across all state and local agencies with health roles, including substance abuse, mental health, and environmental protection agencies. This limitation is especially apparent for environmental health and protection roles. Chapter 6 examines public health expenditures and financial resources from the perspective of the infrastructure of public health. For these reasons, only general information on state health agency expenditures will be discussed.

The organizational placement and specific responsibilities of state health agencies largely determine the size of their budgets and workforce. Figure 4–6

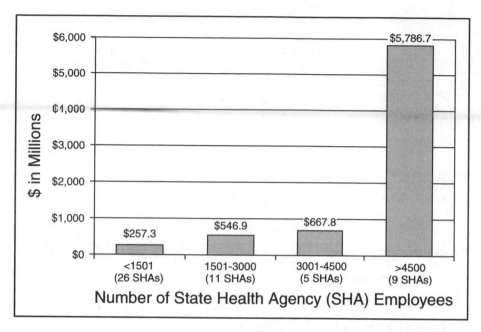

Figure 4–6 State Health Agency Expenditures by Number of State Health Agency Employees, 2002. *Source:* Adapted from Association of State and Territorial Health Officials. *2002 Salary Survey of State and Territorial Health Officials.* Washington, DC: ASTHO; 2003.

provides information on four groups of state health agencies as determined by the number of employees. Just over 50 percent of the state health agencies have 1500 or fewer employees; these agencies have budgets approximating $250 million. This group includes many free-standing agencies that have responsibility for traditional public health services but not for Medicaid, mental health, substance abuse, and environmental regulation. As these other responsibilities are added, the budgets and workforce of state health agencies increases substantially. Nine state health agencies have more than 4500 employees and average expenditures of almost $6 billion.

State health agency expenditures include grants and contracts to local public health agencies, although the current level of these inter-governmental transfers is not known. In 1991 an estimated $2 billion was transferred from state to local public health agencies.[9] As indicated in Figure 4–7, sources of the combined expenditures of state and local health agencies in 1991 were state funds (41 percent), federal funds (32 percent), local funds (12 percent), and fees and reimbursements (10 percent). For state health agencies alone, sources were state funds (55 percent), federal funds for Women, Infants and Children (WIC, 20 percent), federal MCH Block Grant funds (5 percent), and other federal sources (5 percent). Excluding WIC funding, the remaining resources are 69 percent state, 6 percent MCH, and 13 percent other federal funds.

At the federal level, more than a dozen federal departments, agencies, and commissions (Transportation, Labor, Health and Human Services, Commerce, Energy, Defense, EPA, Homeland Security, Interior, Consumer Product Safety

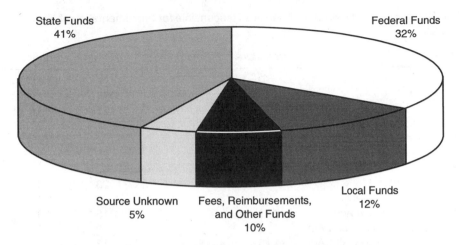

Figure 4–7 Sources of Funds for State and Local Health Departments, 1991. *Source:* Reprinted from *Public Health Macroview*, Vol. 7, No. 1, 1995, Public Health Foundation.

Commission, Agriculture, Nuclear Regulatory Commission, and Housing and Urban Development) have environmental health roles. State and local governments have largely replicated this web of environmental responsibility, creating a complex system often poorly understood by the private sector and general public. Federal statutes have driven the organization of state responsibilities. Key federal environmental statutes include:

- Clean Air Act (CAA)
- Clean Water Act (CWA)
- Comprehensive Environmental Response, Competition, and Liability Act (CERCLA) and Superfund Amendments and Reauthorization Act (SARA)
- Federal Insecticide, Fungicide, and Rodenticide Act (FIFRA)
- Resource Conservation and Recovery Act (RCRA)
- Safe Drinking Water Act (SDWA)
- Toxic Substance Control Act (TSCA)
- Food, Drug, and Cosmetic Act (FDCA)
- Federal Mine Safety and Health Act (MSHA)
- Occupational Safety and Health Act (OSHA)

States, however, have responded in no consistent manner in assigning implementation of federal statutes among various state agencies. The focus of federal statutes on specific environmental media (water, air, waste) has fostered the assignment of environmental responsibilities to state agencies other than official state health agencies, as demonstrated in Table 4–1. The implications of this diversification are important for public health agencies. State health agencies are becoming less involved in environmental health programs; only a handful of states utilize their state health agency as the state's lead agency for environmental concerns. This role has shifted to state environmental agencies, although many other state agencies are also involved. Still, the primary strategy has shifted from a health-oriented approach to a

Table 4–1 Number and Type of State Agencies Responsible for Implementation of Federal Environmental Statutes

Statute	Agriculture	Environment	Health	Labor	Total
Clean Air Act	0	41	10	1	52
Clean Water Act	1	41	11	1	54
CERCLA (Superfund) Act	0	00	26	1	67
Federal Insecticide, Fungicide, and Rodenticide Act	0	41	11	2	54
Resource Conservation and Recovery Act	0	36	33	3	72
Safe Drinking Water Act	0	12	23	3	38
Toxic Substance Control Act	37	4	5	0	46
Food, Drug, and Cosmetic Act	1	1	15	39	56
Federal Mine Safety and Health Act	0	0	0	12	12
Occupational Safety and Health Act	15	1	13	0	29

Source: Reprinted from Health Resources and Services Administration, *Environmental Web: Impact of Federal Statutes on State Environmental Health and Protection—Services, Structure and Funding,* 1995, Rockville, Maryland.

regulatory approach. Despite their diminished role in environmental concerns, state health agencies continue to address a very diverse set of environmental health issues and maintain epidemiologic and quantitative risk assessment capabilities not available in other state agencies. Linking this important expertise to the workings of other state agencies is a particularly challenging task, and there are other implications of this scenario, as well.

The shift toward regulatory strategies is clearly reflected in resource allocation at the state level. In the mid-1990s, about $6 billion was spent on environmental health and regulation by states with only about $1 billion of that total for environmental health (as opposed to environmental regulation) activities.[10] Public health considerations often take a back seat to regulatory concerns when budget decisions are made. In addition, the fact that many environmental health specialists are working in non-health agencies poses special problems for both their training and their practice performance.

The wide variation in organization and structure of state health responsibilities suggests that there is no standard or consistent pattern to public health practice among the various states. An examination of enabling statutes and state public agency mission statements provides further support for this conclusion. Only 11 of 43 state agency mission statements address the majority of the concepts related to public health purpose and mission in the Public Health in America document.[11,12] When state public health enabling statutes are examined for references to the essential public health services (also found in the Public Health in America document), the majority of the essential public health services can be identified in only one-fifth of the states. The most frequently identified essential public health services reflect traditional public health activities, such as enforcement of laws, monitoring of health status, diagnosing and investigating health hazards, and informing and educating the public. The essential public health services least frequently referenced in these enabling statutes reflect more modern concepts of public health practice, including mobilizing community partnerships, evaluating the effects of health services, and research for innovative solutions. Only three states had both enabling statutes and state health agency mission statements highly congruent with the concepts advanced in the Public Health in America document.[11]

In sum, state health agencies face many challenges related to the fragmentation of public health roles and responsibilities among various state agencies. Central to these are two related challenges: how to coordinate public health's core functions and essential services effectively and how to leverage changes within the health system to instill greater emphasis on clinical prevention and population-based services. As the various chapters of this text suggest, these are related aims.

GOVERNMENTAL PUBLIC HEALTH: LOCAL PUBLIC HEALTH ORGANIZATIONS

In the overall structuring of governmental public health responsibilities, local public health agencies (LPHAs) are where the "rubber meets the road." These agencies are established to carry out the critical public health responsibilities embodied in state laws and local ordinances and to meet other needs and expectations of their communities. Although some cities had local public health boards and agencies prior to 1900, the first county health department was not established until 1911. At that time, Yakima County, Washington, created a permanent county health unit, based on the success of a county sanitation campaign to control a serious typhoid epidemic. The Rockefeller Sanitary Commission, through its support for county hookworm eradication efforts, also stimulated the development of county-based LPHAs. The number of LPHAs grew rapidly during the twentieth century, although in recent decades, expansion has been tempered by closures and consolidations.

LPHAs should not be considered separately from the state network in which they operate. It is important to remember that states, through their state legislative and executive branches, establish the types and powers of local governmental units that can exist in that state. In this arrangement, the state and its local subunits, however defined, share responsibilities for health and other state functions. How health duties are shared in any given state depends on a complex set of factors that include state and local statutes, history, need, and expectations.

Local health agencies relate to their state public health systems in one of three general patterns.[4] In most states, LPHAs are formed and managed by local government, reporting directly to some office of local government, such as a local Board of Health, county commission, or city or county executive officer. In this decentralized arrangement, LPHAs often have considerable autonomy although they may be required to carry out specific state public health statutes. Also, there are some states that share oversight of LPHAs with local government through the power to appoint local health officers or to approve an annual budget. In some states with decentralized LPHAs, some areas of the state lack coverage because the local government chooses not to form a local health agency and the state must provide services in those uncovered areas.[13] This mixed arrangement occurs in about 20 percent of the states. Another 30 percent of the states use a more centralized approach in which local health agencies are directly operated by the state or there are no LPHAs and the state provides local health services.

LPHAs are established by governmental units, including counties, cities, towns, townships, and special districts, by one of two general methods. The legislative body may create an LPHA through enactment of a resolution, or the citizens of the jurisdiction may create a local board and agency through a referendum. Both patterns are common. Resolution health agencies are often funded from the general funds of the jurisdiction, whereas referendum health agencies often have a specific tax levy available to them. There are advantages and disadvantages to either approach. Resolution health agencies are simpler to establish and may develop close working relationships with the local legislative bodies that create them. Referendum agencies reflect the support of the local electorate and may have access to specific tax levies that avoid the need to compete with other local government funding sources.

Counties represent the most common form of subdividing states. In general, counties are geopolitical subunits of states that carry out various state responsibilities, such as law enforcement (sheriffs and state's attorneys) and public health. Counties largely function as agents of the state and carry out responsibilities delegated or assigned to them. In contrast, cities are generally not established as agents of the state. Instead, they have considerable discretion through home rule powers to take on functions that are not prohibited to them by state law. Cities can choose to have a health department or to rely on the state or their county for public health services. City health departments often have a wider array of programs and services because of this autonomy. As described previously, the earliest public health agencies developed in large urban centers, prior to the development of either state health agencies or county-based LPHAs. This status also contributes to their sense of autonomy. These considerations, as well as the increased demands and expectations to meet the needs of those who lack adequate health insurance, have made many city-based, especially big city-based, LPHAs qualitatively different from other LPHAs.

Both cities and counties have resource and political bases. Both rely heavily on property and sales taxes to finance health and other services, and both are struggling with the limitations of these funding sources. Political concerns over increasing property taxes are the major limitation for both. Relatively few counties and cities have imposed income taxes, the form of taxation relied upon by federal and state governments. However, both generally have strong political bases, although cities are generally more likely than counties to be at odds with state government on key issues.

Counties play a critical role in the public sector, the extent and importance of which is often overlooked. Three-fourths of all LPHAs are organized at the county level, serving a single county, a city-county, or several counties. As a result, counties provide a substantial portion of the community prevention and clinical preventive services offered in the United States. Counties provide care for about 40 million persons who access LPHAs and other facilities; they spend more than $30 billion of their local tax revenues on health and hospital services annually through some 4,500 sites that include hospitals, nursing homes, clinics, health departments, and mental health facilities. Counties play an explicit role in treatment, are legally responsible for indigent health care in over 30 states, and pay a portion of the nonfederal share of Medicaid in about 20 states. In addition, counties purchase health care for more than 2 million employees.[14]

The National Association of County and City Health Officials (NACCHO) tracks public health activities of LPHAs; the most recent survey of LPHAs took place in 1999.[15] Data provided in this chapter are derived from this 1999 survey, as well as from two other NACCHO profiles of LPHAs completed earlier in the 1990s.[13,16]

One limitation of information on LPHAs is that there is neither a clear nor a functional definition of what constitutes an LPHA. The most widely used definitions call for an administrative and service unit of local government, concerned with health, employing at least one full-time person, and carrying responsibility for health of a jurisdiction smaller than the state. By this definition, more than 3,200 local health agencies operate in 3,042 U.S. counties.[13] The number of local public health agencies varies widely from state to state; Rhode Island has none, whereas neighboring Connecticut and Massachusetts report more than 100 LPHAs (Figure 4–8 and Exhibit 4–4).

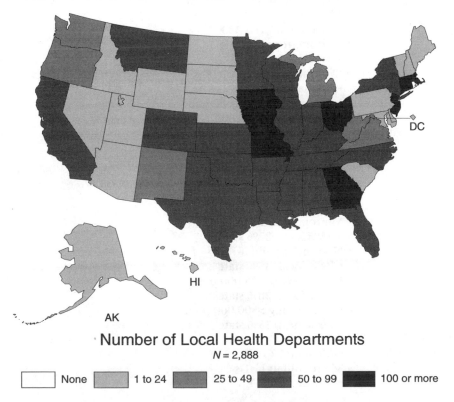

Number of Local Health Departments
N = 2,888

None | 1 to 24 | 25 to 49 | 50 to 99 | 100 or more

Figure 4–8 Number of Local Health Departments by State, 1992–1993. *Source:* Reprinted from National Association of County and City Health Officials and Centers for Disease Control and Prevention, *Profile of Local Health Departments, 1992–1993*, 1995, Washington, DC.

Exhibit 4–4 Vital Statistics for Local Health Departments

Definition	• An administrative and service unit of local government, concerned with health, employing at least one full-time person, and carrying responsibility for health of a jurisdiction smaller than the state
Number	• Approximately 3200 using the above definition • Functional definition would reduce number considerably • Varies from 0 in Rhode Island to more than 100 in seven states
Jurisdiction Type	• 60% single county • 8% multi-county • 7% city-county • 15% town/township • 10% city
Size of Population	• 50% <25,000 • 19% 25,000–49,999 • 13% 50,000–99,999 • 14% 100,000–499,999 • 4% 500,000 and greater

Budget	• All LHDs
	  • 25th percentile: $ 203,905
	  • Median: $621,100
	  • 75th percentile: $2,250,000
	• Metropolitan LHDs
	  • Median: $1,185,433
	• Non-metropolitan LHDs
	  • Median: $509,540
	• LHDs serving <25,000 pop.
	  • Median: $214,658
	• LHDs serving >500,000 pop.
	  • Median: $27,000,000

Source of Funds	• All LHDs
	  • 44% local
	  • 30% state (including federal pass through funds)
	  • 3% federal
	  • 19% reimbursement for services
	  • 3% other
	• Metropolitan LHDs
	  • 58% local, 22% state
	• Non-metropolitan LHDs
	  • 34% local, 35% state
	• LHDs serving <25,000 pop.
	  • 50% local, 28% state
	• LHDs serving >500,000 pop.
	  • 36% local, 35% state

Employees (full time equivalents)	• All LHDs
	  • Median: 17 FTE
	• Metropolitan LHDs
	  • Median: 28 FTE

continues

Exhibit 4–4 continued

	• Non-metropolitan LHDs
	  • Median: 13 FTE
	• LHDs serving <25,000 pop.
	  • Median: 8.5 FTE
	• LHDs serving >500,000 pop.
	  • Median: 437 FTE

Governance	• 81 percent of LHDs relate to a local board of health • 56 percent report to local board of health • 82 percent of boards independent of legislative body
Leadership	• one-half of local health officers are MDs • one-fourth of all local health officers have formal public health training • mean tenure 8 years; median tenure 6 years

Source: National Association of County and City Health Officials.[13,15,16]

Sixty percent of LPHAs are single-county health agencies, and about 75 percent operate out of a county base (single county, multi-county, or city-county).[15] Other LPHAs function at the city, town, or township levels; some state-operated units also serve local jurisdictions. Although the precise number is uncertain, it appears that the number has been increasing, from about 1,300 in 1947 to about 2,000 in the mid-1970s to somewhere over 3,000 today.

Several reports going back more than 50 years have proposed extensive consolidation of small LPHAs because of perceived lack of efficiency and coordination of services, inconsistent administration of public health laws, and inability of small LPHAs to raise adequate resources to carry out their prime functions effectively. Consolidations at the county level would appear to be the most rational approach, but only limited progress has been achieved in recent decades.

Most LPHAs are relatively small organizations; more than two-thirds (69 percent) serve populations of 50,000 or less, whereas less than one in five (18 percent) serves a population of 100,000 or more. Only 4 percent of LPHAs serve populations of 500,000 or more residents.[15]

Some states set qualifications for local health officers or require medical supervision when the administrator is not a physician. About four-fifths of LPHAs employ a full-time health officer. Health officers have a mean tenure of about 8 years and a median tenure of about 6 years. Approximately one-half of all local health officers are physicians, about 15 percent are physicians with formal training in public health, and less than one-fourth have graduate degrees in public health. LPHAs serving larger populations are more likely to have full-time health officers than are smaller LPHAs.

Local boards of health are associated with most LPHAs; in 1997, 81 percent of LPHAs reported working with a local board of health. There are an estimated 3,200 local boards of health; about 85 percent reported an affiliation with an

LPHA. However, 15 percent exist independently of any LPHA; this pattern is most common in Massachusetts, Pennsylvania, New Hampshire, Iowa, and New Jersey. The pattern for size of population, type of jurisdiction, and budget mirrors that for LPHAs. Virtually all local boards of health establish local health policies, fees, ordinances, and regulations. Most also recommend and/or approve budgets, establish community health priorities, and hire the director of the local health agency. Although four-fifths of LPHAs relate to a board of health, only 56 percent report to that board rather than some other office of local government.

Similar to the situation with state health agencies, data on LPHA expenditures lack currency and completeness. Annual LPHA expenditures in 1999 ranged from zero to over $836 million. One-half of LPHAs had budgets of $621,000 or less and 25 percent had budgets over $2,250,000. Total expenditures increase with size of population. LPHAs located in metropolitan areas had substantially higher expenditures than their non-metropolitan area counterparts.

In 1999 LPHAs derived their funding from the following sources: local funds (44 percent), the state (30 percent, including federal funds passing through the state), direct federal funds (3 percent), fees and reimbursements (19 percent), and other sources (4 percent). Metropolitan LPHAs and those serving smaller populations are more dependent on local sources of funding while LPHAs in non-metropolitan areas and those serving larger populations depend more on state sources.

The number of full-time equivalent employees also increases with the size of the population served. Only 10 percent of LPHAs employ 125 or more persons, and 50 percent have 17 or fewer employees. The number of employees and the number of different disciplines and professions are related to LPHA population size. Clerical staff, nurses, sanitarians, physicians, and nutritionists are the most common disciplines (in that order) and are all found in more than one-half of all LPHAs.

There is considerable variety in the services provided by LPHAs. Later chapters will examine in greater detail the functions and services of LPHAs, but several general categories of services are notable. Top priority areas for LPHAs overall are communicable disease control, environmental health, and child health. LPHAs serving both large and small populations report similar priorities, although community outreach replaces environmental health as a top priority for the largest local health jurisdictions (those over 500,000 population). Slight differences in priorities are also apparent between metropolitan and non-metropolitan area LPHAs. LPHAs in metropolitan areas often include inspections as a high priority, while non-metropolitan LPHAs are more likely to include family planning and home health care services as priorities.

Many LPHAs provide a common core battery of services that generally includes adult and childhood immunizations, communicable disease control, community assessment, community outreach and education, environmental health services, epidemiology and surveillance programs, food safety and restaurant inspections, health education, and tuberculosis testing. Less commonly, LPHAs provide services related to primary care and chronic disease, including: cardiovascular disease, diabetes, and glaucoma screening; behavioral and mental health services; programs for the homeless; substance abuse services; and veterinary public health.[15]

LPHAs do not always provide these services themselves; increasingly, they contract for these services or contribute resources to other agencies or organizations in the community. Community partners for LPHAs include state health agencies, other LPHAs, hospitals, other units of government, nonprofit and voluntary organizations, academic institutions, community health centers, the faith community, and insurance companies. LPHAs increasingly interact with managed care organizations, although most do not have either formal or informal agreements governing these interactions.[13] Where agreements existed, they were more likely to be formal, to cover clinical and case management services, and to involve the provision (rather than the purchase) of services. More than one-fourth of LPHAs had formal agreements for clinical services for Medicaid clients in 1996. Chapters 5, 6, and 7 will address other aspects of community public health practice.

INTERGOVERNMENTAL RELATIONSHIPS

In terms of public health roles, no level of government has complete authority and autonomy. Optimal outcomes result from collaborative and complementary efforts. "Public Health Achievements in Twentieth-Century America: Motor Vehicle Safety," presented below, tells the story of improved motor vehicle safety in the United States during the twentieth century; this achievement relied heavily on effective laws and their enforcement by all levels of government.

Example

Public Health Achievements in Twentieth-Century America: Motor Vehicle Safety

State and local health agencies are not the only governmental organizations working to reduce the burden of disease and ill health in society. Motor vehicle-related injuries are a prime example. Federal, state, and local government all play important roles through agencies that are better known for other responsibilities, such as law enforcement and transportation. The complexities of government and its various agencies add an important, but not necessarily the most important, dimension to public health practice.

The reduction of the rate of death attributable to motor vehicle crashes in the United States represents the successful public health response to a great technologic advance of the twentieth century—the motorization of America. Six times as many people drive today as in 1925, and the number of motor vehicles in the country has increased 11-fold since then to approximately 215 million. The number of miles traveled in motor vehicles is 10 times higher than in the mid-1920s. Despite this steep increase in motor vehicle travel, the annual death rate has declined from 18 per 100 million vehicle miles traveled (VMT) in 1925 to 1.7 per 100 million VMT in 1997—a 90 percent decrease (Figure 4–9).

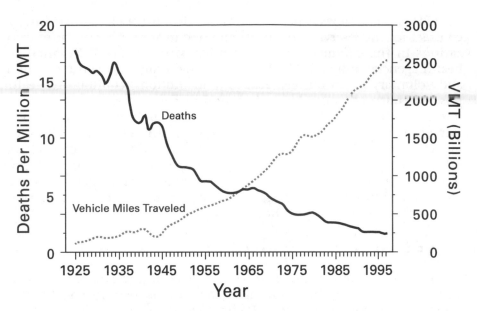

Figure 4–9 Motor Vehicle-Related Death Rates per Million Vehicle Miles Traveled (VMT) and Annual VMT, by Year-United States, 1925–1997. *Source:* Reprinted from Achievements in Public Health, United States, 1900–1999: Motor Vehicle Safety, *Morbidity and Mortality Weekly Report,* Vol. 48, No. 18, pp. 369–374, the Centers for Disease Control and Prevention, 1999.

Systematic motor vehicle safety efforts began during the 1960s. In 1960 unintentional injuries caused 93,803 deaths; 41 percent were associated with motor vehicle crashes. In 1966, after 5 years of continuously increasing motor vehicle-related fatality rates, the Highway Safety Act created the National Highway Safety Bureau (NHSB), which later became the National Highway Traffic Safety Administration (NHTSA). The systematic approach to motor vehicle-related injury prevention began with NHSB's first director, Dr. William Haddon. Haddon, a public health physician, recognized that standard public health methods and epidemiology could be applied to preventing motor vehicle-related and other injuries. He defined interactions between host (human), agent (motor vehicle), and environmental (highway) factors before, during, and after crashes resulting in injuries. Tackling problems identified with each factor during each phase of the crash, NHSB initiated a campaign to prevent motor vehicle-related injuries.

In 1966 passage of the Highway Safety Act and the National Traffic and Motor Vehicle Safety Act authorized the federal government to set and regulate standards for motor vehicles and highways, a mechanism necessary for effective prevention. Many changes in both vehicle and highway design followed this mandate. Vehicles (agent of injury) were built with new safety features, including headrests, energy-absorbing steering wheels, shatter-resistant windshields, and safety belts. Roads

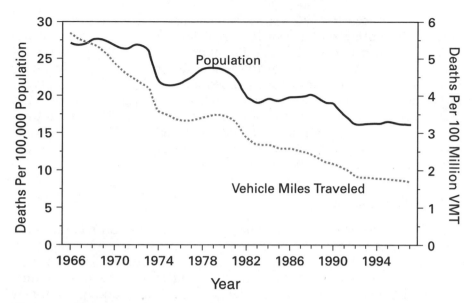

Figure 4–10 Motor Vehicle-Related Death Rates per 100,000 Population and per 100 Million Vehicle Miles Traveled (VMT), by Year—United, States, 1966–1997. *Source:* Reprinted from Achievements in Public Health, United States, 1900–1999: Motor Vehicle Safety, *Morbidity and Mortality Weekly Report,* Vol. 48, No. 18, pp. 369–374, the Centers for Disease Control and Prevention, 1999.

(environment) were improved by better delineation of curves (edge and center line stripes and reflectors), use of breakaway sign and utility poles, improved illumination, addition of barriers separating oncoming traffic lanes, and guardrails. The results were rapid. By 1970, motor vehicle-related death rates were decreasing by both the public health measure (deaths per 100,000 population) and the traffic safety indicator (deaths per VMT) (Figure 4–10).

Changes in driver and passenger (host) behavior also have reduced motor vehicle crashes and injuries. Enactment and enforcement of traffic safety laws, reinforced by public education, have led to safer behavior choices. Examples include enforcement of laws against driving while intoxicated (DWI) and underage drinking, and enforcement of safety belt, child-safety seat, and motorcycle helmet use laws.

Government and community recognition of the need for motor vehicle safety prompted initiation of programs by federal and state governments, academic institutions, community-based organizations, and industry. NHTSA and the Federal Highway Administration within the U.S. Department of Transportation have provided national leadership for traffic and highway safety efforts since the 1960s. The National Center for Injury Prevention and Control, established at CDC in 1992, has contributed public health direction. State and local governments have enacted and enforced laws that affect motor vehicle and highway safety, driver licensing and testing, vehicle inspections, and traffic regulations. Preventing motor vehicle-related injuries has required collaboration among many professional disciplines (e.g., the discipline of biomechanics has been essential to vehicle design and highway safety features). Citizen and community-based advocacy groups have played important prevention roles in areas such as drinking and driving and child-occupant protection. Consistent with the public/private partnerships that characterize motor vehicle safety efforts, NHTSA sponsors "Buckle Up America" week, which focuses on the need always to properly secure children in child-safety seats.

High-Risk Populations

Alcohol-Impaired Drivers: Annual motor vehicle crash-related fatalities involving alcohol have decreased 39 percent since 1982, to approximately 16,000; these deaths account for 38.6 percent of all traffic deaths. Factors that may have contributed to this decline include increased public awareness of the dangers of drinking and driving; new and tougher state laws; stricter law enforcement; an increase in the minimum legal drinking age; prevention programs that offer alternatives, such as safe rides (e.g., taxicabs and public transportation), designated drivers, and responsible alcohol-serving practices; and a decrease in per capita alcohol consumption.

Young Drivers and Passengers: Since 1975, motor vehicle-related fatality rates have decreased 27 percent for young motor vehicle occupants (ages 16–20 years). However, in 1997, the death rate was 28.3 per 100,000 population—more than twice that of the U.S. population (13.3 per 100,000 population). Teenaged drivers are more likely than older drivers to speed, run red lights, make illegal turns, ride with an intoxicated driver, and drive after drinking alcohol or using drugs. Strategies that have contributed to improved motor vehicle safety among young drivers include laws restricting purchase of alcohol among under-aged youths and some aspects of graduated licensing systems (e.g., nighttime driving restrictions).

Pedestrians: From 1975 to 1997, pedestrian fatality rates decreased 41 percent, from 4 per 100,000 population in 1975 to 2.3 in 1997, but still account for 13 percent of motor vehicle-related deaths. Factors that may have reduced pedestrian fatalities include more and better sidewalks, pedestrian paths, playgrounds away from streets, one-way traffic flow, and restricted on-street parking.

Occupant-Protection Systems

Safety Belts: In response to legislation, highly visible law enforcement, and public education, rates of safety belt use nationwide have increased from approximately 11 percent in 1981 to 68 percent in 1997. Safety belt use began to increase following enactment of the first state mandatory-use laws in 1984. All states except New Hampshire now have safety-belt use laws. Primary laws (which allow police to stop vehicles simply because occupants are not wearing safety belts) are more effective than secondary laws (which require that a vehicle be stopped for some other traffic violation). The prevalence of safety belt use after enactment of primary laws increases 1.5–4.3 times, and motor vehicle-related fatality rates decreased 13–46 percent.

Child-Safety and Booster Seats: All states have passed child passenger protection laws, but these vary widely in age and size requirements and the penalties imposed for noncompliance. Child-restraint use in 1996 was 85 percent for children aged less than 1 year and 60 percent for children aged 1–4 years. Since 1975, deaths among children aged less than 5 years have decreased 30 percent to 3.1 per 100,000 population, but rates for age groups 5–15 years have declined by only 11–13 percent. Child seats are misused by as many as 80 percent of users. In addition, parents fail to recognize the need for booster seats for children who are too large for child seats but not large enough to be safely restrained in an adult lap-shoulder belt.

Source: Adapted from Achievements in Public Health, United States, 1900–1999: Motor Vehicle Safety, *Morbidity and Mortality Weekly Report,* Vol. 48, No. 18, pp. 369–374, the Centers for Disease Control and Prevention, 1999.

The relationships between and among the three levels of government have changed considerably over time in terms of their relative importance and influence in the health sector. This is especially true for the federal and local roles. The federal government had little authority and little ability to influence health priorities and interventions until after 1930. Since that time, it has exercised its influence primarily through financial leverage on both state and local government, as well as on the private medical care system. The massive financing role of the federal government has moved it to a position of preeminence among the various levels of government in actual ability to influence health affairs. This is evident in the federal share of total national health expenditures and the federal government's substantial support of prevention activities. However federal public health spending represents only about 1.2 percent of total federal health spending, nearly 75 percent less than in 1965 (Figure 4–11). This suggests that the federal commitment to public health has declined over recent decades. The proportion of the federal component of government spending for population-based public health activities shows a similar pattern (Figure 4–12), declining from 72 percent in 1970 to 29 percent in 2000. Although federal bioterrorism preparedness funds beginning in 2002 may modify this trend, the financial influence of the federal government on public health activities nationally was lower in 2000 than it had been at any point in the second half of the twentieth century.

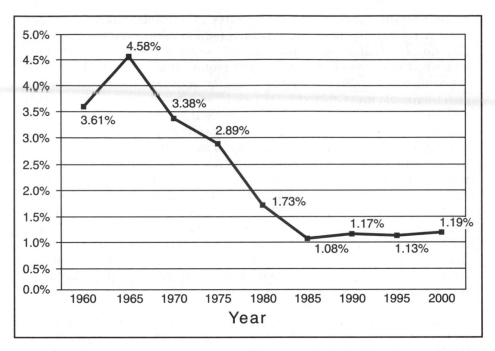

Figure 4–11 Federal Public Health Spending as a Percent of Total Federal Health Spending, United States, 1960–2000. *Sources and Notes:* Data compiled from National Centers for Health Statistics, *Health United States 2002,* PHS, 2002 and Centers for Medicare and Medicaid Services, National Health Accounts (NHA) 1960–2000. The NHA breaks down health spending by source of funding and by activity and type of service provided.

In recent decades political initiatives have sought to diminish the powerful federal role and return some of its influence back to the states. However, little in the form of true transfer of authority or resource control has taken place through 2003. It is likely that the federal government's fiscal muscle will enable it to continue its current dominant role in its relationships with state and local government.

Local government has experienced the greatest and most disconcerting change in relative influence over the twentieth century. Prior to 1900 local government was the primary locus of action, with the development of both population-based interventions for communicable disease control and environmental sanitation and locally-provided charity care for the poor. However, the massive problems related to simultaneous urbanization and povertization of the big cities spawned needs that could not be met with local resources alone. Outside the large cities, local government responses generally took the form of LPHAs organized at the county level at the behest of state governments. This was viewed by states as the most efficient manner of executing their broad health powers. States often viewed local governments in general and LPHAs in particular as their delivery system for important programs and services. In any event, the power of states and the growing influence of financial incentives through grant programs of both federal and state government

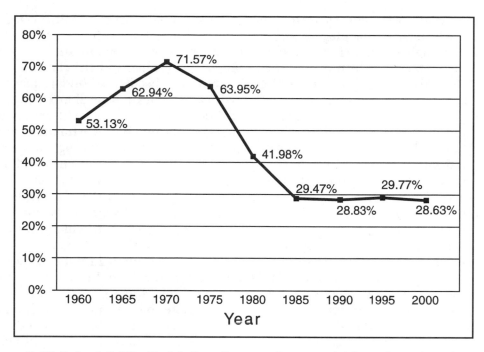

Figure 4–12 Federal Public Health Spending as a Percent of Adjusted Total Public Health Spending, United States, 1960–2000. *Sources and Notes:* Data compiled from National Centers for Health Statistics, *Health United States 2002,* PHS, 2002 and Centers for Medicare and Medicaid Services, National Health Accounts (NHA) 1960–2000. The NHA breaks down health spending by source of funding and by activity and type of service provided.

acted to influence local priorities greatly. Priorities were being established by higher levels of government more often than through local determinations of needs. Although the demands and expectations were being directed at local governments, key decisions were being made in state capitals and in Washington, DC. Unfortunately there are signs that local governments across the country are looking for opportunities to reduce their health roles for both clinical services and population-based interventions where they can. The perception is that the responsibility for clinical services lies with federal and state government or the private sector and that even traditional public health services can be effectively outsourced. How these actions will comport with the widespread belief that services are best provided at the local level raises serious questions regarding new roles of oversight and accountability that are not easily answered. Local governments have lost control over priorities and policies; they bridle under the regulations and grant conditions imposed by state and federal funding sources. As costs increase, grant awards fail to keep pace. However, growing numbers of wholly or partly uninsured individuals now look to local government for services. These rising expectations and increasing costs are occurring at a time when local governments are unable and unwilling to seek additional tax revenues. The complexities of organizing and coordinating community-wide responses to modern public health problems and risks also push local government to look elsewhere for solutions.

States were slow to assume their extensive powers in the health sector, but have been major players since the latter half of the nineteenth century. Although the growing influence of the federal government since 1930 displaced states as the most important level of government, their relative role has strengthened since about 1980. Still, states have become secondary players in the health sector. Most states lack the means, political as well as statutory, to intervene effectively in the portion of the health sector located within their jurisdictional boundaries. This is further complicated by their tradition of imitating the federal health bureaucracy whenever possible through the decentralization of health roles and responsibilities throughout dozens of administrative agencies. Coordination of programs, policies, and priorities has become exceedingly difficult within state government. Outside of state government, it has become virtually impossible. Still, the widely disparate circumstances from state to state make for laboratories of opportunity in which innovative approaches can be developed and evaluated.

The relationship between state and local government in public health has traditionally been tenuous and difficult. Just as the federal government views the states, states themselves have come to view local governments as just another way to get things done. As a result, states have turned to other parties, such as community-based organizations, and have begun to deal directly with them, leaving local government on the sidelines. This undervaluing of LPHAs, when coupled with the declining appreciation among local governments for their health agencies, presents major challenges for the future of public health services in the United States. Instead of becoming stronger allies, these forces are working to pull apart the fabric of the national public health network.

These ever-changing and evolving relationships call into question whether the governmental public health network can be strengthened through a more centralized approach involving greater federal leadership and direction.[17] In decentralized approaches, some states may truly be laboratories of innovation and provide better services than can be achieved through a centralized approach. There are many examples of creative policies and programs at the state level, but there are also many examples of state creativity being stifled by the federal government. The history of state requests for waivers of Medicaid requirements is a case in point. Many states waited two or more years for federal approval of the waivers necessary to begin innovative programs, and some of the more creative proposals were actually rejected. Still, it can be argued that state political processes are more reflective of the different political values that must be reconciled for progressive policies to develop.

CONCLUSION

The structural framework for public health in the United States includes a network of state and local public health agencies working in partnership with the federal government. This framework is precariously balanced on a legal foundation that gives primacy for health concerns to states, a financial foundation that allows the federal government to promote equality and minimum standards across 50 diverse states, and a practical foundation of local public health agencies serving as the point of contact between communities and their three-tiered government. Over time, the relative influence of these partners has shifted dramatically because of changes in needs, resources, and public expectations. The challenges to this organizational structure are many. Those related to the core functions of public health are addressed in the next chapter, and those emerging from the rapid changes within the health system and in the expansion of community public heath practice are addressed in Chapters 3 and 5 of this text. There are increasing calls for the national government to turn over many public programs to private interests and growing concern over the role of government, in general. These developments make it easy to forget that many of the public health achievements of the past century would not have been possible without a serious commitment of resources and leadership by those in the public sector. In any event, it is clear that the organizational structure of public health—its form—intimately reflects the structure of government in the United States. As a result, the success or failure of these public health organizations will be determined by our success in governing ourselves.

DISCUSSION QUESTIONS AND EXERCISES

1. What is the legal basis for public health in the United States, and what impact has that had on the public health powers of federal, state, and local governments?
2. How can the enforcement of nuisance control regulations work for as well as against public health agencies?
3. What is meant by a state's police power, and how is that used in public health?
4. What is the basis for the historical tension between the powers of the federal government and the powers of states in public health matters?
5. Review Appendix 4-A. How extensive is administrative law in public health, and how does it work? Cite a recent example of important public health rules or regulations in the news media.
6. Describe the basic structure of a typical LPHA in the United States in terms of type and size of jurisdiction served, budget, staff, and agency head. (The National Association of County and City Health Officials' website may be useful here!) How does this compare with the typical LPHA in your own state?
7. For the prevention of motor vehicle injuries (see "Public Health Achievements in Twentieth-Century America: Motor Vehicle Safety"), how are responsibilities assigned or delegated among the three levels of government (federal, state, local) and among various agencies of those levels of government? Who is responsible for what?
8. What are the primary federal roles and responsibilities for public health in the United States? How do those roles and responsibilities comport with PHS agency budget requests for federal fiscal year 1999 (see Figure 4–4)?

9. Review both the History of Public Health in Chicago (Appendix 1-A) and History of CDC (Exhibit 4–2). Has the evolution of the local and federal public health agencies taken parallel pathways? How has their development differed in terms of roles and responsibilities? What are the implications of these similarities and differences for public health problems that require more than one level of government?

10. Access the websites of any two U.S. state health departments and compare and contrast the two organizations in terms of their structure, general functions, specific services, resources, and other important features. (The Association of State and Territorial Health Officials' link to state health agency websites may be useful here.)

REFERENCES

1. Centers for Disease Control and Prevention. History of CDC. *Morb Mortal Wkly Rep.* 1996;45:526–528.

2. *Profile of State and Local Public Health Systems 1990.* Atlanta, GA: CDC; 1991.

3. Shonick W. *Government and Health Services: Government's Role in the Development of the U.S. Health Services 1930–1980.* New York: Oxford University Press; 1995.

4. Pickett G, Hanlon JJ. *Public Health Administration and Practice. 9th ed.* St. Louis, MO: Mosby; 1990.

5. *Jacobson v Massachusetts.* 197 US 11 (1905).

6. U.S. Department of Health and Human Services (DHHS). *The Fiscal Year 2004 Budget.* Washington, DC: DHHS; 2003.

7. DHHS. *Healthy People 2000.* Washington, DC: U.S. Public Health Service (PHS); 1990.

8. Association of State and Territorial Health Officials. *2002 Salary Survey of State and Territorial Health Officials.* Washington, DC: ASTHO; 2003.

9. Public Health Foundation. *Public Health Macroview.* 1995;7(1):1–8.

10. Burke TA, Shalauta NM, Tran NL, Stern BS. The environmental web: A national profile of the state infrastructure for environmental health and protection, *J Public Health Manage Pract.* 1997;3(2):1–12.

11. Gebbie KM. State public health laws: An expression of constituency expectations. *J Public Health Manage Pract.* 2000;6(2):46–54.

12. Core Public Health Functions Steering Committee. *Public Health in America.* Washington, DC: DHHS-PHS; 1994.

13. National Association of County and City Health Officials. *Profile of Local Health Departments 1996–1997 Data Set.* Washington, DC: NACCHO; 1997.

14. National Association of County and City Health Officials. Fact Sheet. Washington, DC: National Association of County and City Health Officials (NACCHO); 1991.

15. National Association of County and City Health Officials. *Local Public Health Agency Infrastructure: A Chartbook.* Washington, DC: NACCHO; 2001.

16. National Association of County and City Health Officials. *Profile of Local Health Departments 1992–1993.* Washington, DC: NACCHO; 1995.

17. Turnock BJ and Atchison C. Governmental Public Health in the United States: The Implications of Federalism. *Health Affairs* 2002;6:68–78.

Administrative Law

The most frequently encountered legal interactions for most people, affecting both health professionals and consumers, are not associated with constitutional, judicial, or even statutory laws. Rather they occur through the subsystem of administrative law, which develops and enforces rules and regulations through an administrative agency. Administrative law affects people in their daily lives in many ways. It affects people personally (even in very intimate ways) through such requirements as up-to-date immunizations before entering school or identification of sexual contacts of persons with certain STDs. Administrative law also affects our property. For example specific requirements for septic fields can prevent us from building our dream vacation home on the perfect lakefront lot. It also affects many of us professionally, most notably in the licensing of health and other professions. These are but a few examples of how pervasive administrative law has become in modern American society.

At first glance it appears that administrative law violates, or at least circumvents, one of the most fundamental principles of American government—the separation of powers among the legislative, executive, and judicial branches—with its elaborate system of checks and balances. The development and promulgation of administrative law represents the legislative function. The enforcement of the law, through inspections and other means, represents the executive function. Finally, the determination of compliance, often involving hearings and appeals within the agency before a final decision is rendered by the agency, represents the judicial function. Although the life cycle of administrative rules can be complex, it presents an interesting picture of governmental processes in public health.

The process begins with the enactment of a statute, which provides the administrative agency with the authority to develop rules and regulations to implement the intent of the newly enacted law. This authority may be limited to specific aspects of the statute, or the law may only broadly declare the legislative intent, leaving the agency considerable latitude in terms of the scope and content of rule-making needed for implementation. The

171

agency then initiates its rule-making processes, which involve technical experts from the field or program affected by the statute and legal staff from the agency or from the legal office of government (such as the attorney general's office at the state level, state's attorney office of the county, or corporation counsel office of the city). Increasingly, agency staffs involved in intergovernmental affairs participate in this process, because rule-making requires collaboration with the legislative branch. Interested parties, especially those organizations or industries likely to be affected by the law and regulations, may be involved in early stages of drafting rules and regulations through either standing boards, advisory bodies, or ad hoc groups brought together to gain different perspectives. Draft rules are developed and submitted as proposed rules.

There may be public hearings held on the proposals or a specific period in which interested parties and the public can comment on the proposed rules. The agency then must formally respond to public comments and indicate why proposed rules were or were not changed in response to those comments. Revisions are made to the rules, and, depending on the requirements of that level of government, the revised rules are submitted to a legislative oversight commission or committee, which then has its opportunity to comment on whether the proposed rules are consistent with the intent of the legislative body and whether the scope of the rules exceeds the authority conferred in the statute. The oversight commission also reviews the agency's response to the comments received. This presents another opportunity for interest groups and affected constituencies to influence the shape of the final regulations. After the legislative oversight comments and objections are made, the agency finalizes the rules and begins enforcement. If the agency chooses not to make changes suggested by the legislative oversight body, it faces the possibility of more specifically worded amendments to the statute or an adversarial relationship between the agency and the legislature. When final rules are adopted, they are widely circulated to the affected groups, and enforcement begins as specified in the new rules. These can be lengthy processes, taking 6–18 months (or longer) after enactment of a statute.

Implementation and enforcement of rules often rest with specific program staff of the agency. For licensing programs, these staff may be surveyors or inspectors. For other programs, they may be professional or administrative personnel. For many licensing programs, evidence of compliance with statutory and regulatory requirements is compiled through routine or complaint-related inspections. Based on the seriousness and, to a lesser extent, on the number of violations, a determination of noncompliance may lead to demands that specific actions take place to correct violations and that specific sanctions (as provided in the law or rules) be imposed. There is generally an opportunity for these decisions and actions to be challenged before they become final. If they are challenged, a hearing is held before a hearing officer within the administrative agency, and testimony and evidence are presented. The legal staff of the agency (or of that level of government) serve as the prosecutors. Program staff, some of whom may have been involved with the development of the rules in question, serve as witnesses. A formal record is compiled, and the hearing officer makes a recommendation to the agency head, who issues the final decision.

Several factors justify the circumvention of the principle of separation of powers. The basic rationale for permitting one agency to carry out these functions is that these agencies often operate in a narrow and discrete area that requires a high level of technical expertise to ensure that the intent of the legislative body is fulfilled. With the rapid expansion of science and technology in many areas, and certainly in the health system, there is an increasing need for technologic and professional expertise to develop and apply the details needed to implement the legislative intent. The growth of regulatory responsibilities for government has also served to expand the need for administrative law because it is becoming increasingly unwise for legislative bodies to attempt to put extensive details into statutes. Often these details reflect technical or practice standards that are updated or revised periodically, otherwise necessitating revisions and amendments to existing laws. All of these reasons relate to the growing complexity of society and the need for special expertise to be applied in narrow discrete areas in a timely and professional manner.

However, administrative law is not completely exempt from checks and balances, as illustrated in Figure 4–A1. Control points exist both for the rule-making process and for judicial review of final administrative decisions. In general, a committee or commission of legislators oversees the development and promulgation of rules to ensure that the legislative intent is being addressed and that the agency is not going beyond the authority provided to it in the statute. This oversight often includes provisions for public notice as to proposed rules and regulations and for written agency responses to public comments received as a result of hearings or public postings of proposed rules. Proposed rules can then be modified or withdrawn, if necessary. The legislative oversight also serves to alert the agency that actual or perceived transgressions may be met with more explicit statutes that would limit the agency's autonomy in developing rules and regulations in a particular area.

The second control point involves judicial review of final agency decisions. Any decision of the agency that adversely affects a party can be challenged through judicial review. This brings the agency's actions and decisions into the formal court system, where administrative actions, including fines and other sanctions, are either upheld or overturned by the courts and appeals are possible to even higher levels of review. These proceedings generally focus on procedural as opposed to evidentiary issues, relying on the record of facts and findings from the agency adjudication process. Most challenges brought for judicial review argue that the agency did not properly follow its own rules. There are instances in which judicial review is sought to require the agency to make a decision when it has not done so. However, these claims are more difficult to sustain unless the agency has completely failed to act in a situation specifically mandated by the legislative body. Agencies are granted considerable discretion in determining when and where to exercise their authorities and responsibilities, and courts are reluctant to step

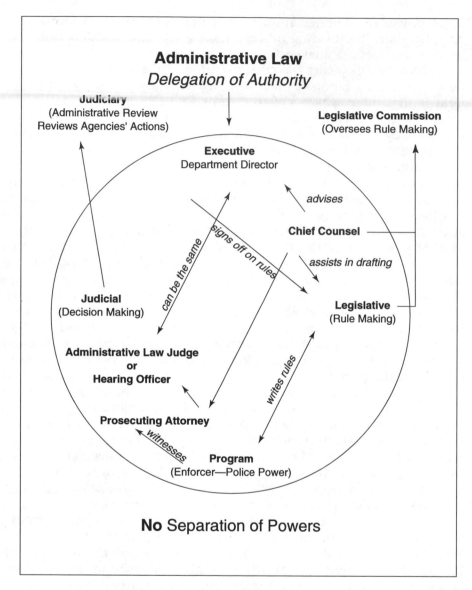

Figure 4–A1 Administrative Law and the Separation of Powers

in and second-guess the experts. The net result is that the courts often presume that the agency's actions are proper and prefer to focus, instead, on issues of procedural propriety. This suggests that those involved with compliance decisions, from inspectors to administrative hearing officers, must be as concerned over procedural matters as they are with factual issues of health and safety. After the initial judicial review makes its determination, appeals and higher appeals can bring these issues to state and federal supreme courts.

Chapter 5

Core Functions and Public Health Practice

The Institute of Medicine's (IOM) landmark report in 1988[1] initiated important changes in the U.S. public health system. The report rearticulated the mission, substance, and core functions of public health and challenged the public health community to think more strategically, plan more collectively, and perform more effectively. Exciting opportunities afforded by broader participation in community-wide health planning and better integration of public health and medical care activities have energized these efforts, accompanied by new hope for achieving improved health outcomes through the public health system.

These developments have clearly brought change to the public health system and public health practice over the past decade. It is not clear, however, whether these developments have improved public health practice and, more importantly, the results of the public health system—health outcomes. This chapter will examine the linkage between public health's functions and public health practice, including different understandings as to what constituted public health functions at various points in time over the past century. It also traces efforts to measure the performance of these functions. These tracings help us to understand how well public health addresses its main functions and which of its aspects needs improvement. Key questions to be addressed in this chapter are:

- What have been public health's main functions over the past century?
- What are the core functions of public health today?
- How are these functions translated into practice?
- How well are these functions being carried out by the public health system?
- How can public health practice performance be improved?

Continuous quality management (CQM) concepts argue that results reflect the systems that produce them. In other words, every system is perfectly designed to achieve the exact results it gets. This somewhat elliptical wisdom identifies a major challenge confronting efforts to enhance the results of public health practice: Improving health outcomes calls for improving the basic processes of public health practice. However, as some additional reasoning from the CQM movement warns, to improve something, we must be able to control it; to control it, we must be able to understand it; and to understand it, we must be able to measure it. Measurement relies on operational definitions for the concepts under study. Improving the performance of public health functions calls for an agenda that defines, measures, understands, and controls the processes that constitute public health practice.

For more than 90 years, the public health community has been grappling with this agenda, with only limited success along the way.[2] Over much of the twentieth century, an adequate conceptual framework for defining the public health system was lacking. As a result, past efforts generally focused on measuring aspects of the public health system that only indirectly or partially characterized the functions carried out in public health practice. This limited opportunities for understanding, controlling, and improving public health practice and health outcomes. Nonetheless, these efforts set the stage for developments since the 1988 IOM report and the opportunities that lie ahead.

PUBLIC HEALTH FUNCTIONS AND PRACTICE BEFORE THE IOM REPORT

Over much of the past century, the mission and purpose of public health (what it is) and its functions (how it addresses its mission) were viewed as synonymous with the provision of public health services. In fact, public health's services were frequently characterized as its functions. Public health was known more by its deeds than its intent. As a result, early efforts to describe and measure public health practice focused primarily on measuring aspects of important public health services.

The earliest attempts to define and measure public health practice in the United States date back to 1914. Prior to that time, public health functions were primarily those identified in the broad statutes of state and local governments, centering on the prevention and control of infectious diseases. In 1914, however, a survey catalogued the various services of state health agencies, as well as their role in fostering the development of local public health agencies. This study concluded that, even though public health agencies were carrying out a wide variety of programs and services, they were missing their mark. Much of what was being done through public health agencies had little effect on community health status, and there was actually much that these agencies could have been doing that would have reduced mortality and morbidity.[3] Public health practice was evaluated using a scoring system that placed greater weight on some public health activities and services than on others, allowing a basis for comparisons across agencies. Key elements of this approach were soon incorporated into local public health assessment initiatives orchestrated by the American Public Health Association (APHA).

In 1921 the first report of APHA's Committee on Municipal Health Department Practice called for the systematic collection and analysis of information on local public health practice to support the development of standards for local public health agencies (LHPAs) serving the nation's largest municipalities. The committee had determined that LHPAs and the communities they served would benefit from standards that would ensure a consistent level of public health services from jurisdiction-to-jurisdiction. The committee also sought to identify characteristics of LHPA practice that produce the best results. An elaborate survey instrument and process were established; more than 80 big-city health departments were reviewed in the initial effort.

The need to examine public health practice outside the nation's large cities, especially in the growing number of county-based LHPAs, was soon apparent. In 1925 the committee was reconstituted as the Committee on Administrative Practice to more broadly assess the status of public health practice in the United States. The new committee developed the first version of an "Appraisal Form" to be used as a self-assessment tool by local health officers. The intent was to measure the immediate results attained from local public health services. Examples of these immediate results follow:

- birth and death records adequately catalogued and analyzed
- various vaccinations provided for specific age groups
- health problems in school-aged children identified and treated
- tuberculosis cases hospitalized and treated
- laboratory tests performed[4]

Successive iterations of the Appraisal Form appeared through the 1920s and 1930s; these were well received by the public health community, although there were occasional concerns that quantity was being emphasized over quality. Local health officers were able to compare their ratings with those of other public health agencies. The basis for comparison was a numerical rating score, based on aggregated points awarded across key administrative and service areas. Comparative ratings were used to improve health programs, advocate for resources, summarize health agency activities in annual reports, and engage other health interests in the community. Agency ratings often attracted considerable public interest, resulting in both good and bad publicity for local agencies. Despite the initial intent to emphasize immediate results, however, the major focus of the ratings remained on measuring the more concrete aspects of public health practice, such as staff, clinic sites, patient visits, and the number of services rendered.

In 1943 a new instrument, the "Evaluation Schedule," which was scored centrally by the APHA Committee on Administrative Practice, replaced the self-assessment approach used in the Appraisal Form. The scores for health agencies of varying size and type were widely disseminated so that individual LHPAs could directly compare their performance in meeting community needs with that of their peers. Exhibit 5–1 illustrates some of the key performance measures included in the 1947 version of the Evaluation Schedule.

To develop a blueprint for a national network of local public health agencies that would provide every American with coverage by an LHPA, the Committee on Administrative Practice established a Subcommittee on Local Health Units. The subcommittee's major report (widely known as the Emerson Report) in 1945 was a landmark for recommendations regarding local public health practice. The Emerson Report became the postwar plan for public health in the United States. The report's far-reaching recommendations called for a minimum population base of 50,000 people for each LHPA and included state-by-state proposals for networks of LHPAs that would cover all Americans while reducing the number of LHPAs by about 50 percent through consolidation of smaller units.[5]

Exhibit 5–1 Public Health Practice Performance Measures from 1947 Evaluation Schedule

1. Hospital beds: percentage in approved hospitals
2. Practicing physicians: population per physician
3. Practicing dentists: population per dentist
4. Water: percentage of population in communities over 2,500 served with approved water
5. Sewerage: percentage of population in communities over 2,500 served with approved sewerage systems
6. Water: percentage of rural school children served with approved water supplies
7. Excreta disposal: percentage of rural school children served with approved means of excreta disposal
8. Food: percentage of food handlers reached by group instruction program
9. Food: percentage of restaurants and lunch counters with satisfactory facilities
10. Milk: percentage of bottled milk pasteurized
11. Diphtheria: percentage of children under 2 years given immunizing agent
12. Smallpox: percentage of children under 2 years given immunizing agent
13. Whooping cough: percentage of children under 2 years given immunizing agent
14. Tuberculosis: newly reported cases per death, 5-year period
15. Tuberculosis: deaths per 100,000 population, 5-year period
16. Tuberculosis: percentage of cases reported by death certificate
17. Syphilis: percentage of cases reported in primary, secondary, and early latent stage
18. Syphilis: percentage of reported contacts examined
19. Maternal: puerperal deaths per 1,000 total births, 5-year rate
20. Maternal: percentage of antepartum cases under medical supervision seen before 6th month
21. Maternal: percentage of women delivered at home under postpartum nursing supervision
22. Maternal: percentage of births in hospital
23. Infant: deaths under 1 year of age per 1,000 live births, 5-year rate
24. Infant: deaths from diarrhea and enteritis under 1 year per 1,000 live births, 2-year rate
25. Infant: percentage of infants under nursing supervision before 1 month
26. School: percentage of elementary children with dental work neglected
27. Accidents: deaths from motor accidents per 100,000 population, 5-year rate
28. Health department budget: cents per capita spent by health department

Source: Data from American Public Health Association, Committee on Administrative Practice, *Evaluation Schedule for Use in Study and Appraisal of Community Health Programs*, 1947, New York, New York.

The Emerson Report gave increased prominence to six basic services believed to represent local government's public health responsibilities to its citizens: vital statistics, environmental sanitation, communicable disease control, maternal and child health services, public health education, and public health laboratory services.[5] This was not a new formulation for local public health services. Rather, it was essentially the same package of services that had been considered the standard of practice among LHPAs for several decades and that had been assessed since the early years of the Appraisal Form. Over time, these services had become widely known as the six basic functions of public health ("Basic Six"); Exhibit 5–2 describes the Basic Six. With the added impetus of

Exhibit 5–2 Basic Six Services of Local Public Health

1. Vital statistics—collection and interpretation
2. Sanitation
3. Communicable disease control, including immunization, quarantine, and other measures, such as identifying communicable disease carriers and distributing vaccines to physicians, as well as doing immunizations directly
4. Maternal and child health (MCH), consisting of prenatal and postpartum care for mothers and babies and supervision of the health of school children; in some places, immunization of children was handled by the MCH program
5. Health education, including instruction in personal and family hygiene, sanitation, and nutrition, given in schools, at neighborhood health center classes, and in home visits
6. Laboratory services to physicians, sanitarians, and other interested parties

Source: Data from W. Shonick, *Government and Health Services: Government's Role in the Development of US Health Services 1930–1980,* © 1995, Oxford Press.

the Emerson Report, they became the cornerstone for structuring local public health practice. Although the report's extensive recommendations never became national public policy, they promoted positive changes in many states.

The Committee on Administrative Practice stimulated considerable interest in local public health practice. After about 1950 and continuing into the 1980s, there were repeated efforts to reexamine and redefine the boundaries of local public health practice. This search for mission redefinition is evident in a series of APHA policy statements from 1950 to 1970.[6] In a 1950 APHA statement on LHPA services and responsibilities, the Basic Six were presented as desirable minimal services, and several new "optimal" responsibilities were identified: recording and analysis of health data, health education and information, supervision and regulation, provision of direct environmental health services, administration of personal health services, and coordination of activities and services within the community. Another APHA policy statement in 1963 added the seventh and eighth services to the Basic Six: operation of health facilities and area-wide planning and coordination. Then, in 1970, APHA adopted yet another policy statement, expanding on these concepts and calling for increased involvement of state and local public health agencies in coordinating, monitoring, and assessing the adequacy of health services in their jurisdictions. The evolution of these various characterizations of public health practice is traced in Exhibit 5–3.

After World War II, important new expectations for local public health practice emerged. Lack of medical care was increasingly identified as a significant impediment to promoting and improving community health. This resulted in LHPAs increasingly serving a safety-net function. This expanded direct service provision role moved LHPAs into new territory, beyond the boundaries of the expanded Basic Six model. There was considerable debate as to whether this new role was appropriate, as well as whether LHPAs were serving leadership roles within their communities in integrating medical and

Exhibit 5–3 Expansion of the Basic Six Public Health Services, 1920–1980

Initial "Basic Six"
  • Vital statistics
  • Sanitation
  • Communicable disease control
  • Maternal and child health
  • Health education
  • Laboratory services
"Optimal" Services in 1950s
  • Basic Six as minimal level
  • Analysis and recording of health data
  • Health education and information
  • Supervision and regulation
  • Provision of direct environmental health services
  • Administration of personal health services
  • Coordination of activities and services within the community
Added in 1960s
  • Operation of health facilities
  • Area-wide planning and coordination
Added in the 1970s
  • Coordinating, monitoring, and assessing the adequacy of health services

Source: Data from W. Shonick, *Government and Health Services: Government's Role in the Development of US Health Services 1930–1980,* © 1995, Oxford Press.

---

community health services. The movement into medical care was controversial from its inception. Hanlon, in examining the future of LHPAs in 1973, called for official public health agencies to withdraw from the business of providing personal health services (whether preventive or therapeutic) and instead to "concentrate upon [their] important and unique potential as community health conscience and leader"[7(p901)] in promoting the establishment of sound social policy. Despite these admonitions, direct medical care services increased among LHPAs throughout the 1960s, 1970s, and 1980s, as a result of new federal and state grant programs. LHPAs were becoming significant providers of safety-net medical services, joining public hospitals and community health centers in this important role.

Slowly evolving through these developments was a unique concept that began to shift the emphasis from the services of public health to its mission and functions. This concept, often characterized as "a governmental presence at the local level" (AGPALL),[8] emerged in the 1970s in the process of fashioning "model standards" for communities to participate in achievement of the 1990 national health objectives (Exhibit 5–4). AGPALL means that local government, acting through various means, is ultimately responsible and accountable for ensuring that minimum standards are met in the community. Every locality is served by a unit of government that has responsibility for the health of that locality and population. This responsibility can be executed through an organization other than the official public health agency, but government,

Exhibit 5–4 Governmental Presence at the Local Level

This concept is based upon a multifaceted, multitiered governmental responsibility for ensuring that standards are met—a responsibility that often involves agencies in addition to the public health agency at any particular level. Regardless of the structure, every community must be served by a governmental entity charged with that responsibility, and general-purpose government must assign and coordinate responsibility for providing and assuring public health and safety services. Where services in any area covered by standards are readily available, government may also (but need not) be involved the responsibility of government to have, or to develop, the capacity to deliver such services. Where county and municipal responsibilities overlap, agreements on division of responsibility are necessary.

In summary, government at the local level has the responsibility for ensuring that a health problem is monitored and that services to correct that problem are available. The State government must monitor the effectiveness local efforts to control health problems and act as a residual guarantor of services where community resources are inadequate—recognizing, of course, that state resources are also limited.

Source: Reprinted from Preamble to Original Model Standards, US Public Health Service.

through its presence and interest in health, is responsible to see that necessary, agreed-upon services are available, accessible, acceptable, and of good quality.

The AGPALL concept emphasizes the leadership and change-agent aspects of community public health practice. However, exercising leadership to serve the community's health is neither simple nor straightforward. The complexities of health problems and their contributing factors call for collaborative, rather than command-and-control solutions. Key to identifying and solving important community health problems is the ability to deal with diverse interests and build constituencies. The AGPALL concept suggests that public health practice involves more than the provision of services. This broader view of public health's functions was powerfully reinforced by the IOM report.

PUBLIC HEALTH PRACTICE AND CORE FUNCTIONS
AFTER THE IOM REPORT

The picture of the state of the public health system painted in the 1988 IOM report[1] was more dismal than many had expected. After all, the infrastructure of the national public health system had grown substantially throughout the century, especially in terms of LHPA coverage of the population. There was widespread acceptance that appropriate community services should include chronic disease prevention and medical care, in addition to the Basic Six. Also, notably, health status had never been better. Yet, the HIV/AIDS epidemic had emerged and there was no shortage of intractable health and social issues now being placed on the public health agenda. Resources to meet these challenges were greatly limited, due in part to the insatiable appetite of the medical care delivery system for every available health dollar. These forces acted together to dissipate public appreciation and support for public health, and the IOM feared that public health would not be able to meet these challenges without a new vision that would engender the support of the public, policy makers, the media, the medical establishment, and other key stakeholders.

The vision articulated in the IOM report was founded in a broader view of public health functions than had existed in the past. Throughout earlier decades, the services provided by public health agencies had come to be viewed by many as public health's "functions." In characterizing three core functions, the IOM report suggested that the function "to serve"—whether described in terms of specific services or as the more abstract concept of "assurance"—inadequately characterizes the unique role of public health in our society. Public health interventions represent the products of carrying out public health's core functions, rather than the functions themselves. The IOM examination described three public health core functions: (1) assessment, (2) policy development, and (3) assurance:[1]

1. Assessment Calls for Public Health: to regularly and systematically collect, assemble, analyze, and make available information on the health of the community, including statistics on health status, community health needs, and epidemiologic and other studies of health problems. Not every agency is large enough to conduct these activities directly; intergovernmental and interagency cooperation is essential. Nevertheless each agency bears the responsibility for seeing that the assessment function is fulfilled. This basic function of public health cannot be delegated.[1(p7)]

2. Policy Development Calls for Public Health: to serve the public interest in the development of comprehensive public health policies by promoting the use of the scientific knowledge base in decision-making about public health and by leading in developing public health policy. Agencies must take a strategic approach, developed on the basis of a positive appreciation for the democratic political process.[1(p8)]

3. Assurance Calls for Public Health: to assure their constituents that services necessary to achieve agreed upon goals are provided, either by encouraging actions by other entities (private or public), by requiring such action through regulation, or by providing services directly . . . Each public health agency is to involve key policy makers and the general public in determining a set of high-priority personal and communitywide health services that government will guarantee to every member of the community. This guarantee should include subsidization or direct provision of high-priority personal health services for those unable to afford them.[1(p8)]

The core functions were widely accepted within the public health community;[9] its broader characterization of the important functions of public health led to the definition and measurement of their operational aspects, permitting assessment of their performance. Several key aspects of the assessment, policy development, and assurance functions are processes that identify and address health problems; others are processes (e.g., services and other interventions) generated to assure that these problems are addressed. To explicate the core functions and provide a framework for characterizing modern public health practice, a workgroup representing the national public health organizations developed the *essential public health services* framework.[10] Since 1995 virtually all national and state public health initiatives have used the essential public health services framework in efforts to characterize, measure and improve the performance of public health core functions. Unfortunately, the use of the term services in the essential public health services framework can be a source of confusion. Although they are not services in the same sense that most people view clinical services (e.g., immunizations) or community preventive services (e.g., fluoridated water), the essential public health services are important processes that operationalize the core functions—assessment, policy development, and assurance—into measurable processes of public health practice.

Public health functions involve identifying health problems and their causative factors, developing strategies to address these problems, and seeing that these strategies are implemented in a way that achieves the desired goals. In this light, public health practice is the development and application of preventive strategies and interventions to promote and protect the health of the public. Whereas the complete description for public health practice is yet to be agreed upon, the best depiction of what contemporary public health practice is all about can be found in the mission, vision, and functions outlined in the *Public Health in America* statement.[11] This one-page document includes a vision (healthy people in healthy communities), a mission (promoting physical and mental health and preventing disease, injury, and disability) and statements of what public health practice does and how it accomplishes these ends. As presented in Exhibit 5–5, these statements establish high standards for public health practice and a framework for measuring the attainment of those standards. The processes embodied in the essential public health services and their links to the three core functions are critical to an understanding of public health practice.

Assessment in Public Health

Two important processes (or essential public health services) characterize the assessment function of public health: (1) monitoring health status to identify community health problems and (2) diagnosing and investigating health problems and health hazards in the community.

Monitoring health status to identify community health problems includes:

- Accurate, ongoing assessment of the community's health status;
- Identification of threats to health;
- Determination of health service needs;
- Attention to the health needs of groups that are at higher risk than the total population;
- Identification of community assets and resources that support the public health system in promoting health and improving quality of life;
- Utilization of appropriate methods and technology to interpret and communicate data to diverse audiences; and
- Collaboration with other stakeholders, including private providers and health benefit plans, to manage multi-sectoral integrated information systems.

Exhibit 5–5 Relationship of Public Health in America Statement to Public Health Practice

Public Health in America Elements*	**Relationship to Public Health Practice**
Healthy people in healthy communities	Vision and mission statements for public health practice
Promote physical and mental health, and prevent disease, injury, and disability	
Public Health	
• prevents epidemics and the spread of disease • protects against environmental hazards • prevents injuries • promotes and encourages healthy behaviors • responds to disasters and assists communities in recovery • assures the quality and accessibility of health services	*Statements of the broad categories of outcomes affected by public health practice, sometimes viewed as what public health does*
Essential Public Health Services 1. monitor health status to identify community health problems 2. diagnose and investigate health problems and health hazards in the community 3. inform, educate, and empower people about health issues 4. mobilize community partnerships to identify and solve health problems 5. develop policies and plans that support individual and community health efforts 6. enforce laws and regulations that protect health and ensure safety 7. link people with needed personal health services and assure the provision of health care when otherwise unavailable 8. assure a competent public health and personal health care work force 9. evaluate effectiveness, accessibility, and quality of personal and population-based health services 10. research for new insights and innovative solutions to health problems	*Statements of the processes of public health practice that affect public health outcomes, sometimes viewed as how public health does what it does*

Source: *Reprinted from *Public Health in America,* Public Health Functions Steering Committee, Public Health Service, 1994.

Diagnosing and investigating health problems and health hazards in the community include:

- Access to a public health laboratory capable of conducting rapid screening and high-volume testing;
- Active infectious disease epidemiology programs; and
- Technical capacity for epidemiologic investigation of disease outbreaks and patterns of infectious and chronic diseases and injuries and other adverse health behaviors and conditions.

Policy Development for Public Health

The assessment function and its related processes provide a foundation for policy development and its key processes, including (1) informing, educating, and empowering people about health issues, (2) mobilizing community partnerships to identify and solve health problems, and (3) developing policies and plans that support individual and community health efforts.

Informing, educating, and empowering people about health issues include:

- Community development activities;
- Social marketing and targeted media public communication;
- Providing of accessible health information resources at community levels;
- Active collaboration with personal health care providers to reinforce health promotion messages and programs; and
- Joint health education programs with schools, churches, worksites, and others.

Mobilizing community partnerships to identify and solve health problems includes:

- Convening and facilitating partnerships among groups and associations (including those not typically considered to be health related);
- Undertaking defined health improvement planning process and health projects, including preventive, screening, rehabilitation, and support programs; and
- Building a coalition to draw upon the full range of potential human and material resources to improve community health.

Developing policies and plans that support individual and community health efforts includes:

- Leadership development at all levels of public health;
- Systematic community-level and state-level planning for health improvement in all jurisdictions;
- Development and tracking of measurable health objectives from the community health plan (CHP) as a part of continuous quality improvement strategy plan;
- Joint evaluation with the medical health care system to define consistent policy regarding prevention and treatment services; and
- Development of policy and legislation to guide the practice of public health.

Assurance of the Public's Health

Whereas assessment and policy development set interventions into motion, the assurance function keeps them on track through five important processes: (1) enforcing laws and regulations that protect health and ensure safety; (2) linking people to needed personal health services and assuring the provision of health care when otherwise unavailable; (3) assuring a competent public health and personal health care work force; (4) evaluating effectiveness, accessibility, and quality of personal and population-based health services; and (5) researching for new insights and innovative solutions to health problems.

Enforcing laws and regulations that protect health and ensure safety includes:

- Enforcement of sanitary codes, especially in the food industry;
- Protection of drinking water supplies;
- Enforcement of clean air standards;
- Animal control;
- Follow-up of hazards, preventable injuries, and exposure-related diseases identified in occupational and community settings;
- Monitoring quality of medical services (e.g., laboratories, nursing homes, and home health care providers); and
- Review of new drug, biologic, and medical device applications.

Linking people to needed personal health services and assuring the provision of health care when otherwise unavailable (sometimes referred to as outreach or enabling services) include:

- Assurance of effective entry for socially disadvantaged people into a coordinated system of clinical care;
- Culturally and linguistically appropriate materials and staff to assure linkage to services for special population groups;
- Ongoing "care management";
- Transportation services; and
- Targeted health education/promotion/disease prevention to high-risk population groups.

Assuring a competent public and personal health care work force includes:

- Education, training, and assessment of personnel (including volunteers and other lay community health workers) to meet community needs for public and personal health services;
- Efficient processes for licensure of professionals;
- Adoption of continuous quality improvement and lifelong learning programs;
- Active partnerships with professional training programs to assure community-relevant learning experiences for all students; and
- Continuing education in management and leadership development programs for those charged with administrative/executive roles.

Evaluating effectiveness, accessibility, and quality of personal and population-based health services includes:

- Assessing program effectiveness and
- Providing information necessary for allocating resources and reshaping programs.

Researching for new insights and innovative solutions to health problems includes:

- Full continuum of innovation, ranging from practical field-based efforts to fostering change in public health practice to more academic efforts to encourage new directions in scientific research;
- Continuous linkage with institutions of higher learning and research; and
- Internal capacity to mount timely epidemiologic and economic analyses and conduct health services research.

The important processes embodied in the essential public health services framework underscore the complexities of public health practice. These processes are important aspects to both problem identification and problem solving. In this sense, the essential public health services framework is relevant, both inside and outside the programs and services that many people continue to view as the main function of public health ("to serve"). These processes are evident in virtually any public health intervention (although in different degrees) and constitute what might be considered generic public health practice. They argue that public health practice is more than a collection of programs and services; it is something that embodies the AGPALL concept and the tools to carry out that role. The remarkable advances made in reducing cardiovascular disease mortality during the twentieth century relied on public health practice efforts of both a general and categorical nature, as illustrated in "Public Health Achievements in Twentieth-Century America, 1900–1999: Cardiovascular Disease Mortality."

Example

Public Health Achievements in Twentieth-Century America, 1900–1999: Cardiovascular Disease Mortality

Cardiovascular disease has a complex web of causation, with contributing factors, including physiologic, behavioral, environmental, and social factors. Intervention strategies that focus on only some of these factors will have only limited success. The gains achieved during the twentieth century reflect a multi-pronged assault on this health problem across the gamut of assessment, policy development, and assurance functions of public health.

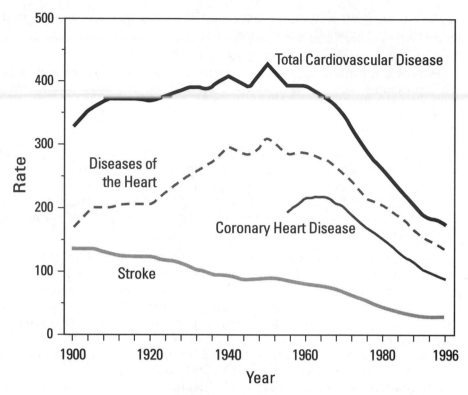

Figure 5-1 Age-Adjusted Death Rates for Total Cardiovascular Disease, Diseases of the Heart, Coronary Heart Disease, and Stroke by Year—United States, 1900–1996. *Source:* Reprinted from Achievements in Public Health, United States, 1900–1999: Decline in Deaths for Heart Disease and Strokes. *Morbidity and Mortality Weekly Report,* Vol. 48, No. 36, pp. 649–656, the Centers for Disease Control and Prevention, 1999.

Heart disease has been the leading cause of death in the United States since 1921, and stroke has been the third leading cause since 1938; together they account for approximately 40 percent of all deaths. Since 1950 age-adjusted death rates from cardiovascular disease (CVD) have declined 60 percent, representing one of the most important public health achievements of the twentieth century.

Age-adjusted death rates per 100,000 persons (standardized to the 1940 U.S. population) for diseases of the heart (i.e., coronary heart disease, hypertensive heart disease, and rheumatic heart disease) have decreased from a peak of 307.4 in 1950 to 134.6 in 1996, an overall decline of 56 percent (Figure 5–1). Age-adjusted death rates for coronary heart disease (the major form of CVD contributing to mortality) continued to increase into the 1960s, then declined. In 1996, 621,000 fewer deaths occurred from coronary heart disease than would have been expected, had the rate remained at its 1963 peak.

Age-adjusted death rates for stroke have declined steadily since the beginning of the century. Since 1950 stroke rates have declined 70 percent, from 88.8 in 1950 to 26.5 in 1996. Total age-adjusted CVD death rates have declined 60 percent since 1950 and accounted for approximately 73 percent of the decline in all causes of deaths during the same period.

Intensive investigation into the CVD epidemic largely began in the 1940s following World War II, although causal hypotheses about CVD and recognition of geographic differences in disease rates occurred earlier. Landmark epidemiologic investigations, such as the Framingham Heart Study and others, established the major risk factors of high blood cholesterol, high blood pressure, and smoking and dietary factors (particularly dietary cholesterol, fat, and sodium). The risk factor concept—that particular biologic, lifestyle, and social conditions were associated with increased risk for disease—developed out of CVD epidemiology. In addition to the major risk factors (i.e., high blood pressure, high blood cholesterol, and smoking), other important factors include socioeconomic status, obesity, and physical inactivity. Striking regional differences were noted, particularly for stroke mortality, with the highest rates observed in the southeastern United States. Cross-national and cross-cultural studies highlighted the importance of social, cultural, and environmental factors in the development of CVD.

Coronary heart disease and stroke, the two major causes of CVD-related mortality, are not influenced to the same degree by the recognized risk factors. For example, elevated blood cholesterol is a major risk factor for coronary heart disease, and hypertension is the major risk factor for stroke. Physical activity, smoking cessation, and a healthy diet, which can lower the risk for heart disease, also can help lower the risk for stroke.

Early intervention studies in the 1960s sought to establish whether lowering risk factor levels would reduce risk for CVD. During the 1970s and 1980s, along with numerous clinical trials demonstrating the efficacy of antihypertensive and lipid-lowering drugs, community trials sought to reduce risk at the community level. Public health interventions to reduce CVD have benefited from a combination of the "high risk" approach—aimed at persons with increased risk for CVD—and the population-wide approach—aimed at lowering risk for the entire community. National programs that combine these complementary approaches and that are aimed at health-care providers, patients, and the general public include the National High Blood Pressure Education Program, initiated in 1972, and the National Cholesterol Education Program, initiated in 1985. Although earlier Centers for Disease Control and Prevention (CDC) community demonstration projects focused on cardiovascular health, CDC established its National Center for Chronic Disease Prevention and Health Promotion in 1989 with a high priority of promoting cardiovascular health.

Table 5–1 Estimated Change in Risk Factors and Correlates for Heart Disease and Stroke, by Selected Characteristics—United States

Characteristic	Baseline year	Baseline estimate	Follow-up year	Follow-up estimate
Adults aged 20–74 years with hypertension	1960–1962	37%	1988–1994	23%
Persons with hypertension who are taking action to control their blood pressure (eg, medication, diet, reducing salt intake, and exercise)	1985	79%	1990	90%
Persons with hypertension whose blood pressure is controlled	1976–1980	11%	1988–1991	29%
Adults aged 20–74 with high blood cholesterol	1960–1962	32%	1988–1994	19%
Mean serum cholesterol levels mg/dL of adults aged > 18 years +	1960–1962	220	1988–1994	203
Adults aged ≥ 18 years who are current smokers	1965	42%	1995	25%
Persons who are overweight	1960–1962	24%	1988–1994	35%
Percentage of calories in the diet from fat	1976–1980	36%	1988–1994	34%
Percentage of calories in the diet from saturated fat	1976–1980	13%	1988–1994	12%
Number of physicians indicating cardiovascular diseases as their primary area of practice	1975	5,046	1996	14,304

Source: Reprinted from Achievements in Public Health, United States, 1900–1999: Decline in Deaths for Heart Disease and Strokes, *Morbidity and Mortality Weekly Report,* Vol. 48, No. 36, pp. 649–656, the Centers for Disease Control and Prevention, 1999.

Reasons for the declines in heart disease and stroke may vary by period and across region or socioeconomic group (e.g., age, sex, and racial/ethnic groups). Prevention efforts and improvements in early detection, treatment, and care have resulted in a number of beneficial trends (Table 5–1), which may have contributed to declines in heart disease and stroke. These trends include:

- a decline in cigarette smoking among adults aged greater than or equal to 18 years from approximately 42 percent in 1965 to 25 percent in 1995. Substantial public health efforts to reduce tobacco use began soon after recognition of the association between smoking and CVD and between smoking and cancer and the first Surgeon General's report on smoking and health, published in 1964
- a decrease in mean blood pressure levels in the U.S. population
- an increase in the percentage of persons with hypertension who have the condition treated and controlled

- a decrease in mean blood cholesterol levels
- changes in the U.S. diet. Data based on surveys of food supply suggest that consumption of saturated fat and cholesterol has decreased since 1909. Data from the National Health and Nutrition Examination surveys suggest that decreases in the percentage of calories from dietary fat and the levels of dietary cholesterol coincide with decreases in blood cholesterol levels
- improvements in medical care, including advances in diagnosing and treating heart disease and stroke, development of effective medications for treatment of hypertension and hyper cholesterolemia, greater numbers of specialists and health-care providers focusing on CVD, an increase in emergency medical services for heart attack and stroke, and an increase in coronary care units. These developments have contributed to lower case-fatality rates, lengthened survival times, and shorter hospital stays for persons with CVD.

Source: Adapted from Achievements in Public Health, United States, 1900–1999: Decline in Deaths for Heart Disease and Strokes, *Morbidity and Mortality Weekly Report,* Vol. 48, No. 36, pp. 640–656, the Centers for Disease Control and Prevention, 1999.

POST-IOM REPORT INITIATIVES

The delineation of core functions and essential public health services provided a new foundation for public health practice.[12] In the decade following the appearance of the IOM report, new tools for public health practice came onto the scene to build on this foundation.

APEXPH and MAPP

Among the post-IOM report initiatives, the Assessment Protocol for Excellence in Public Health (APEXPH), developed by the National Association of County and City Health Officials (NACCHO), in collaboration with other national public health organizations, has had the most extensive and positive influence on public health practice. Even more promising is the second generation of this tool, Mobilizing for Action through Planning and Partnerships (MAPP).

The original APEXPH was a tool for organizational self-assessment and improvement for LHPAs, as well as a simple and effective community needs assessment process. APEXPH provided a means for LHPAs to enhance their organizational capacity and strengthen their leadership role in their community. APEXPH guided health department officials in two principal areas of activity: (1) assessing and improving the organizational capacity of the agency and (2) working with the local community to improve the health status of its citizens. There were three principal parts to this process.[13]

- Organizational Capacity Assessment—self-assessed key aspects of operations, including authority to operate, community relations, community health assessment, public policy development, assurance of public health services, financial management, personnel management, and program management, resulting in an organizational action plan that set priorities for correcting perceived weaknesses.
- Community Process—guided formation of a community advisory committee that identified health problems requiring priority attention, then set health status goals and programmatic objectives. The aim was to mobilize community resources in pursuit of locally relevant public health objectives consistent with the Healthy People objectives.
- Completing the Cycle—ensured that the activities from the organizational and community processes were effectively carried out and that they accomplished the desired results through policy development, assurance, monitoring, and evaluation activities.

After its appearance in 1991, APEXPH gradually became well accepted; more than one-half of all LHPAs used all or part of APEXPH during the 1990s. Although the decade's experience with APEXPH was highly positive, opportunities for strengthening the process were apparent. Heightened interest in community health improvement efforts, widespread acceptance of the essential public health services as the framework for public health practice, the need to strategically engage a wider range of community interests, and the opportunity to formalize and activate local public health systems converged to suggest that a strategic approach to community health improvement was needed.

The development of MAPP addressed these needs, envisioning and designing a robust tool of public health practice to be used by communities with effective local public health agency leadership to create a local system that assures the delivery of health services essential to protecting the health of the public.[14] Distinguishing features of MAPP include:

- Incorporation of strategic planning concepts—to assist LHPAs in more effectively engaging their communities, securing resources, and managing the process of change. Visioning, contextual environment assessment, strategic issue identification, and strategy formulation principles are among the strategic planning concepts embedded in MAPP.
- Grounding in local public health practice—to assure that the process is practical, flexible, and user friendly. The instruments rely heavily on relating the experiences and successes of typical communities through vignettes, case studies, and other examples.
- A focus on local public health system—to broaden community health improvement efforts by recognizing and including all public and private organizations contributing to public health at the local level.

Public health involves more than what public health agencies do; MAPP provides a framework for actualizing this assertion through:

- A common approach for assessing local public health systems—to promote consistent quality of public health practice from community-to-community and state-to-state. The essential public health services framework provides the measures used to assess local public health systems consistent with other national and state efforts to promote a basic set of public health performance standards.
- Expansion of the basic indicators for health status—to reflect better the demographic and socioeconomic determinants of health, community assets, environmental and behavioral risks, and quality of life. MAPP includes a core set of measures for all communities and an extended menu of additional measures for use, where appropriate.
- Recognition that community themes and strengths play an important role in community health improvement efforts—to balance over-reliance on data and expert opinion, provide new insights into factors affecting community health, and increase buy-in and active participation as stakeholders feel their concerns and opinions are important to the process.

The model developed for MAPP involves interrelated and interactive components. To be practical for use in widely diverse communities and to meld basic strategic planning concepts with public health and community health improvement concepts, MAPP is both simple and complex, as illustrated in Figure 5–2. There is no fixed or even preferred sequencing of these components. The boundaries of the model identify the four assessments that comprise the MAPP process; these are usually completed after visioning has taken place but before strategic issues are identified in the steps indicated in the center of the model. Each element of the model is briefly described below:

- Organizing for Success/Partnership Development—involves establishing values and outcomes for the process and determining the scope, form, and timing for planning process, as well as its participants.
- Visioning—involves developing a shared vision of the ideal future for the community, which serves to provide the process with focus, purpose, direction, and buy-in.
- Four MAPP Assessments—these inform the planning process and drive the identification of strategic issues. All are critical to the success of the process, although there is no prescribed order in which they need to be undertaken. The four strategic assessments are:
  1. Community Themes and Strengths—involves the collection of inputs and insights from throughout the community in order to understand issues that residents feel are important.
  2. Local Public Health Assessment—involves an analysis of mission, vision, and goals through the use of performance measures for the essential public health services. Both strengths and areas for improvement are identified.

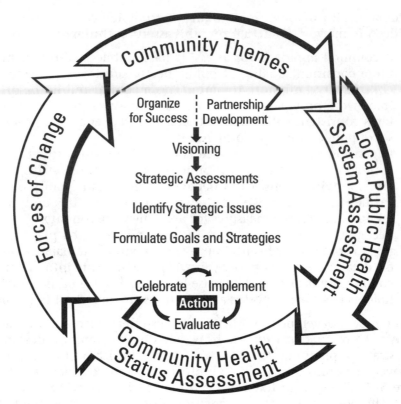

Figure 5–2 Mobilizing for Action through Planning and Partnerships (MAPP) Model. *Source:* Reprinted from National Association of County and City Health Officials, 2000.

3. Community Health Status Assessment—involves an extensive assessment of indicators in 11 domains, including asset mapping and quality of life; environmental health; socioeconomic, demographic, and behavioral risk factors; infectious diseases; sentinel events; social and mental health; maternal and child health; health resource availability; and health status indicators.
4. Forces of Change—identifies broader forces affecting the community, such as technology and legislation.
- Identify Strategic Issues—involves fundamental policy questions for achieving the shared vision, arising from the information developed in the previous phases. Some are more important than others and require action.
- Formulate Goals and Strategies—involves developing and examining options for addressing strategic issues, including questions of feasibility and barriers to implementation. Preferred strategies are selected.
- The Action Cycle—involves implementation, evaluation, and celebration of achievements after strategies are selected and agreed upon.

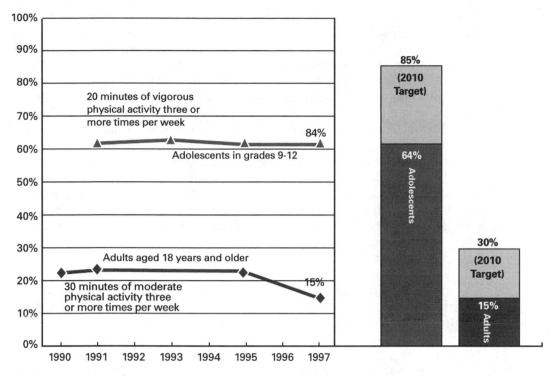

Figure 5–3 Participation in Regular Physical Activity, United States, 1990–1997. *Source:* Reprinted from *Healthy People 2010: Understanding and Improving Health,* U.S. Department of Health and Human Services, Public Health Service, 2000.

Widespread use of MAPP began in 2001. Although its impact on the performance of public health core functions will not be known for several years, its success will depend, in part, on its links to other important post-IOM report initiatives.

Planned Approach to Community Health, Model Standards, and Community Health Improvement Processes

In addition to the essential public health services framework and the APEXPH/MAPP processes, the IOM report stimulated several other important initiatives to promote core function-related performance, especially for the assessment and policy development functions. As described in Chapter 2, new national health objectives were established for the year 2010, based on two decades of experience with the year 1990 and year 2000 national health objectives. The panel of leading health indicators introduced in Healthy People 2010 covers a wide variety of important health risks, such as those related to physical activity (Figure 5–3). Broader participation in their design and more concerted strategies for their implementation in community settings distinguish the year 2010 objectives from the two earlier efforts.

One of the first community health planning tools to be widely used was the Planned Approach to Community Health (PATCH), a process for community organization and community needs assessment that emphasizes community mobilization and constituency building. PATCH focuses on orienting and training community leaders and other community participants in all aspects of the community needs assessment process and includes excellent documentation and resource materials. Although originally developed by the CDC to focus on chronic health conditions and stimulate health promotion and disease prevention interventions, PATCH is flexible enough to be used in a wide variety of community health needs assessment applications.

Another important tool for addressing public health core functions and their associated processes is Model Standards, Healthy Communities.[8] The steps outlined for implementation of the Model Standards process in the community link many of the various core function-related tools; they represent, in effect, a path way for organizations to participate in community health improvement activities.

1. Assessment of Organizational Role—Communities are organized and structured differently. As a result, the specific roles of local public health organizations will vary from community-to-community. An essential first step is to reexamine organizational purpose and mission and develop a long-range vision through strategic planning involving its internal and external constituencies. The resulting mission statement and long-range vision serve to guide the organization (leadership and board, as well as employees) and to define it for its community partners. This critical step should be completed before the remaining steps can be successfully addressed. Part I of APEXPH and the expanded strategic planning elements of MAPP are useful in accomplishing this task.

2. Assessment of Organizational Capacity—After mission and role have been defined, it is necessary to examine an organization's capacity to carry out its role in the community. This calls for an assessment of the major operational elements of the organization, including its structure and performance for specific tasks. This type of organizational and local public health system self-assessment is best carried out through broad participation from all levels. Both APEXPH and MAPP include hundreds of indicators that can be used in this capacity assessment. These indicators can be modified or eliminated if deemed inappropriate and additional indicators can also be used. This step serves to identify strengths and weaknesses relative to mission and role.

3. Development of a Capacity-Building Plan—The development of a capacity-building plan incorporates the organization's strengths and prioritizes its weaknesses so that the most important are addressed first. As in any plan, specific objectives for addressing these weaknesses are developed, responsibilities are assigned, and a process for tracking progress over time is established. Again, APEXPH and MAPP are valuable tools for accomplishing this task.

4. Assessment of Community Organizational Structure—Having looked internally at its capacity and ability to exercise its leadership role for identifying and addressing priority health needs in the community, the public health organization must assess the key stakeholders and necessary participants for a community-wide needs assessment and intervention initiative. This is often a long-term and continuous process in which the relationship of all important community stakeholders and partners (e.g., the health agency, community providers of health-related services, community organizations, community leaders, interest groups, the media, and the general public) is assessed. This step determines how and under whose auspices community health planning will take place within the community. Both APEXPH/MAPP and PATCH processes support the successful completion of this step.

5. Organization of Community—This step calls for organizing the community so that it represents a strong constituency for public health and will participate collaboratively in partnership with the health agency. Specific strategies and activities will vary from community-to-community but will generally include hearings, dialogues, discussion forums, meetings, and collaborative planning sessions. The specific roles and authority of community participants should be clarified so that the process is not perceived as one driven largely by the health agency and so-called experts. Both APEXPH/MAPP and PATCH are useful for completing this step.

6. Assessment of Community Health Needs—The actual process of identifying health problems of importance to the community is one that must carefully balance information derived from datasets with information derived from the community's perceptions of which problems are most important. Often, community readiness to mitigate specific problems greatly increases the chances for success, as well as support for the overall process within the community. In addition to generating information on possible health problems, this step gathers information on resources available within the community. This step serves to provide the information necessary for the community's most important health problems to be identified. The community needs assessment tools provided in both APEXPH/MAPP and PATCH can be used to accomplish this step.

7. Determination of Local Priorities and Community Health Resources—After important health problems are identified, decisions must be made as to which are most important for community action. This step requires broad participation from community participants in the process so that priorities will be viewed as community rather than agency-specific priorities. Debate and negotiation are essential for this step, and there are many approaches to coming to consensus around specific priorities. Both APEXPH/MAPP and PATCH support this step.

8. Selection of Outcome Objectives—After priorities are determined, the process must establish a target level to be achieved for each priority problem. For this step, the Model Standards process is especially useful

in linking community priorities to national health objectives and establishing targets that are appropriate for the current status and improvement possible from a community intervention. This step also calls for negotiation within the community because deployment and reallocation of resources may be needed to achieve the target outcomes that are agreed upon. In addition to Model Standards, both APEXPH/MAPP and PATCH can be useful in accomplishing this step.

9. Development of Intervention Strategies—This step is one of determining strategies and methods of achieving the outcome objectives established for each priority health problem. This can be quite difficult and, at times, contentious. For some problems, there may be few or even no effective interventions. For others, there may be widely divergent strategies available, some of which may be deemed unacceptable or not feasible. After agreement is reached as to strategies and methods, responsibilities for implementing and evaluating interventions will be assigned. With community-wide-interventions, overall coordination of efforts may also need to be addressed as part of the intervention strategy.

10. Implementation of Intervention Strategies—After the establishment of goals, objectives, strategies, and methods, specific plans of action for the intervention are developed and specific tasks and work plans developed. Clear delineation of responsibilities and time lines are essential for this step.

11. Continuous Monitoring and Evaluation of Effort—The evaluation strategy for the intervention will track performance related to outcome objectives, as well as process objectives and activity measures over time. If activity measures and process objectives are being accomplished, there should be progress toward achieving the desired outcome objectives. If this does not occur, the selected intervention strategy needs to be reconsidered and revised.

Since 1990 numerous communities have used PATCH, Model Standards, and other tools (such as Healthy Cities and Healthy Communities, two similar community needs assessment processes) in community health improvement initiatives.

In 1996 the IOM revisited issues addressed in the Future of Public Health, concluding that different organizations, leadership, and political and economic realities were transforming how public health carried out its core functions and essential services.[15] On the one hand, market-driven health care was forcing public health to clarify and strengthen its public role in a predominately private system. On the other, public health was increasingly identifying and working with a variety of entities within the community that shape community health and well-being. A third important IOM report[16] in 1997 advanced an expanded community health improvement process (CHIP) model that extends the tools developed earlier in the decade and the steps described above. Its main features are its expanded perspective on the wide variety of factors that influence health, its support for broad participation by community stakeholders, and its emphasis on the use of performance measures to assure accountability of partners and track progress over time.

Table 5–2 Percent of Local Health Jurisdictions Performing 20 Core Function-Related Measures of Local Public Health Practice, 1995 and 1999

LHJ Strata (by Population Size and Jurisdiction Type)	% Performing Community Health Assessment	% Completing Community Health Improvement Plan	% Using Established Tools for Assessment
<25,000 population	44	41	47
25,000–49,999 population	63	59	51
50,000–99,999 population	65	68	57
100,000–499,999 population	66	69	55
>500,000 population	72	76	48
County	61	56	54
City	50	57	51
City-County	68	62	60
Township	19	27	26
Multi-County	71	63	54
Metropolitan	53	54	48
Non-Metropolitan	56	52	52
All	55	53	51

Source: Reprinted from Turnock BJ, Handler AS, Miller CA. Core Function-Related Local Public Health Performance. *Journal of Public Health Management & Practice* 1998;4(5):26–32. © 1998, Lippincott, Williams & Wilkins.

Community health assessments leading toward community health improvement plans have increased in quantity as well as quality during the 1990s. A survey conducted by NACCHO found that, by 1999, 55 percent of local health jurisdictions (LHJs) nationwide had already conducted a community health assessment and 75 percent or more were expected to be involved within the next three years.[17] Those not planning to conduct assessments were primarily the smallest local health jurisdictions with few full time employees. Similar patterns were identified for community health improvement plans, as demonstrated in Table 5–2. The most widely used tools for assessment and planning were APEXPH/MAPP (47 percent) and state-specific tools (25 percent, some patterned after APEXPH/MAPP). Model Standards were used by 6 percent, PATCH was used by 4 percent, and other tools were used by 18 percent. Metropolitan LHJs were more likely to develop their own assessment tools while non-metropolitan LHJs were somewhat more prone to use tools developed at the state level. The expanded use of these tools underscores the importance of community health improvement indicatives as a hallmark of twenty-first century community public health practice.

TWENTY-FIRST CENTURY COMMUNITY PUBLIC HEALTH PRACTICE

Communities are the battlefields on which public health threats will be met, and public health challenges will be addressed in the new century. There has been steady growth in the armamentarium of community public health practice during the late twentieth century. This movement gained pace in the 1990s and promises to be the new public health of the early twenty-first century. It is grounded in the notion that more doctors, more clinics, and more sophisticated diagnostic and treatment advances will not alleviate the major health problems facing Americans. Instead, the greatest gains will come from what people do or don't do for themselves, collectively. Acting collectively can take place at many levels; at the community level, it often works best. This section will examine the approaches, tools, and opportunities of modern community public health practice.

The notion of community is an elusive concept. Generally, communities are aggregates of individuals who share common characteristics or other bonds. One person can be part of many different communities. One definition views community as the associative, self-generated gathering of common people who have sufficient resources in their lives to cope with life's demands and not suffer ill health. This definition of community focuses on the capacity of communities to achieve their health goals through the effective use of their own assets. It differs considerably from the view of communities as the location in which health services are delivered. Rather than focusing on the level of individual actions and behaviors, it recognizes the importance of social determinants of health and of the environmental and policy levels for public health responses. Community public health practice revolves around engaging communities to work collectively on their own behalf. Community engagement is the process of working collaboratively with groups of people who are affiliated by geographic proximity, special interests, or similar situations, with respect to issues affecting their well-being. For public health workers in government agencies, health care organizations, educational institutions, voluntary organizations, or corporate settings, community engagement is essential.

Although community engagement is a relatively recent phenomenon for many governmental public health organizations, health education specialists have been utilizing these principles for more than four decades, based on the fundamental admonition to start where the people are. The early experience of community health educators is well expressed in the "Ten Commitments for Community Health Education"[18] (Exhibit 5–6).

This positive approach emphasizes that all communities have assets. This may sound obvious, but all too often communities have been viewed solely in terms of their needs and problems. The implication of these different perspectives is important. If communities are viewed from their needs, the policies and interventions will be based on needs. If they are to be viewed from their assets, the policies and interventions will be based on the community's capacities, skills, and assets. Community health improvement seldom occurs from the actions of outside interests alone; the most successful community development efforts are driven by the commitment of those investing themselves and their resources in the effort. Identifying community assets is possible through approaches that catalog and actually map the basic building blocks that will be used to address important community health problems.[19] Primary building blocks include those community assets that are most readily available for community health improvement, including both individual and organizational assets. Individual assets include the skills, talents, and experiences of residents, individual businesses, and home-based enterprises, as well as per-

Exhibit 5–6 Ten Commitments for Community Health Education

---

1. Start where the people are
2. Recognize and build on community strengths
3. Honor thy community, but do not make it holy
4. Foster high-level community participation
5. Laughter is good medicine and good health education
6. Health education is educational, but is also political
7. Thou shall not tolerate the bad "isms," (such as racism, sexism, agism)
8. Think globally, act locally
9. Foster individual and community empowerment
10. Work for social justice

Source: Reprinted from Mikler M. Ten Commitments for Community Health Education. *Health Education Research Theory & Practice* 1994;9(4):527–534 by permission of Oxford University Press.

---

sonal income. Organizational assets include associations of businesses, citizen associations, cultural organizations, communications organizations, and religious organizations. Secondary building blocks are private, public, and physical assets, which can be brought under community control and used for community improvement purposes. These include private and nonprofit organizations (higher educational institutions, hospitals, social service agencies), public institutions and services (public schools, police, libraries, fire department, parks), and physical resources (vacant land, commercial and industrial structures, housing, energy, and waste resources).

In addition to community engagement and asset-mapping strategies, performance measurement offers another tool for community health improvement activities. Performance measures are also not new to public health practice. The use of performance measures to track progress toward community or national health objectives and to monitor programs has long been standard practice. The community health improvement processes (CHIP) proposed by the IOM in its report on performance monitoring, however, take performance measurement to a new level. In these processes, performance measures serve to hold communities (acting through stakeholders and partnerships) accountable for actions for which they have accepted responsibility.[16] This supports the development of a shared vision and a collaborative and integrative approach to community problem solving for the purpose of improving health status. It offers a pathway for stakeholders and partners to assume responsibility collectively and to marshal their resources and assets in pursuit of agreed-upon objectives.

The CHIP model includes a problem identification and prioritization cycle, followed by an analysis and implementation cycle. This second cycle develops, implements, and evaluates health intervention strategies that address priority community health problems. The distinguishing feature of this approach is the emphasis on measurement to link performance and accountability on a community-wide basis, rather than solely on the local public health agency or another public entity. Several recommendations were developed to operationalize the community health improvement concept:[16]

- Communities should base a health improvement process on a broad definition of health and a comprehensive conceptual model of how health is produced within the community.
- A community health improvement process should develop its own set of specific, quantitative performance measures, linking accountable entities to the performance of specific activities expected to lead to the production of desired health outcomes in the community.
- A community health improvement process should seek a balance between strategic opportunities for long-term health improvement and goals that are achievable in the short term.
- Community conditions guiding community health improvement processes should strive for strategic inclusiveness, incorporating individuals, groups, and organizations that have an interest in health outcomes, can take actions necessary to improve community health, or can contribute data and analytic capabilities needed for performance monitoring.
- A community health improvement process should be centered in a community health coalition or similar entity.

To enable the widespread adoption of the community health improvement process concept, the IOM made additional recommendations.[16]

- State and local public health agencies should assure that an effective community health improvement process is in place in all communities. These agencies should, at a minimum, participate in community health improvement process activities and, in some communities, should provide the leadership and/or organizational home.
- In support of community-level health improvement processes, state health agencies, in cooperation and collaboration with local public health agencies, should assure the availability of community-level data needed for health profiles.
- States and the federal government, through health departments or other appropriate channels, should require that health plans, indemnity insurers, and other private entities report standard data on the characteristics and health status of their enrolled populations, on services provided, and on outcomes of those services, as necessary for performance monitoring in the community health improvement process.

Numerous useful tools and guides have been published and made available via the Internet (including the website resources for this book) to support the expanded community health improvement efforts in models such as CHIP, Mobilizing for Action through Planning and Partnerships (MAPP), and similar initiatives. Prominent among these tools are CDC's Principles of Community Engagement,[20] the Community Tool Box (developed by the University of Kansas),[21] and the Healthy People 2010 Tool Kit (produced by the Public Health Foundation).[22] Geographic information systems, an example of which is provided in Figure 5–4, are emerging as an important technique for assessment of community health problems, needs, and assets.

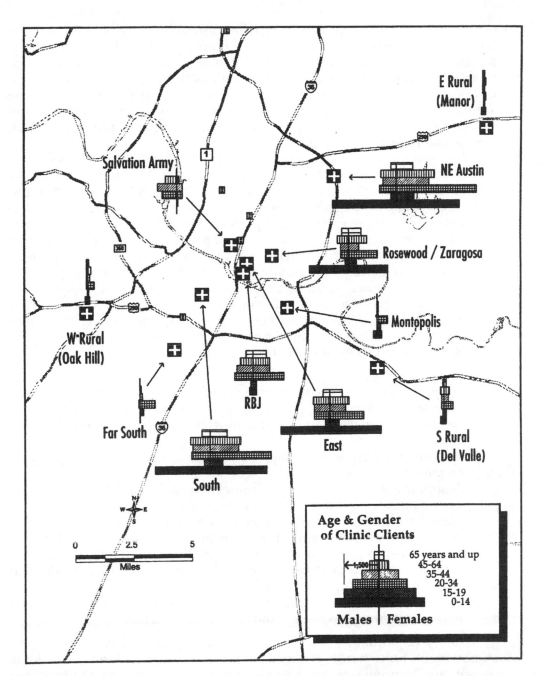

Figure 5–4 Client Demographics (Age and Gender) at Low-Income Clinics in Austin/Travis County, Texas, 1995–1996. The population pyramids in this geographic information system (GIS)-produced map quickly convey the very different populations seen at low-income clinics in Austin/Travis County, Texas. For example, the Salvation Army Clinic in the downtown area deals mostly with homeless men between the ages of 20 and 64, whereas the North East Austin Clinic mainly serves women 20–34 and their children. The challenges in running clinics with such different profiles are apparent. *Source:* Reprinted from G. F. White and K. C. Cerny, Client Demographics at Low-Income Clinics in Austin/Travis County, Texas, 1995–1996, *Journal of Public Health Management and Practice,* Vol. 5, No. 2, p. 48, © 1999, Aspen Publishers, Inc.

Governmental public health agencies, especially LHPAs, have steadily increased their partnerships with business, nonprofit, and other governmental organizations. Data from the 1996–1997 profile of LHPAs[23] demonstrate that 8 of 10 LHPAs have partnerships with state health agencies, and 7 of 10 collaborate with other LHPAs. More than two-thirds partner with other state agencies and hospitals, and more than half collaborate with academic institutions, professional associations, community organizations, and civic groups. Almost half have business sector partners.

The need for new community-driven models of public health practice is also reflected in the National Turning Point Initiative.[24] Funded jointly by the Kellogg and Robert Wood Johnson Foundations, Turning Point seeks to transform and strengthen the public health infrastructure at the state and local levels, in effect, reforming public health practice. More than 21 states participate in Turning Point through statewide and local partnerships that bring together a broad spectrum of health interests to develop a shared vision and strategic plans to improve statewide public health systems. Community health improvement processes, performance measurement, and health statute reform are receiving special attention as Turning Point states move from planning into implementation. The collaborations in the various Turning Point sites vary significantly, nurturing and developing many different models for systems change. Broad strategies include:

- Developing sustainable and appropriate capacity and infrastructure to support a population-based approach to health improvement.
- Developing sustainable partnerships for decision making and policy development related to health improvement at the community and state levels.
- Creating ongoing evaluation processes that will highlight best practices in public health systems design.
- Emphasizing prevention, health protection, and health promotion programs and activities that focus on the broad health determinants.
- Building systems that will engage proactive and aggressive actions to direct and protect the population from emerging threats to health.
- Clearly defining roles and responsibilities for the public health core functions and essential services of all state and community entities that contribute to health.
- Focusing on community health improvement models at the local level and using system-level health improvement models at the state level.

Healthy Communities is another successful model for community health improvement, using health as a metaphor for a broader approach to building community.[25] Since health cuts across lines of race, ethnicity, class, culture, and sector, the focus on a healthy community enables the entire community to collaborate in community renewal. Healthy Communities believes that only when people act together to participate directly in the public work of our society will change in our public policies and problems occur. A key to success involves community institutions using their organizational skills, relationships, in-kind resources, and credibility to engage the rest of the community in mobilizing the creativity and resources of the community to improve health and well-being. Focusing on systems change, Healthy Communities seeks to build broad citizen participation that encourages new players and honors diversity. It looks to build true collaborations between business, government, nonprofit organizations, and citizens stimulating the community and political will to act together.

Community-based health policy development is also receiving greater attention in these collaborations and partnerships. Public policy serves as a guide to influence governmental decisions and action at any jurisdictional level, thereby affecting what would otherwise occur.[26] For the health and well being of communities, policies indicate broad directions toward important goals, cutting across many different stakeholders and affecting large populations. Policies focus on both goals and the means to achieve those goals, often affecting the policies of individual organizations. At the community level, health policy has many options, such as more and better health services to address unmet needs in the community or advocacy for broader support to improve the conditions influencing health in the community. Increasingly, community-driven public health initiatives are tackling the broader social and community factors, even as they seek to assure that gaps in services are somehow met. The experiences are many and varied, although one accounting of key lessons learned to date includes:[26]

- the need to monitor the policy environment continuously because every issue exists in a historical context, involving past experiences on similar issues and current circumstances that limit possibilities;
- the importance of choosing appropriate frames, forums, and channels for debate, so that issues are framed in the public interest in ways that are sensitive to the current environment;
- the art of designing policy proposals that offer clear gains, even after tradeoffs are made with other stakeholders in the process;
- the value of negotiating with allies and opponents alike because both are major stakeholders in the policy development process; and
- the necessity of influencing the social climate of the community through effective use of public opinion and the media.

Little research is available to illuminate the value of community-driven health policy development initiatives. There is some evidence that widespread initiation of community health improvement processes increases the frequency that key policy development components take place. Policy development may be the public health core function most heavily impacted by community health improvement processes. The increase in performance of specific practices related to the core functions has been greatest for those related to policy development and, generally, the baseline level of measures of policy development lags behind that of assessment and assurance where community health improvement processes have not been implemented.

Together, these strategies, initiatives, and tools can make substantial contributions to improving public health practice in the United States. In addition, there is reason to believe that improvement is needed in view of assessments of performance that were completed in the 1990s.

CORE FUNCTION PERFORMANCE THROUGH 2002

Much of what is known about public health performance in the United States has been developed within the context of initiatives established after the appearance of the IOM report. Unfortunately, many of these experiences remain unpublished, and few are readily transported and replicated elsewhere. However, more than a dozen reports on various aspects of public health performance were published during the 1990s. Using somewhat different panels of performance measures, they provided significant insight into the performance of public health core functions and essential public health services.

Public health practice performance data, focused on process performance (including outputs), were reported by NACCHO in four surveys of local health jurisdictions undertaken during the 1990s.[17,23,27,28] For 48 questions associated with the three core functions from the 1990 NACCHO survey, mean LHPA performance was 50 percent. For 96 questions linked with the core functions in the 1992/1993 NACCHO survey, mean performance was similar, at 46 percent. Other studies, using practice measures based on the core functions, reported performance scores of 57 percent performance for 14 LHPAs in 1992, 56 percent for 370 LHPAs in 1993, and 50 percent for 208 LHPAs in 1993.[29-32] When similar performance measures were used on a statewide basis in Iowa in 1995, the overall performance score was 61 percent.[33]

Based on a variety of field tests and performance studies completed in the early 1990s, a consensus set of 20 practice performance measures (Exhibit 5–7) was established by leading researchers in the field. Using these 20 measures with a random sample of 298 LHPAs stratified by population size and type of jurisdiction,[34] an effort was made to assess the extent to which the U.S. population in 1995 was being effectively served by the public health core functions identified in the IOM report (assessment, policy development, and assurance). Performance of these 20 measures ranged from 23 to 94 percent. The most frequently performed measures were investigating adverse health events, maintaining necessary laboratory services, implementing mandated programs, maintaining a network of relationships, and regularly providing information to the public. The least frequently performed measures were assessing use of preventive and screening services in the community, conducting behavioral

Exhibit 5–7 Core Function-Related Practice Performance Measures, 1995

Assessment
1. For the jurisdiction served by your local health department, is there a community needs assessment process that systematically describes the prevailing health status in the community?
2. In the past three years in your jurisdiction, has the local public health agency surveyed the population for behavioral risk factors?
3. For the jurisdiction served by your local health agency, are timely investigations of adverse health events, including communicable disease outbreaks and environmental health hazards, conducted on an ongoing basis?

continues

Exhibit 5–7 continued

4. Are the necessary laboratory services available to the local public health agency to support investigations of adverse health events and meet routine diagnostic and surveillance needs?
5. For the jurisdiction served by your local public health agency, has an analysis been completed of the determinants and contributing factors of priority health needs, adequacy of existing health resources, and the population groups most impacted?
6. In the past three years, in your jurisdiction, has the local public health agency conducted an analysis of age-specific participation in preventive and screening services?

Policy Development

7. For the jurisdiction served by your local public health agency, is there a network of support and communication relationships that includes health-related organizations, the media, and the general public?
8. In the past year, in your jurisdiction, has there been a formal attempt by the local public health agency at informing elected officials about the potential public health impact of decisions under their consideration?
9. For the jurisdiction served by your local public health agency, has there been a prioritization of the community health needs that have been identified from a community needs assessment?
10. In the past three years, in your jurisdiction, has the local public health agency implemented community health initiatives consistent with established priorities?
11. For the jurisdiction served by your local public health agency, has a community health action plan been developed with community participation to address priority community health needs?
12. During the past three years, in your jurisdiction, has the local public health agency developed plans to allocate resources in a manner consistent with the community health action plan?

Assurance

13. For the jurisdiction served by your local public health agency, have resources been deployed as necessary to address the priority health needs identified in the community health need assessment?
14. In the past three years, in your jurisdiction, has the local public health agency conducted an organizational self-assessment?
15. For the jurisdiction served by your local public health agency, are age-specific priority health needs effectively addressed through the provision of or linkage to appropriate services?
16. In the past three years, in your jurisdiction, has there been an instance in which the local public health agency has failed to implement a mandated program or service?
17. For the jurisdiction served by your local public health agency, have there been regular evaluations of the effect that public health services have on community health status?
18. In the past three years, in your jurisdiction, has the local public health agency used professionally recognized process and outcome measures to monitor programs and to redirect resources as appropriate?
19. For the jurisdiction served by your local public health agency, is the public regularly provided with information about current health status, health care needs, positive health behaviors, and health care policy issues?
20. In the past year, in your jurisdiction, has the local public health agency, provided reports to the media on a regular basis?

risk factor surveys, regularly evaluating the effect of services in the community, allocating resources consistent with community action plans, and deploying resources to meet identified needs (Table 5–3). The overall weighted mean performance score for all 20 measures was 56 percent. Sub-scores for assessment, policy development, and assurance measures were similar to the overall mean. City and county-based LHPA jurisdictions with populations greater than 50,000 performed these measures more frequently (65 percent) than did other LHPAs in this study (Table 5–4).

Another study[35] using the same 20 measures in 1998 found similar levels of performance (65 percent) in 356 jurisdictions with populations of 100,000 or more. These jurisdictions include only about 20 percent of LHPAs but serve about 70 percent of the U.S. population. Although the performance of the more populous jurisdictions was somewhat higher than the combination of large and small jurisdictions included in the 1995 national study, both the relative rankings and the population size-specific scores were quite similar in these two studies.

The most extensive use of these 20 measures took place as part of the Department of Justice's initial efforts to assess national bioterrorism preparedness. More than 2000 local jurisdictions provided information relative to these 20 measures between mid-2000 and early 2002. The overall score for all jurisdictions was 65 percent with scores varying by jurisdiction population and type. Jurisdiction serving populations of less than 25,000 had a mean score of 58 percent while jurisdictions serving populations of more than 500,000 had a mean score of 74 percent. Scores for local health jurisdictions organized at the city or municipal level score lower than those organized at the city/county, county, district, regional, or state levels.[36]

Although the various studies conducted between 1992 and 2002 used somewhat different methods and measures, they appear to show steady improvement in public health practice performance. These studies also consistently demonstrate practice (process and outputs) performance in the 50–70 percent range and paint a picture of less than optimal functioning of the public health system nationally and in many states. Interestingly, this range is consistent with conclusions of the Emerson Report a half-century earlier as to effective public health coverage of the nation, based on an assessment of capacity factors. Although the precise status is not known, it is clear that the United States fell well short of its year 2000 target of having 90 percent of the population residing in jurisdictions in which public health's core functions are being effectively addressed. Two studies of practice performance conducted nationally in the 1990s concluded that only about one-third of the U.S. population was effectively served.[32,34]

In addition to the extent of performing core functions and essential services, several other dimensions of performance are important. One relates the level of adequacy and characterizes how well communities are served. Another characterizes the contribution made by the local public health agency and other community partners. The limited information available on these dimensions of performance, also summarized in Table 5–3, says much about the current state of public health practice.

Table 5–3 Mean Performance Scores for Local Health Jurisdictions by Population Size and Jurisdiction Type, 1995

Core Function-Related Performance Measures	% LHJs Performing Activity, 1995*	% LHJs >100,000 pop. Performing Activity, 1998**	% Perceived Adequacy of Performance**	% Perceived Share of Effort Contributed by LPHA**
1. Community needs assessment process	53.0	71.5	35.3	54.5
2. Behavioral risk factor surveys	29.2	45.8	21.0	51.0
3. Timely investigations of adverse health events	93.6	98.6	75.1	75.7
4. Necessary laboratory services available	89.3	96.3	72.9	49.5
5. Analysis of determinants, resources, and populations most impacted	45.0	61.3	29.4	52.8
6. Analysis of preventive and screening services	22.8	28.4	12.1	59.3
7. Network of relationships	82.6	78.8	42.3	46.2
8. Inform elected officials	73.2	80.9	37.7	73.8
9. Prioritization of community health needs	52.7	66.1	33.8	57.6
10. Implemented community health initiatives	68.8	81.9	34.7	58.0
11. Community health action plan	39.6	41.5	16.2	49.6
12. Plans for resource allocation	36.6	26.2	10.5	57.1
13. Resources deployed to meet needs	37.3	48.6	18.4	50.1
14. Organizational self-assessment	50.3	56.3	31.3	87.6
15. Provision/linkage of services for priority needs	64.1	75.6	35.9	47.9
16. Implemented all mandated programs	82.9	91.4	91.4	N/A
17. Evaluations of effect of services in the community	30.5	34.7	15.9	67.8
18. Programs monitored and resources redirected	42.3	47.3	21.6	70.9
19. Public provided information regularly	78.8	75.4	32.5	58.7
20. Provide reports to media regularly	68.5	75.2	39.5	76.8
Average: Assessment Measures (#1–#6)	54.9	66.7	40.8	59.9
Average: Policy Development Measures (#7–#12)	58.2	60.2	27.5	57.7
Average: Assurance Measures (#13–#20)	55.4	64.4	37.7	80.0
Average: All Activities	56.1	63.8	35.4	67.1

Source: *Reprinted from Turnock BJ, Handler AS, Miller CA. Core Function-Related Local Public Health Performance. *Journal of Public Health Management & Practice* 1998;4(5):26–32. © 1998, Lippincott, Williams & Wilkins.
**Mays GP, Miller CA, Halverson PK, Stevens R, Vann JJ. Availability and Perceived Effectives of Public Health Activities in the Nation's Most Populous Communities (in press).

Table 5–4 Mean Performance Scores for Local Health Jurisdictions by Population Size* and Jurisdiction Type, 1995

LHD Strata (by Population Size and Jurisdiction Type)	Mean Performance Score (%)
City ≤ 50,000 (n = 12)	47.9
City > 50,000 (n = 10)	77.0
County ≤ 50,000 (n = 80)	56.4
County > 50,000 (n = 43)	66.9
City-County ≤ 50,000 (n = 34)	57.1
City-County > 50,000 (n = 24)	59.2
Multicounty ≤ 50,000 (n = 6)	60.8
Multicounty > 50,000 (n = 7)	60.7
All other LHDs (all population sizes) (n = 26)	36.9
Jurisdiction Unknown (n = 56)	54.8
Weighted Sample Total	56.1

*n = 298

Source: Reprinted from B.J. Turnock, A.S. Handler, and C.A. Miller, Core Function-Related Local Public Health Performance, *Journal of Public Health Management and Practice*, Vol. 4, No. 5, pp. 26–32, © 1998, Aspen Publishers, Inc.

The perceived adequacy for 20 measures of public health practice was 35 percent in the nation's most populous health jurisdictions in 1998. Assessment activities and assurance activities were rated higher (41 percent and 38 percent respectively) than policy development activities (28 percent). The highest rated activities were implementation of mandated programs (91 percent), investigations of adverse health events (75 percent), and laboratory services (73 percent). The lowest rated activities were plans for resource allocation (10 percent), analysis of preventive services (12 percent), evaluation of services (16 percent), community action plans (16 percent), and allocating resources for priorities (18 percent).

The perceived share of effort contributed by LPHAs for 20 measures of public health practice was 67 percent in the nation's most populous health jurisdictions in 1998. LPHAs were responsible for 80 percent of the total effort for assurance activities, 60 percent for assessment activities, and 58 percent for policy development activities. LPHAs contributed most heavily to organizational self-assessment (87 percent), provision of information to the media (77 percent), investigations of adverse health events (76 percent), information for elected officials (74 percent), and monitoring and evaluation of programs (71 percent). LPHAs contributed least to support and communication networks (46 percent) provision or linkage of services (48 percent) allocating resources for priority needs (50 percent), community action plans (50 percent), and laboratory services (50 percent).

Many different organizations partner with LPHAs in carrying out public health's core functions and essential services. These include state health agencies, hospitals, nonprofit agencies, other agencies of local government, private healthcare providers, universities, health centers, managed care plans, and federal agencies. The participation of these partners varies from activity to activity. Overall, they contribute about one-third of the activities that comprise local public health practice in LHJs with populations over 100,000.

Together these findings suggest that performance of core functions and essential public health services can be greatly improved. Because the concepts used to assess performance were basically standards of public health practice, these measurement and surveillance activities served to promote their adoption by the public health community. These same performance expectations are also advanced in several other initiatives that trace their roots to the IOM report.

Public Health Standards Based on Core Functions

Standards are basically performance expectations. Public health standards, when used prior to 1990, primarily related to capacities and the output aspects of public health practice, rather than the key processes necessary to carry out the public health core functions characterized in the IOM report. Standards for public health practice developed after 1990 have focused both on key processes and outputs and have proven useful in a variety of applications, including agency self-assessment for capacity building, measures of performance in state/local public health systems, and state and national surveillance of practice performance. Still, these standards are in an early stage of development.

The 1990s witnessed many public health organizations conducting organizational self-assessments, identifying strengths and weaknesses, and channeling this information into organizational capacity building plans. The panel of performance expectations for local public health practice in APEXPH served as a blueprint for many public health agencies seeking to focus and strengthen their roles in their communities. APEXPH adoption and implementation experience has been substantial, although not universal. Where APEXPH has been implemented widely, public health practice performance has been found to be substantially higher than where it is less frequently used. However, few self-assessment tools other than APEXPH have been widely used within the public health community and even APEXPH has lacked a strategic planning component and a focus on community public health systems. States are using a variety of approaches based on core functions and the essential public health services framework to establish standards for public health practice in order to improve performance. The following examples from Washington State and Illinois illustrate some of these approaches.

The state legislature in Washington adopted a framework for a statewide public health improvement plan in 1994 and directed the public health community to identify the capacities needed to carry out core functions, the total cost associated with these capacities, the extent to which the capacities were in place, the difference between current and necessary capacity, and the funding needed to close the gap. Capacity categories needed to address public health core functions were identified, and capacity standards were developed. Subsequent concerns emerged that these capacity standards were overly subjective and not equally applicable for local health jurisdictions with different characteristics. This prompted the development of process and output standards for state and local public health agencies organized around community health assessment and four broad output-related categories (preventing illness and injury, protecting against environmental risks, promoting healthy behaviors, and assuring quality health services).[37] These performance standards are described in Exhibit 5–8; they are to be used as the basis for contracts between the state and its local public health agencies.

Local public health agencies in Illinois have been subject to performance standards established by the state since the 1970s. After a series of strategic planning activities, beginning about 1985, these performance standards were revised, effective in 1993, changing the basis of certification by the state to standards based on processes (including outputs) related to public health core functions[38,39] (Exhibit 5–9). The revised certification requirements call for LHPAs to implement an adaptation of APEXPH known as Illinois Plan for Local Assessment of Needs (IPLAN), including both the organizational self-assessment and community health improvement planning components of APEXPH. This produced substantial change in patterns of performance of core function-related practices, nearly doubling performance scores over a two-year period from 1992

Exhibit 5–8 Washington State Public Health Standards, 2001

Understanding Health Issues
1. Public health assessment skills and tools are in place in all public health jurisdictions and their level is continuously maintained and enhanced.
2. Information about environmental threats and community health status is collected, analyzed, and disseminated at intervals appropriate for the community.
3. Public health program results are evaluated to document effectiveness.
4. Health policy decisions are guided by health assessment information, with involvement of representative community members.
5. Health data is handled so that confidentiality is protected and health information systems are secure.

Protecting People from Disease
1. A surveillance and reporting system is maintained to identify emerging health threats.
2. Response plans delineate roles and responsibilities in the event of communicable disease outbreaks and other health risks that threaten the health of people.
3. Communicable disease investigation and control procedures are in place and actions are documented.
4. Urgent public health messages are communicated quickly and clearly and actions are documented.
5. Communicable disease and other risk responses are routinely evaluated for opportunities for improving public health system response.

Assuring a Safe, Healthy Environment for People
1. Environmental health education is a planned component of public health programs.
2. Services are available throughout the state to respond to environmental events or natural disasters that threaten the public's health.
3. Both environmental health risks and environmental health illnesses are tracked, recorded, and reported.
4. Compliance with environmental health regulations is sought through enforcement actions.

---

continues

Exhibit 5–8 continued

Prevention Is Best: Promoting Healthy Living
1. Policies are adopted that support prevention priorities and that reflect consideration of scientifically-based public health literature.
2. Active involvement of community members is sought in addressing prevention priorities.
3. Access to high quality prevention services for individuals, families, and communities is encouraged and enhanced by disseminating information about available services and by engaging in and supporting collaborative partnerships.
4. Prevention, early intervention, and outreach services are provided directly or through contracts.
5. Health promotion activities are provided directly or through contracts.

Helping People Get the Services They Need
1. Information is collected and made available at both the state and local level to describe the local health system, including existing resources for public health protection, health care providers, facilities, and support services.
2. Available information is used to analyze trends which, over time, affect access to critical health services.
3. Plans to reduce specific gaps in access to critical services are developed and implemented through collaborative efforts.
4. Quality measures that address the capacity, process for delivery, and outcomes of critical health care services are established, monitored, and reported.

Example of Local and State Performance Measures
Protecting People from Disease and Injury: Standard 3—Communicable disease investigation and control procedures are in place and actions documented.

Local measures:
1. Lists of private and public sources for referral to treatment are accessible to LHJ staff.
2. Information is given to local providers through public health alerts and newsletters about managing reportable conditions.
3. Communicable disease protocols require that investigations begin within 1 working day, unless a disease-specific protocol defines an alternate time frame. Disease-specific protocols identify information about the disease, case investigation steps, reporting requirements, contact and clinical management (including referral to care), use of emergency biologics, and the process for exercising legal authority for disease control (including non-voluntary isolation). Documentation demonstrates staff member actions are in compliance with protocols and state statutes.
4. An annual evaluation of a sample of communicable disease investigations is done to monitor timeliness and compliance with disease specific protocols.
5. LHJs identify key performance measures for communicable disease investigation and enforcement actions.
6. Staff members conducting disease investigations have appropriate skills and training as evidenced in job descriptions and resumes.

State measures:
1. Consultation and staff time are provided to LHJs for local support of disease intervention management during outbreaks or public health emergencies, as documented by case write-ups. Recent research findings relating to the most effective population-based methods of disease prevention and control are provided to LHJs. Labs are provided written protocols for the handling, storage, and transportation of specimens.

continues

Exhibit 5–8 continued

2. DOH leads statewide development and use of a standardized set of written protocols for communicable disease investigation and control, including templates for documentation. Disease-specific protocols identify information about the disease, case investigation steps, reporting requirements, contact and clinical management (including referral to care), use of emergency biologics, and the process for exercising legal authority for disease control (including non-voluntary isolation). Documentation demonstrates staff member actions are in compliance with protocols and state statutes.
3. An annual evaluation of a sample of state communicable disease investigations and consultations is done to monitor timeliness and compliance with disease specific protocols.
4. DOH identifies key performance measures for communicable disease investigations and consultation.
5. Staff members conducting disease investigations have appropriate skills and training as evidenced in job descriptions and resumes.

Source: Reprinted from *Standards for Public Health in Washington State,* Washington State Department of Health, 2001.

Exhibit 5–9 Requirements for Certification of Local Health Departments in Illinois before and after July 1993

Before July 1993, To Be Certified as a Local Health Department in Illinois	*After July 1993, to Be Certified as a Local Health Department in Illinois*
A local health agency must carry out the following programs:	A local health agency must:
1. food sanitation	1. assess health needs of the community
2. potable water	2. investigate health effects and hazards
3. maternal health/family planning	3. advocate and build community support
4. child health	4. develop policies and plans to address needs
5. communicable disease control	5. manage resources
6. private sewage	6. implement programs
7. solid waste	7. evaluate and provide quality assurance
8. nuisance control	8. inform and educate the public
9. chronic disease	
10. administration	

to 1994.[40] Performance measures for Illinois LHPAs are similar to those described in Exhibit 5–7. There is explicit authority in state law for the state health agency to establish performance standards for LHPAs. The standards are promulgated through the state rulemaking process, with compliance reviews conducted every five years by the state health agency. Longitudinal assessments of performance of these practices in 1992, 1994, and 1999 have been linked with selected capacity factors, as well as with outcomes related to community health priorities identified in the first round of IPLAN implementation.

Experiences such as those found in these states, as well as Missouri, California, Oregon, Florida, Michigan, South Carolina, and others, have laid the foundation for development of a national public health performance standards program. The overall lack of uniformity and consistency among these various state efforts reflects the different needs, values, and circumstances of the relatively autonomous state/local public health networks across the United States. In part due to this diversity in type and focus of performance standards, the CDC's Public Health Practice Program Office has promoted the development of national public health performance standards for use in several complementary applications. These applications include:

1. self-assessment and continuous improvement of local public health systems as part of the MAPP process;
2. surveillance of the public health system nationally and longitudinally;
3. accreditation of public health organizations; and
4. performance standards for use in state/local systems.

The National Public Health Standards Program represents a partnership among national and state public health organizations to improve the public health delivery system through the development of local and state-based performance standards focused on capacity and processes, the systematic collection and analysis of performance-based data, and a national leadership effort to improve system-wide performance. NACCHO has coordinated the development of standards for local public health systems, the Association of State and Territorial Health Officials (ASTHO) has led the development of standards for state health agencies, and the National Association of Local Boards of Health (NALBOH) has guided the development of governance standards for local boards of health. Exhibit 5–10 provides examples of performance measures for local public health practice derived from this process. Complementary to these standards is an extensive panel of national health objectives for the public health infrastructure,[41] which is included in Healthy People 2010 (see Chapter 6). Primary goals for both these efforts are to improve quality, enhance accountability, and strengthen the science base of public health practice.

A variety of salutary effects has been cited as potential benefits of a nationwide public health performance standards initiative. These include: improved accountability; better resource deployment; enhanced capacity building for community, state, and national public health systems; widespread use of best practices; and greater focus on mission and goals.[42] Depending on the lens used, each of these can be viewed as quality improvement, although widespread implementation of national public health performance standards presents formidable challenges.

The establishment of a national accreditation or certification initiative for LHPAs, through either the national public health organizations or the Joint Commission on Accreditation of Healthcare Organizations (JCAHO), has recently received serious consideration. Absent a federal initiative to support and fund core functions and essential public health services in state/local public health systems through block grants to states, a voluntary national accreditation program for LHPAs may emerge as the most realistic approach to promoting widespread adoption of practice standards related to the core functions.

Exhibit 5–10 Example of Public Health Performance Standards from Local Public Health Systems Instrument, 2003

Essential Service 2
Diagnose and Investigate Health Problems and Health Hazards in the Community

Indicators:
2.1 Identification and surveillance of health threats
2.2 Plan for public health emergencies
2.3 Investigate and respond to public health emergencies
2.4 Laboratory support for investigation of health threats

Standard for Indicator 2.3
In order to investigate public health emergencies, the local public health system:
2.3.1 Designates an emergency response coordinator
2.3.2 Develops written epidemiological case investigation protocols for immediate investigations of:
  • Communicable disease outbreaks,
  • Environmental health hazards,
  • Potential chemical and biological agent threats,
  • Radiological threats, and
  • Large scale disasters.
2.3.3 Maintains written protocols to implement a program of source and contract tracing for communicable diseases or toxic exposures
2.3.4 Maintains a roster of personnel with the technical expertise to respond to potential biological, chemical, or radiological public health emergencies
2.3.5 Evaluates past incidents for effectiveness and opportunities for improvement

Measures for Indicator and Standard 2.3
2.3.1   Has the local public health system designated an Emergency Response Coordinator?
If so,
2.3.1.1 Is there coordination with the local public health agency's Emergency Response Coordinator?
2.3.2   Does the local public health system have current epidemiological case investigation protocols to guide immediate investigations of public health emergencies?
If so, do these protocols address:
2.3.2.1 Communicable disease outbreaks?
2.3.2.2 Environmental heath threats?
2.3.2.3 Chemical threats?
2.3.2.4 Biological agent threats?
2.3.2.5 Radiological threats?
2.3.2.6 Large-scale natural disasters?
2.3.2.7 Possible terrorist incidents?
2.3.3   Does the local public health system maintain written protocols for implementing a program of source and contact tracing for communicable disease or toxic exposures?
If so, are protocols in place for:
2.3.3.1 Animal and vector control?
2.3.3.2 Exposure to food-borne illness?

continues

Exhibit 5–10 continued

2.3.3.3   Exposure to water-borne illness?
2.3.3.4   Exposure to lead levels?
2.3.3.5   Exposure to asbestos?
2.3.3.6   Exposure to other toxic chemicals?
2.3.3.7   Communicable diseases?
2.3.3.8   Radiological health threats?
2.3.4   Does the local public health system maintain a roster of personnel with the technical expertise to respond to potential biological, chemical, or radiological public health emergencies?
If so, does the local public health system have access to the following personnel within one hour? If so, are protocols in place for:
2.3.4.1   Chemists?
2.3.4.2   Emergency management?
2.3.4.3   Environmental health scientists?
2.3.4.4   State epidemiologists?
2.3.4.5   Hazardous materials response teams?
2.3.4.6   Health physicists?
2.3.4.7   Industrial hygienists?
2.3.4.8   Infectious disease specialists?
2.3.4.9   Law enforcement?
2.3.4.10 Medical examiners/coroner?
2.3.4.11 Microbiologists?
2.3.4.12 National Guard?
2.3.4.13 Occupational health physicians?
2.3.4.14 State public health laboratory director?
2.3.4.15 Toxicologists?
2.3.4.16 Veterinarians?
2.3.4.17 Funeral/Mortuary directors?
2.3.5   Does the local public health system evaluate public health emergency response incidents for effectiveness and opportunities for improvement?

Note: Responses for Indicators 2.3.1–2.3.5 (and their various sub-indicators) allow for four possible responses:
• Yes
• High partially
• Low partially
• No

2.3.6   How much of this local public health system standard is achieved by the local public health system collectively? (0–25%, 26–50%, 51–75%, 76–100%)
2.3.6.1   What percent of the response reported in 2.3.6 is the direct contribution of the local public health agency? (0–25%, 26–50%, 51–75%, 76–100%)

Source: Reprinted from Centers for Disease Control and Prevention, Public Health Practice Program Office. *The National Public Health Performance Standards: Guiding Collaborative Work to Strengthen Public Health Systems.* Atlanta GA; CDC-PHPPO; 2003.

Progress toward accrediting local public health agencies may accelerate with the implementation of a national certification program, NACCHO's Public Health Ready initiative, which focuses on bioterrorism and emergency readiness standards for local public health agencies (see Chapter 8).

NEW OPPORTUNITIES FOR IMPROVING PUBLIC HEALTH PRACTICE

Measuring performance of public health core functions and essential public health services is necessary but not sufficient to understand, control, and improve public health practice. Figure 5–5 expands the simple model presented in Chapter 1 (Figure 1–2), illustrating a more comprehensive approach to describing and measuring key aspects of the public health system. Because a system is a set of interdependent elements with a common purpose, the interdependencies are as much a part of the system as are the elements themselves. Interest in a system's "results" requires attention to the interdependencies generating that result. Measures of core function performance further an understanding of the relationships between and among key dimensions of the public health system when linked with measures of capacity and outcomes. This understanding is essential to improve public health practice.

A few studies have already shed light on some of these relationships. For example, the relationship between capacity and process performance (including outputs) has been examined in two studies. One study linked practice performance measures from a 1993 national survey with NACCHO Profile information for 264 LHPAs. Capacity factors linked to higher levels of practice performance included full-time agency head, larger annual expenditures, greater number of total and part-time staff, budgets derived from multiple funding sources, private health insurance as a significant budget component, and female agency heads.[43]

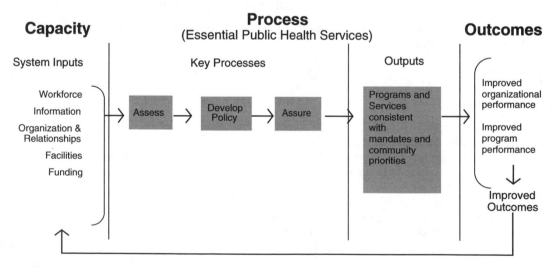

Figure 5–5 Framework for Measuring Public Health System Performance

A 1998 study of LHPAs in the most populous jurisdictions identified several capacity factors associated with higher levels of core function performance. These were population size, presence of a local board of health, existence of mixed or shared arrangements with state health agency, and participation in public health activities by managed care plans and universities.[35] This study also documented the substantial contribution (one-third of the total effort) to practice performance made by parties other than the governmental health agency in these jurisdictions. The most important contributors to process performance were state agencies, hospitals, local government agencies, nonprofit organizations, physicians and medical groups, universities, federally funded community health centers, managed care plans, and federal agencies.

The link between key processes and programs and services (outputs) offered by LHPAs can also be examined. One study linked higher levels of performance of key processes with a greater percentage of services directly provided, as well as with the following specific services: personal preventive treatment in maternal and child health, chronic disease personal prevention, health education, injury control, dental health, case management services, and HIV/AIDS testing.[43] In another study, only the provision of behavioral health services was linked with higher levels of performance of key public health processes.[35]

CONCLUSION

Several lessons are apparent after more than 90 years of trial and error. Early efforts to characterize and measure public health practice were limited by a narrower view of public health's core functions than that articulated in the IOM report. Performance of six specific services—components of the assurance function—was emphasized over more basic public health processes, such as community assessment and constituency building, linked to the assessment and policy development functions. In part, this was due to the lack of a comprehensive conceptual framework that links public health practice to capacity, process, and outcome measures.

The IOM report identified assessment and policy development functions to complement the longstanding view that public health's role is one of assurance. The essential public health services framework provides operational definitions for these concepts and establishes new standards for public health practice. Additional strategies and tools are now available to promote these practice standards and to measure their performance in public health systems. Despite these advances, there is little evidence of significant improvement in core function-related performance since the appearance of the IOM report and little progress toward a comprehensive examination of the links among capacity, processes, and outcomes and their relationship to an effective governmental presence. The clearest lesson after nine decades of efforts is that it has always been easier to measure specific aspects of public health practice and its core functions than to develop consensus as to what these measurements tell us about public health performance.

DISCUSSION QUESTIONS AND EXERCISES

1. What are the three core functions of public health, and how are these operationalized by public health organizations?
2. Explain the relationships among capacity, processes, and outcomes in Figure 5–5.
3. What features are similar among MAPP, PATCH, and Model Standards? What features are different?
4. Determine whether your LHPA has completed APEXPH or MAPP. If it has, what were the results? If it has not, why? What other approaches or tools were used?
5. Obtain the community health plan (or a summary) for your city or county and review the process that developed it for consistency with the 11 steps of Model Standards and with the essential public health services framework. In what ways did the process and plan differ from these frameworks?
6. Review the organization of health responsibilities in the state of your choice and describe how the three core functions of public health are delegated and carried out among various offices and agencies of state government beyond the state health department. The URL for a state is usually <http://www.state.stateinitials.us>. For example, Illinois would be <http://www.state.il.us>.
7. What role do tools such as PATCH, APEXPH, and MAPP play in carrying out public health's core functions at the local level?
8. How do current community-driven health planning models differ from resource-based planning models of the past?
9. You are the administrator of a typical county-based local health department in a midwestern state. Your newly elected county board president has ordered you to come up with new health-related initiatives that will improve the health of the county's residents. How would you approach this charge?
10. Review the progress of the past century related to reducing the toll from cardiovascular diseases ("Public Health Achievements in Twentieth-Century America, 1900–1999 Cardiovascular Disease Mortality") and related year-2010 objectives and leading indicators (Figure 5–3). To what extent is there a constituency group for these issues? Why would it be beneficial to the public's health to build or strengthen a constituent group for these issues?
11. What arguments can be made in support of national standards for public health organizations and systems? What arguments can be made against them?

REFERENCES

1. Institute of Medicine (IOM), Committee on the Future of Public Health. *The Future of Public Health*. Washington, DC: National Academy Press; 1988.
2. Turnock BJ, Handler AS. From measuring to improving public health practice. *Annu Rev Public Health*. 1997;18:261–282.
3. Vaughan HF. Local health services in the United States: The story of CAP. *Am J Public Health*. 1972;62:95–108.
4. American Public Health Association, Committee on Administrative Practice. Appraisal form for city health work. *Am J Public Health*. 1926;16(Suppl.):1–65.
5. Emerson H, Luginbuhl M. *Local Health Units for the Nation*. New York: Commonwealth Fund; 1945.
6. Shonick W. *Government and Health Services: Government's Role in the Development of U.S. Health Services 1930–1980*. New York: Oxford University Press; 1995.
7. Hanlon JJ. Is there a future for local health departments? *Health Serv Rep*. 1973;88:898–901.
8. American Public Health Association. *Healthy Communities 2000: Model Standards*. Washington, DC: American Public Health Association; 1991.
9. Scutchfield FD, Hiltabiddle SE, Rawding N, Violante T. Compliance with the recommendations of the IOM report, the future of public health: A survey of local health departments. *J Public Health Policy*. 1997;18:155–166.
10. Harrell JA, Baker EL. The essential services of public health. *Leadership in Public Health*. 1994;3(3):27–31.
11. Public Health Functions Steering Committee. *Public Health in America*. Washington, DC: U.S. Public Health Service (PHS); 1994.
12. Corso LC, Wiesner PJ, Halverson PK, Brown CK. Using the essential services as a foundation for performance measurement and assessment of local public health systems. *J Public Health Manage Pract*. 2000;6(5):1–18.
13. National Association of County and City Health Officials (NACCHO). *Assessment Protocol for Excellence in Public Health*. Washington, DC: NACCHO; 1991.
14. National Association of County and City Health Officials. *Mobilizing for Action through Planning and Partnerships*. Washington, DC: NACCHO; 2000.
15. Institute of Medicine. *Healthy Communities: New Partnerships for the Future of Public Health*. Washington, DC: National Academy Press; 1996.
16. Institute of Medicine. *Improving Health in the Community: A Role for Performance Monitoring*. Washington, DC: National Academy Press; 1997.
17. National Association of County and City Health Officials. *Local Public Health Agency Infrastructure: A Chartbook*. Washington, DC: NACCHO; 2001.
18. Minkler M. Ten commitments for community health education. *Health Edu Res Theory Pract*. 1994;9(4):527–534.
19. McKnight JL, Kretzmann J. Mapping community capacity. *New Designs*. 1992;Winter:9–15.
20. CDC/ATSDR Committee on Community Engagement. *Principles of Community Engagement*. Atlanta, GA: CDC; 1997.
21. University of Kansas. Community Tool Box. <http://ctb.lsi.ukans.edu>. Accessed 12 March 2003.
22. Public Health Foundation. *Healthy People 2010 Tool Kit*. Washington, DC: American Public Health Foundation; 1999.
23. National Association of County and City Health Officials (NACCHO). *Profile of Local Health Departments, 1996–1997 Data Set*. Washington, DC: NACCHO; 1997.
24. Berkowitz B. Collaboration for health improvement: Models for state, community, and academic partnerships. *J Public Health Manage Pract*. 2000;6(1):67–72.
25. Norris T. Healthy Communities. *Natl Civic Rev*. 1997;86(1):3–10.

26. Milio N. Priorities and strategies for promoting community-based prevention policies. *J Public Health Manage Pract.* 1998;4(3):14–28.

27. National Association of County and City Health Officials. *1990 National Profile of Local Health Departments.* Washington, DC: NACCHO; 1992.

28. National Association of County and City Health Officials. *1992–1993 National Profile of Local Health Departments.* Washington, DC: NACCHO; 1995.

29. Miller CA, Moore KS, Richards TB, Monk JD. A proposed method for assessing the performance of local public health functions and practices. *Am J Public Health.* 1994;84:1743–1749.

30. Richards TB, Rogers JJ, Christenson GM, Miller CA, Gatewood DD, Taylor MS. Assessing public health practice: Application of ten core function measures of community health in six states. *Am J Prev Med.* 1995;11(Suppl. 6):36–40.

31. Richards TB, Rogers JJ, Christenson GM, Miller CA, Taylor MS, Cooper AD. Evaluating local public health performance at a community level on a statewide basis. *J Public Health Manage Pract.* 1995;1(4):70–83.

32. Turnock BJ, Handler AS, Hall W, Potsic S, Nalluri R, Vaughn EH. Local health department effectiveness in addressing the core functions of public health. *Public Health Rep.* 1994;109:653–658.

33. Rohrer JE, Dominguez D, Weaver M, Atchison CG, Merchant JA. Assessing public health performance in Iowa's counties. *J Public Health Manage Pract.* 1997;3(3):10–15.

34. Turnock BJ, Handler AS, Miller CA. Core function-related local public health performance. *J Public Health Manage Pract.* 1998;4(5):26–32.

35. Mays GP, Miller CA, Halverson PK, Baker EL, Stevens R, Vann JJ. Availability and perceived effectiveness of public health activities in the nation's most populous communities. *Am J Public Health.* 2003 (in press).

36. Suen J, Gadsden-Knowles K, Sohani M. Public Health Jurisdiction Capabilities: Assessment of Core Function Related Performance. APHA 130th Annual Meeting Abstract Session 4109, 2002.

37. Washington State Department of Health. *Standards for Public Health in Washington State.* Olympia, WA: Washington State Department of Health; 2001.

38. Illinois Roadmap Implementation Task Force. *Improving the Public Health System: The Road to Better Health for All of Illinois.* Springfield, IL: Illinois Department of Public Health; 1990.

39. Illinois Local Health Liaison Committee. *Project Health: The Reengineering of Public Health in Illinois.* Springfield, IL: Illinois Department of Public Health; 1994.

40. Turnock BJ, Handler AS, Hall W, Lenihan DP, Vaughn EH. Capacity-building influences on Illinois local health departments. *J Public Health Manage Pract.* 1995;1(3):50–58.

41. U.S. Department of Health and Human Services (DHHS). *Healthy People 2010: Understanding and Improving Health.* Chapter 23 Public Health Infrastructure. Washington, DC: DHHS-PHS; 2000.

42. Halverson PK, Nicola RM, Baker EL. Performance measurement and accreditation of public health organizations: A call to action. *J Public Health Manage Pract.* 1998;4(4):5–7.

43. Handler AS, Turnock BJ. Local health department effectiveness in addressing the core functions of public health: Essential ingredients. *J Public Health Policy.* 1996;17:460–483.

Chapter 6

The Infrastructure
of Public Health

After the violin virtuoso had finished her concert presentation and was attempting to slip out of the orchestra hall through the delivery entrance, some adoring fans mobbed her. One particularly aggressive young man pushed his way to the front of the throng and grabbed the musician's hand, shaking it furiously. "Maestro, you played those notes just brilliantly tonight," he said. Taken a little aback by these circumstances, the violinist replied, "Young man, anyone can play the notes correctly. It's the spaces between the notes that present the real challenge."

Similar to the maestro's music, public health derives its effectiveness from both its notes and how they are blended together. This chapter will examine the basic ingredients of public health that are integrated to carry out its work. This ground-level view of public health focuses on infrastructure, a concept that is more easily understood outside the field of public health. When we think of infrastructure, we routinely think of roads, bridges, sewers, power lines, and water supplies. It is not easy to see the similarities between these concrete and visible structures in our communities and their counterparts in public health, although it can be useful to picture the public health infrastructure as a bridge over which trucks delivering public health services must pass. Needs and expectations are met by using more and bigger trucks to deliver more and better public health services, as illustrated in Figure 6–1. However, this approach has limitations in terms of the ability of the infrastructure to accommodate those trucks, just as the state of the nation's roads, bridges, and tunnels limits the effectiveness of the national transportation system. Attention to the infrastructure is essential for public health services to be delivered effectively.[1] There are, however, different views as to what the concept of public health infrastructure actually represents.

Infrastructure can be described in terms of both static and dynamic attributes. In a static representation, such as the bridge described previously, public health infrastructure is the basic foundation for public health activities; this foundation consists of building blocks and other basic materials. In a more dynamic representation, infrastructure is the capacity or capability of that foundation to carry out its main functions. Both of these views—what the infrastructure is and what the infrastructure does—provide useful insights into

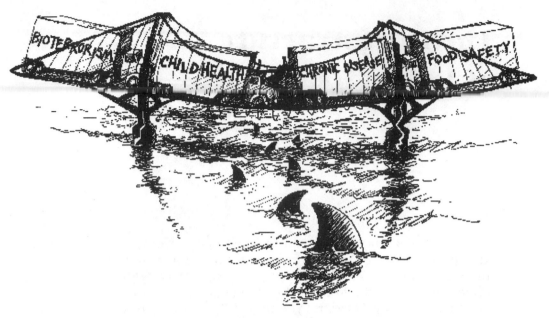

Figure 6–1 Public Health Infrastructure. *Source:* Reprinted from Public Health Practice Program Office, the Centers for Disease Control and Prevention, 1999.

the public health system and derive from the governmental presence in health concept described in Chapter 5. Importantly, both also portray infrastructure as essential for carrying out public health's core functions and essential public health services.

The public health infrastructure serves as the nerve center of the public health system, representing the capacity necessary to carry out public health's core functions. But it is also a composite that can be broken down to reveal the basic building blocks of the public health system. What makes the system's infrastructure difficult to describe fully is that public health itself is not neatly partitioned within our complex society. Nonetheless, this chapter will present a broad description of the public health infrastructure as it exists at the dawn of the new century. The key questions addressed are:

- What are the critical components of public health's infrastructure?
- What is the current status of these components?
- How can public health's infrastructure be enhanced?

INFRASTRUCTURE, INGREDIENTS, AND INPUTS

In simple terms, the public health infrastructure consists of the resources and relationships necessary to carry out the core functions and essential services of public health. Contributing to the system's capacity are some relatively recognizable resources: human, informational, financial, and organizational, including aspects of organizational relationships (such as statutes, leadership, and partnerships) that specify how the building blocks relate to each other—similar to the spaces between the notes in the maestro's response.

It is no simple task to separate the elements of the public health infrastructure into discrete categories. For example, drawing lines between the knowledge and skills of the workforce and information resources calls for an arbitrary distinction between what people do and what they are able to do after accessing information that is readily available to them. Other distinctions between organizational relationships within a community and individual leadership skills also lack clear boundaries. Financial resources can be considered as system resources or as a means of measuring the other resources in economic terms. Still, it is useful to categorize the elements of the public health infrastructure, realizing that they can be lumped or split in many different ways.

Human resources include the workforce of public health and the knowledge, skills, and abilities of public health workers. Organizational resources include the relationships among the various system participants—public and private—and the mechanisms that manage the system practices, including their statutory aspects, leadership components, and collaborative strategies. Information resources include various data, information, and communication systems. Fiscal resources are the funding levels and sources for the work of public health. Each of these elements contributes to the system's capacity to perform, and each will be examined in turn. Physical resources, such as equipment and physical facilities, are also necessary to carry out the work of public health. However, these will not be examined here.

HUMAN RESOURCES IN PUBLIC HEALTH

The human resources involved in carrying out the core functions and essential services of public health constitute the public health workforce. This definition links public health professionals to public health practice. Unfortunately, this does not simplify the task of determining who is, and who is not, part of the public health workforce. There has never been any specific academic degree or unique set of experiences that distinguish public health's workers from those in other fields. Many, if not most, public health workers have a primary professional discipline in addition to their attachment to public health. Physicians, nurses, dentists, social workers, nutritionists, health educators, anthropologists, psychologists, architects, sanitarians, economists, political scientists, engineers, epidemiologists, biostatisticians, managers, lawyers, and dozens of other professions and disciplines contribute to the field of public health. This multidisciplinary workforce, with somewhat divided loyalties to multiple professions, blurs the distinctiveness of public health as a profession. At the same time, however, it facilitates interdisciplinary approaches to community problem identification and problem solving.

Workforce Size and Composition

Although the precise size of the public health workforce is uncertain, it is small in comparison to the estimated 12 million workers in the entire health system at the turn of the new century. The overall health workforce has more than doubled in size since 1975 and has increased by more than 25 percent since 1990.[2] The Health Resources and Services Administration (HRSA) estimates that about seven million health workers can be classified as health professionals.[3] Nurses and allied health professionals constitute more than 75 percent of these professionals.

Enumerations and estimates of public health workers in general and public health professionals in particular suffer from several limitations: the definition of a public health professional is unclear; public health professionals working outside governmental public health agencies are difficult to identify; and not all employees of governmental public health agencies have public health responsibilities associated with their jobs. Identifying specific types of public health professionals is also difficult because many have other professional affiliations. Due to these limitations, a clear picture of the public health workforce is not available. Best estimates, however, suggest that the number of public health workers is approximately 500,000, representing only a small proportion (about 4 percent) of all health workers. About half of the public health workforce fit into various classifications of health professionals.

A definitive enumeration of the public health workforce does not exist, although an HRSA-commissioned estimate identified 458,000 public health workers in 2000.[4] Included in this total were approximately 86,000 federal employees, 156,000 state workers, 151,000 local government workers, and 64,000 individuals not working for any level of government.

Prior to 1990, HRSA had estimated the size of the public health workforce at about 500,000 workers,[5] suggesting a moderate reduction in the size of the public health workforce during the 1990s. That may not have been the case, however, as the methods used for the enumeration in the late 1980s differed from those used in 2000. Also, data from the national employment census indicate that the number of full time equivalent (FTE) workers in state and local health agencies has been increasing steadily throughout the 1990s, more than offsetting a slight reduction in the number of federal health workers.[6] The number of FTE employees working for governmental health agencies was about 480,000 FTEs in 1993 (128,000 federal, 163,000 state, 189,000 local). By 2001, the total was 535,000 (120,000 federal, 179,000 state, 236,000 local).

In the 1980s, according to HRSA estimates, the public health workforce was about equally divided among the three levels of government. Slightly more than one-third were employed by federal agencies, slightly less than one-third were employed in state agencies, and the remaining one-third worked in local public health agencies and other local settings, spread among private, voluntary, community, and academic organizations.[5] The public health workforce enumeration completed in 2000 also found about equal one-third shares at the state and local levels, but less than 20 percent at the federal level and about 14 percent outside government entirely. Government employment census data, which excludes non-governmental workers, also classify about one-third as state workers, but 45 percent as employees of local government and 22 percent working for federal agencies. It is likely that the HRSA enumeration in 2000 slightly overestimates federal public health workers and moderately undercounts local and non-governmental public health workers. The governmental employment census data includes workers who do not perform public health work and, by definition, excludes non-governmental public health workers. These findings are not altogether inconsistent in that the HRSA 2000 enumeration probably undercounted workers of local public

Exhibit 6–1 The Necessity for Trained and Educated Health Officials

There has probably been no time in the history of this country when trained, competent and efficient health officers were needed so much as they are now. The average health officer is appointed without any special training or qualification. . . . His tenure of office is so slight that very few feel warranted in qualifying themselves for such duties. . . . No one is eligible to such appointment in Great Britain without special training and his qualification having been established by examination; his position is then assured and he is not subject to removal with change in administration. It ought to be axiomatic that no health officer, no health commissioners, no executive officer of a board of health, should anywhere be appointed, until after thorough examination, or training in a subordinate capacity, and until he had evinced special aptitude for and interest in that line of work. A great misfortune in this country is that whenever a change of administration is brought about, it is considered necessary to change officers of health. . . . Instances frequently occur, involving great responsibility, where the appointee is wholly incompetent, and is dependent upon the subordinates in his office for information and advice; in short, is compelled to learn the duties incumbent upon him at the expense of the life and treasure of the public. . . .

In all civilized countries, except the United States, there are some special qualifications required for this office, and just in proportion as they are exacted, in the same proportion is the community protected from preventable diseases; from unnecessary panics with the suffering incident thereto, and from the economic loss caused thereby. . . . It is unfortunate that in the absence of epidemics or pestilence, too little attention is paid to the protection of the public health, and as a necessary consequence, to the selection of those whose duties require them to guard the public health. Laws should be passed in all the States defining the qualifications necessary for eligibility for appointment of health officers. This is the direction of a civil service reform much needed.

Source: Reprinted from the *Journal of the American Medical Association,* Vol. 20, p. 189, © 1893, American Medical Association. All rights reserved.

health agencies whose increase likely reflects the changes in community public health practice described in Chapter 5. Together these data sources suggest that the actual total approximates 500,000 full time workers.

Although recent decades have witnessed an increase in the number of public health workers employed by non-governmental agencies due to expanded partnerships for public health priorities, governmental public health workers are often considered the primary public health workforce. Their number, distribution, training, and competence are issues of public concern. Some of these concerns have persisted since the late nineteenth century, as suggested by an editorial appearing in the Journal of the American Medical Association more than 110 years ago. (see Exhibit 6–1)

The HRSA 2000 enumeration categorized 4 percent of public health workers in administrative positions, 45 percent in professional positions, 9 percent in technical positions, and 18 percent in various clerical/support positions (Figure 6–2). However, 25 percent could not be assigned to one of these categories. As a result the proportion of professionals within the public health workforce cannot be determined with precision.

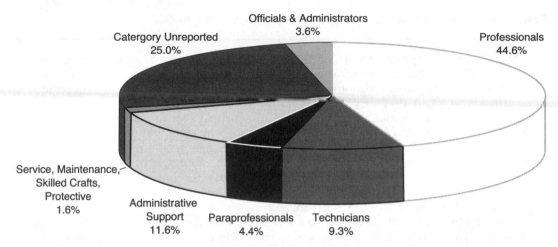

Figure 6–2 Percent of Public Health Workers in Selected Occupational Categories, United States, 2000. *Source:* Health Resources Services Administration, U.S. Department of Health and Human Services. *Public Health Enumeration 2000.* Washington, DC: Government Printing Office, December 2000.

Studies of local public health agencies indicate that three positions are found in more than two-thirds of all local public health agencies (LPHAs)—public health nurse, administrator, and sanitarian/environmental health specialist.[7,8] These positions are present in large and small agencies alike. The next most frequent positions (registered nurse, dietitian/nutritionist, licensed practical nurse, nurse practitioner, health educator, and social worker) are filled in only 20–33 percent of LPHAs. There is considerable variation in the proportion of LPHAs, with these positions depending on agency size. For example, health educators are employed in only 10 percent of LPHAs serving populations under 50,000 persons, but in 85 percent of agencies serving 500,000 or more. Two general patterns of LPHA staffing exist around a core set of employees. One pattern focuses on clinical services; the other on more population-based programs.[9] The core employees consist of dietitian/nutritionists, sanitarians/ environmental specialists, administrators, lab specialists, and health educators. The clinical pattern adds physicians, nurses, and dental health workers. The population-based pattern includes epidemiologists, public health nurses, social workers, and program specialists.

The availability of information on public health workers at the state and local level varies from state-to-state and is often inconsistent and incomplete. Detailed information from the official state health departments has not been available since the late 1980s and even then did not include public health workers employed by other state agencies. The periodic profiles of LPHAs completed by the National Association of County and City Health Officials (NACCHO) provide only general data on the proportion of responding agencies that employ specific public health job titles, either directly or through contracted services.[7,8] This information does not distinguish between those who are trained in public health and those who are not. Also, the total number of public health workers in the various job categories cannot be determined.

Table 6–1 Estimated Number and Percent of Public Health Professionals Employed in Agencies That Provide Population-Based Public Health Services, by Occupational Title, Texas, 1995

Title	Number	Percent
Nurse	1,180	15.3
Auditor, inspector, surveyor	1,078	13.9
Environmental health worker	988	12.8
Environmental health engineer	622	8.1
Health services administrator	597	7.7
Program specialist	394	5.1
Microbiologist	336	4.3
Social worker	307	4.0
Physician	273	3.5
Nutritionist	203	2.6
Chemist	175	2.3
Health educator	135	1.8
Behavioral or social scientist	135	1.8
Health planner/policy analyst	109	1.4
Other laboratory scientist	103	1.3
Disease investigator	96	1.2
Dental worker	94	1.2
Epidemiologist	86	1.1
Safety specialist	79	1.0
Industrial hygienist	71	0.9
Other laboratory worker	70	0.9
Biostatistician	68	0.9
Pharmacist	58	0.7
Veterinarian	34	0.4
Other	335	4.3
Title not specified	105	1.4
Total	7,731	99.9

Source: Reprinted from Kennedy et al., Public Health Workforce Information: A State Level Study, *Journal of Public Health Management & Practice,* 1999;5(3)10–19. © 1999, Lippincott, Williams & Wilkins.

There has been little progress toward clarifying and resolving these issues in recent years; a notable exception is a series of public health workforce studies in Texas.[10-12] An estimated 17,700 public health professionals in Texas represent about 3 percent of the total health workforce in that state. Only 7 percent had formal public health education. About 55 percent worked for population-based health agencies (mainly state and local public health departments); the other 45 percent worked in institutional public health settings (mainly as school health nurses and occupational health nurses). The largest occupational titles were nurses (15 percent), although several environmental titles combined (inspectors, workers, engineers) represented 35 percent of the public health workforce in 1995. A complete list of occupational titles is presented in Table 6–1. The percent of the public health workforce involved with each essential public health service varied, from 22 percent involved with researching for new insights to 60 percent involved with developing policies and plans that support individual and community health efforts[11] (Table 6–2).

Table 6–2 Estimated Number and Percentage of Public Health Professionals Employed in Agencies that Provide Population-Based Health Services, Texas, 1995

Essential Public Health Service	Number	Percentage
Monitor health status to identify community health problems	2,548	33.0
Diagnose and investigate health problems and health hazards in the community	2,175	28.1
Inform, educate, and empower people about health issues	2,809	36.3
Mobilize community partnerships to identify and solve health problems	2,319	30.0
Develop policies and plans that support individual and community health efforts	4,654	60.2
Enforce laws and regulations that protect health and ensure safety	3,053	39.5
Link people with needed personal health services and assure the provision of health care when otherwise unavailable	2,683	34.7
Ensure a competent public health and personal health care work force	3,009	38.9
Evaluate effectiveness, accessibility, and quality of personal and population-based health services	1,663	21.5
Research for new insights and innovative solutions to health problems	1,660	21.5

Source: Reprinted from Kennedy et al., Public Health Workforce Information: A State Level Study, *Journal of Public Health Management & Practice,* 1999;5(3)10–19. © 1999, Lippincott, Williams & Wilkins.

The criteria for defining the professional public health workforce used in a series of Texas studies overcome a number of previously cited obstacles by examining the public health workforce in several dimensions. These criteria represent the most useful operational description of the professional public health workforce developed to date. Key dimensions include:

- Employment setting—the individual must be employed by an organization engaged in an organized effort to promote, protect, and preserve the health of a defined population group. The group may be public or private, and the effort may be secondary or subsidiary to the principal objectives of the organization.
- Work content—the individual must perform work involving one or more of the essential public health services.
- Position—the individual must occupy a position that conventionally requires at least one year of post-secondary specialized public health training and that is (or can be) assigned a professional occupational title.[12]

Workforce Preparation

Information from public health agencies indicates that more than three-quarters of the public health workforce lack formal education and training in public health. While the proportion of those who have formal training varies by category of worker, the lack of formal training is striking in even some of the most critical categories. For example, a National Association of County and City Health Officials (NACCHO) survey in 1997 found that 78 percent of local health department leaders have had no formal public health education or training.[13] A survey of Illinois local health jurisdictions in 2000 yielded similar results, with 79 percent of local health agency administrators lacking formal preparation in public health.[14]

Only 44 percent of the 500,000 individuals in the public health workforce in 1989 had formal training in public health,[5] and the bulk of this training focused on a specific aspect of public health practice such as environmental health and public health nursing. These two groups comprised about 60 percent of those trained in public health; administrators and health educators comprised another 30 percent. Even among those with formal training in public health, public health workers with graduate degrees from schools of public health or other graduate public health programs represent only a small fraction. In view of the number of master's-level graduates of schools of public health and other graduate-level public health degree programs, about 7,000 in 2004, this is not surprising.

The lack of formal public health training is prevalent throughout the public health workforce. For example, the environmental health workforce included about 235,000 professionals in its total workforce of about 715,000 in the late 1980s, but only about 80,000 had received formal education in the environmental health sciences.

Evidence of the lack of formal training within this workforce, however, doesn't necessarily lead to the conclusion that public health workers are unprepared. On the contrary, public health workers enter the field having earned a wide variety of degrees and professional training credentials from non-public health academic programs and institutions. Often overlooked, these institutions produce the bulk of the public health workforce and represent major assets for addressing unmet needs. On-the-job training and work experience contribute substantially to the overall competency and preparedness of the public health workforce. For example, public health workers are frequently involved in responses to earthquakes, floods, and other disasters and have increasingly acquired and demonstrated skills in assessing community health needs and devising community health improvement plans. These are skills that most public health workers acquired through real world work experience rather than through their formal training.

Continuing Education

Continuing education for public health workers has long been a cottage industry involving many different parties. Academic institutions have certainly been contributors, but public health agencies at the state and local level, public health associations (national, state, and local), and other voluntary-sector health organizations have participated as well. Many different entities offer credits for continuing education, including professional organizations, academic institutions, and hospitals, among others. Public health workers value continuing education credits as a means to satisfy requirements of their core disciplines in order to maintain some level of credentialing status (such as licensed physicians and nurses, certified health education specialists, etc.). A few states, such as New Jersey, have adopted continuing education requirements for the public health disciplines licensed by that state. There is no formal system of public health-specific continuing education units (CEUs).

Workforce Development

The dearth of information on the public health workforce prompted the Public Health Functions Steering Committee to develop an ambitious set of recommendations in a 1997 report titled *Public Health Workforce: An Agenda for the 21st Century*,[15] calling for:

- Continued national oversight and planning for development of a public health workforce capable of delivering the essential public health services across the nation,
- Establishment of mechanisms to support workforce planning and training in all states and local jurisdictions,
- Greater use of a standard taxonomy to identify the size and distribution of the public health workforce in official agencies and private and voluntary organizations,
- Refinement and validation of public health practice competencies associated with each of the various professions that make up the workforce to improve basic, advanced, and continuing education curricula for the public health workforce and strategies to certify competencies among practitioners, and
- Strengthening of distance-learning strategies and technologies.

HRSA has long been the primary federal health agency supporting development of the various health professions, although the public health workforce has never been a priority for that agency. Since many public health workers come from other health disciplines, however, HRSA support for training other health professionals also benefits the public health workforce. Throughout the 1990s HRSA training activities for public health have focused increasingly on strengthening links between schools of public health (SPH) and public health agencies. Toward that end, HRSA funded a handful of schools to support fairly substantial projects while also providing minimal discretionary funding for all accredited SPHs. Early in the 1990s HRSA initiated support for the Council on Linkages between Academia and Practice, which has grown to include representation from many prominent public health academic and practice organizations. Since 1999 HRSA has funded Public Health Training Centers, which are multi-state training collaborations involving SPHs and health agencies, with 14 such centers (with approximately $5 million in annual funding) operating in late 2003. Beginning in 2002, HRSA also funded states and several large cities to support hospital bioterrorism planning and provides funds for curriculum development and training for health care professionals and for community-wide planning related to bioterrorism and other public health emergencies.

During the 1990s the Centers for Disease Control and Prevention (CDC) became increasingly engaged in supporting capacity development and improving state-based public health systems. The Public Health Practice Program Office (PHPPO) within CDC spearheaded these efforts, which included the establishment of national and regional leadership development projects in the early 1990s and direct financial assistance to state public health systems for emergency preparedness later in that decade. CDC encouraged states and large cities to utilize this funding to improve the basic capacities of their public health infrastructure in order to respond to a wide range of both emergency and routine threats, including bioterrorism preparedness. CDC increasingly emphasized and supported developing the public health workforce as the cornerstone of infrastructure improvement. Between October 2000 and October 2002, through its Cooperative Agreement with the Association of Schools of Public Health, CDC awarded substantial grants (approximately $1 million per center per year) to 22 academic Centers for Public Health Preparedness. The institutions funded and geographic regions served are strikingly similar to that of the HRSA-funded network of Public Health Training Centers. Preparedness Centers collaborate with CDC in the development and deployment of training activities consistent with a planning process facilitated by CDC through a series of national workshops beginning in the year 2000.[16] Progress slowed after September 2001 as CDC refocused its resources on bioterrorism preparedness and response as a national security priority. The process re-engaged in early 2003 with growing consensus on the broad strokes of that plan, although many key issues remain unresolved, including the relative roles and responsibilities of the federal agencies, national public health organizations, and academic institutions under any national plan.

Initial strategic planning for national public health workforce development focused on six basic strategies, which provided an initial roadmap for public health workforce preparedness efforts. The strategic elements convey a logical, but incomplete, series of steps that begin with identifying the public health workforce and monitoring its composition over time and then developing and deploying relevant training interventions through integrated delivery systems. Various forms of incentives, such as credentialing, would be established to increase the demand for effective training interventions. These efforts, taken together, would better serve the needs of public health organizations and systems, which would serve to assure the availability of adequate resources. As illustrated in Figure 6–3, competencies are the heart of these public health workforce development systems.[17] Realizing that the diverse public health workforce has widely varying training needs, several priority categories have been identified, although demarcations among categories are not always clear: frontline public health workers, senior professional staff, highly specialized professional staff, and public health leaders.

Despite the lack of a final and agreed-on national plan, CDC- and HRSA-funded training centers generally organize their efforts around this matrix of strategies and workforce categories. Since 1998 funding for public health workforce development through SPHs has increased dramatically, from under a million dollars (primarily from HRSA) in 1997 to more than $25 million (mainly from CDC) in 2003. Approximately $90 million more for public health training is available in the bioterrorism grants awarded to states and several large cities, an estimated 10 percent of those grants. A total of more than $100 million is being programmed specifically for public health workforce development in 2003, in addition to resources that prepare other health professionals to participate in responses to public health emergencies.

1. Assess Competency Using
   Consistent Methods and Tools

2. Enhance Specific Competencies
   Based on Assessment

3. Verify Competent Performance in
   Workplace via Human Resource
   Management

4. Recognize Competent Performance
   via System Incentives such as
   Credentialing

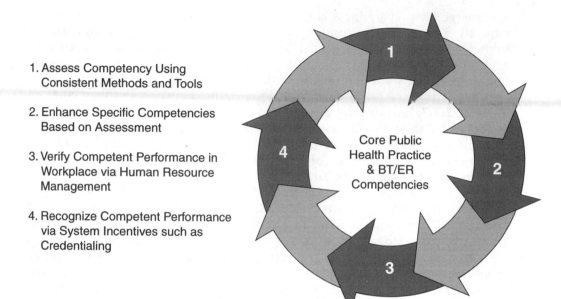

Figure 6–3 Components of a Public Health Workforce Preparedness Management System

There is only piecemeal information as to the extent of organized workforce development activities within state and local health departments and other public health organizations. Nonetheless, virtually all public health organizations provide some form of orientation, training, and support of continuing education for their workers. Costs for these activities are often buried in agency budgets as human resources, administrative support, and employee travel expenditures encompassing both direct and indirect, or opportunity, costs for time spent away from performing official duties. Aggregating these costs would likely demonstrate that they represent a significant pool of resources.

Anecdotal information, historical as well as current, suggests that there are acute shortages of specific categories of public health workers, such as epidemiologists and public health nurses. There also appears to be increasing demand for graduate-level education in public health, as evidenced by the steady increase in the number of schools of public health and public health graduates. It is not clear whether these perceptions are accurate and whether they will eventually translate into an expanding professional public health workforce.

Public Health Practitioner Competencies

In comparison to the modest progress in identifying and enumerating the public health workforce, there has been considerably greater progress over recent years in delineating the competencies and skills necessary for public health practice. Many of these initiatives have their roots in the Institute of Medicine (IOM) report of 1988.[18] A key development was the convening of public health practitioners and academics in 1990 through a Public Health Faculty/Agency Forum to outline a set of core competencies for public health professionals.[19] These core competencies were expanded and revised by the Council on Linkages between Academia and Public Health Practice in 2001 and adopted by the national public health practice organizations as the basis for assessing and enhancing the skills of public health workers (Exhibit 6–2). These core competencies have been linked with the essential public health services framework[20] as demonstrated in Exhibit 6–3. The core competencies also serve as a useful benchmark for competency frameworks developed to serve state or local public health systems or to guide the development of more focused skills, such as in public health law, informatics, genomics, and emergency preparedness.

Exhibit 6–2 Core Competencies for All Public Health Workers

Analytical and Assessment Competencies
- Defines a problem
- Determines appropriate uses of both quantitative and qualitative data
- Selects and defines variables relevant to defined public health problems
- Identifies relevant and appropriate data and information sources
- Evaluates the integrity and comparability of data and identifies gaps in data sources
- Applies ethical principles to the collection, maintenance, use, and dissemination of data and information
- Partners with communities to attach meaning to collected quantitative and qualitative data
- Makes relevant inferences from quantitative and qualitative data
- Obtains and interprets information regarding risks and benefits to the community
- Applies data collection processes, information system technology applications, and computer systems storage/retrieval strategies
- Recognizes how the data illuminates ethical, political, scientific, economic, and overall public health issues

Policy and Program Competencies
- Collects, summarizes, and interprets information relevant to an issue
- States policy options and writes clear and concise policy statements
- Identifies, interprets, and implements public health laws, regulations, and policies related to specific programs
- Articulates the health, fiscal, administrative, legal, social, and political implications of each policy option
- States the feasibility and expected outcome of each policy option
- Utilizes current techniques in decision analysis and health planning
- Decides on the appropriate course of action
- Develops a plan to implement the policy, including goals, outcome and process objectives, and implementation steps
- Translates policy into organizational plans, structures, and programs
- Prepares and implements emergency response plans
- Develops mechanisms to monitor and evaluate programs for their effectiveness and quality

continues

Exhibit 6–2 continued

Communication Competencies
- Communicates effectively both in writing and orally (unless a handicap precludes one of these forms of communication)
- Solicits input from individuals and organizations
- Advocates for public health programs and resources
- Leads and participates in groups to address specific issues
- Uses the media, advanced technologies, and community networks to communicate information
- Effectively presents accurate demographic, statistical, programmatic, and scientific information for professional and lay audiences
- Listens to others in an unbiased manner, respects points of view of others, and promotes the expression of diverse opinions and perspectives

Cultural Competencies
- Utilizes appropriate methods for interacting sensitively, effectively, and professionally with persons from diverse cultural, socioeconomic, educational, racial, ethnic, and professional backgrounds, and persons of all ages and lifestyle preferences
- Identifies the role of cultural, social, and behavioral factors in determining the delivery of public health services
- Develops and adapts approaches to problems that take into account cultural differences
- Understands the dynamic forces contributing to cultural diversity
- Understands the importance of a diverse public health workforce

Community Practice Competencies
- Establishes and maintains linkages with key stakeholders
- Utilizes leadership, team building, negotiation, and conflict resolution skills to build community partnerships
- Collaborates with community partners to promote the health of the population
- Identifies how public and private organizations operate within a community
- Accomplishes effective community engagements
- Can identify community assets and available resources
- Develops, implements, and evaluates a community public health assessment
- Describes the role of government in the delivery of community health services

Basic Public Health Competencies
- Identifies the individual's and organization's responsibilities within the context of the Essential Public Health Services and core functions
- Defines, assesses, and understands the health status of populations, determinants of health and illness, factors contributing to health promotion and disease prevention, and factors influencing the use of health services
- Understands the historical development, structure, and interaction of public health and health care systems
- Identifies and applies basic research methods used in public health
- Applies the basic public health sciences including behavioral and social sciences, biostatistics, epidemiology, environmental public health, and prevention of chronic and infectious diseases and injuries
- Identifies and retrieves current relevant scientific evidence
- Identifies the limitations of research and the importance of observations and interrelationships
- Develops a lifelong commitment to rigorous critical thinking

continues

Exhibit 6–2 continued

Management Competencies
- Develops and presents a budget
- Manages programs within budget constraints
- Applies budget processes
- Develops strategies for determining budget priorities
- Monitors program performance
- Prepares proposals for funding from external sources
- Applies basic human relations skills to the management of organizations, motivation of personnel, and resolution of conflicts
- Manages information systems for collection, retrieval, and use of data for decision-making
- Negotiates and develops contracts and other documents for the provision of population-based services
- Conducts cost-effectiveness, cost-benefit, and cost utility analyses

Leadership Competencies
- Creates a culture of ethical standards within organizations and communities
- Helps create key values and shared vision and uses those principles to guide action
- Identifies internal and external issues that may impact delivery of essential public health services (i.e. strategic planning)
- Facilitates collaboration with internal and external groups to ensure participation of key stakeholders
- Promotes team learning and organizational learning
- Contributes to development, implementation, and monitoring of organizational performance standards
- Uses the legal and political system to effect change
- Applies theory of organizational structures to professional practice

Source: Council on Linkages between Academia and Public Health Practice.

Exhibit 6–3 Core Public Health Competencies Related to Essential Public Health Practice

Analytical and Assessment Competencies
- Defines a problem
- Determines appropriate uses of both quantitative and qualitative data
- Selects and defines variables relevant to defined public health problems
- Identifies relevant and appropriate data and information sources
- Evaluates the integrity and comparability of data and identifies gaps in data sources
- Applies ethical principles to the collection, maintenance, use, and dissemination of data and information
- Partners with communities to attach meaning to collected quantitative and qualitative data
- Makes relevant inferences from quantitative and qualitative data
- Obtains and interprets information regarding risks and benefits to the community
- Recognizes how the data illuminates ethical, political, scientific, economic, and overall public health issues

continues

Exhibit 6–3 continued

Policy and Program Competencies
- Collects, summarizes, and interprets information relevant to an issue
- States policy options and writes clear and concise policy statements
- Articulates the health, fiscal, administrative, legal, social, and political implications of each policy option
- States the feasibility and expected outcome of each policy option
- Decides on the appropriate course of action

Communication Competencies
- Communicates effectively both in writing and orally (unless a handicap precludes one of these forms of communication)
- Solicits input from individuals and organizations
- Leads and participates in groups to address specific issues
- Uses the media, advanced technologies, and community networks to communicate information
- Effectively presents accurate demographic, statistical, programmatic, and scientific information for professional and lay audiences
- Listens to others in an unbiased manner, respects points of view of others, and promotes the expression of diverse opinions and perspectives

Cultural Competencies
- Utilizes appropriate methods for interacting sensitively, effectively, and professionally with persons from diverse cultural, socioeconomic, educational, racial, ethnic, and professional backgrounds, and persons of all ages and lifestyle preferences
- Understands the dynamic forces contributing to cultural diversity

Community Practice Competencies
- Accomplishes effective community engagements
- Can identify community assets and available resources
- Develops, implements, and evaluates a community public health assessment
- Defines, assesses, and understands the health status of populations, determinants of health and illness, factors contributing to health promotion and disease prevention, and factors influencing the use of health services

Basic Public Health Competencies
- Identifies and applies basic research methods used in public health
- Applies the basic public health sciences including behavioral and social sciences, biostatistics, epidemiology, environmental public health, and prevention of chronic and infectious diseases and injuries

Management Competencies
- Develops and presents a budget
- Manages programs within budget constraints
- Applies budget processes
- Develops strategies for determining budget priorities
- Monitors program performance
- Prepares proposals for funding from external sources
- Applies basic human relations skills to the management of organizations, motivation of personnel, and resolution of conflicts
- Manages information systems for collection, retrieval, and use of data for decision-making

Leadership Competencies
- Creates a culture of ethical standards within organizations and communities
- Identifies internal and external issues that may impact delivery of essential public health services (i.e. strategic planning)

Source: Council on Linkages between Academia and Public Health Practice.

The Public Health Faculty/Agency Forum also formulated strategies to facilitate the expansion of these competencies within the public health workforce. Key recommendations called for:

- Strengthening relationships between the practice and academic sectors of the public health community,
- Improving the teaching, training, and practice of public health, and
- Establishing firm practice links between schools of public health and public health agencies.

In part, these strategies were a response to conclusions of the IOM report that the education of public health professionals had become isolated from the practice of public health. Both the delineation of competencies and the recommended implementation strategies have had a substantial impact on public health education and training since 1990. For example, most schools of public health have established public health practice offices to interface with practitioners and practice agencies and have developed ongoing affiliations agreements to cover faculty appointments, joint research agendas, technical assistance, and practice placements, among other activities.[21]

At the federal level, both HRSA and the Centers for Disease Control and Prevention (CDC) have sought to strengthen the bonds between education and practice. Both agencies served as co-sponsors of the Public Health Faculty/Agency Forum, and each has supported initiatives that would implement the forum's various recommendations. Educational resources contributing to this national network include 32 schools of public health (a number that has grown steadily over the past three decades), nearly 90 additional graduate training programs in public health, and as many as 300 other graduate-level training programs in areas related to public health, such as health administration, public health nursing, and environmental engineering.

The first school of public health was established in 1916 at Johns Hopkins School of Hygiene and Public Health with the support of the Rockefeller Foundation. By 1969 there were only 12 schools of public health, but that number grew to 32 by the year 2003, with about a half-dozen new schools in the pipeline. Before about 1970 students in public health training were primarily physicians or other disciplines with professional degrees; however, during the final decades of the twentieth century, more than two-thirds of the students entered public health training to obtain a primary postgraduate degree. Public health training evolved from a second degree for medical professionals to a primary health discipline. Schools of public health initially emphasized the study of hygiene and sanitation; subsequently, the basic public health curriculum has expanded into five core disciplines: biostatistics, epidemiology, health services administration, health education/behavioral science, and environmental science.

Reports from the Pew Health Professions Commission have also generated discussion and debate as to approaches that would expand public health competencies among other health professions within the health sector. The commission concluded that current trends within the health system would result in substantial surpluses of physicians, nurses, and even pharmacists and that the proliferation of allied health professions would reverse itself with the growth of multi-skilled professions as the health sector reengineered its service delivery activities. For public health, however, the commission projected a growth in demand for public health professionals also linked to the needs of an increasingly market-driven health system.[22] The expansion of public health skills within the health sector workforce can be addressed through additional public health education programs in schools of public health and other sites, through the provision of public health education and training to other health professionals, or both. In any event, the core competencies represent the educational products to be marketed and provided to new audiences of health professionals.

Large scale assessments of the need for education and training toward these core competencies are lacking. However, on the basis of assessments to date of the core function-related performance (using measures related to the essential public health services framework such as those presented in Chapter 5), great need exists for enhancing competencies of the workforce associated with the core functions and essential services of public health. For education and training of the public health workforce to be taken seriously, both academic and practice interests must merge into state or regional alliances or consortia. These aspirations appear achievable due to heightened interest in public health worker preparedness and an infusion of federal funding. As demonstrated in Figure 6–4, comprehensive workforce development strategies must focus not only on the worker, but on the organizations in which the work is performed.[12,23]

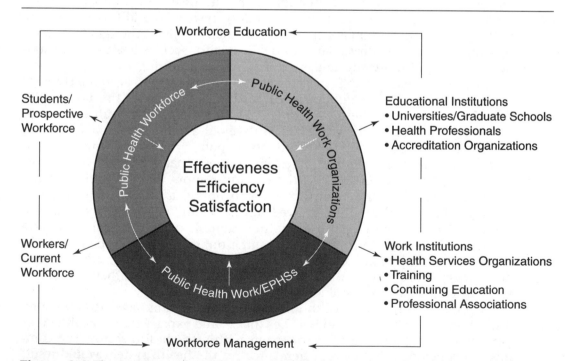

Figure 6–4 The Structure of a Public Health Work-Doing System. *Source:* Office of Workforce Policy and Planning, Public Health Practice Program Office, Centers for Disease Control and Prevention, 2002.

ORGANIZATIONAL RESOURCES

Organizational resources in public health include the complex web of federal, state, and local public health agencies described in Chapter 4, as well as mechanisms for linking public, private, and voluntary organizations through collaborative relationships. Before collaboration patterns are addressed, several organizational aspects of public health agencies merit discussion.

Organizational Aspects of Public Health Systems

Organizations are groups of individuals linked by common goals and objectives. This implies that each organization has a specific mission or purpose, resources appropriate to work toward that purpose, the ability to determine progress toward its goals and objectives, and a defined process for making decisions that change the direction or speed of the organization in pursuit of its goals. Each organization takes on a structure to delegate its activities to specific units or individuals and to coordinate the tasks among them. Communication pathways facilitate the accomplishment of the organization's goals and objectives. In one respect, communication channels define the organization, even as the organizational structure defines the communication pathways. A variety of forces shape an organization's ability to succeed, including its ability to survive in a changing environment. These include the organization's mission and leadership, as well as key aspects of its operations, such as planning, collaboration, and communications. The specifics of these organizational arrangements are best left to texts in health administration and organizational behavior; only selected pertinent issues will be addressed in this section.

Public-sector organizations differ in many important respects from their private- and voluntary-sector counterparts. The most obvious, and perhaps most important, difference is apparent in their bottom lines. The bottom line of public health agencies is measured in health outcomes, with efficiency and effectiveness valued, but not nearly as much. For the private sector, the bottom line is often profits and customer satisfaction, and efficiency and effectiveness are viewed as means to those ends. Many community and voluntary organizations address missions that resemble those of public agencies. However, public agencies often have political and bureaucratic environments that are unique among organizations. It should not be forgotten that employment itself is an important public objective, although the public sector lacks the ability to expand or contract its workforce rapidly in response to market conditions. In fact, public-sector jobs and services become even more important during times of economic recession.

The presence of a civil service-based workforce in many public health agencies is often cited as an impediment to getting things done, although the real problem may be more related to inadequate management practices than to institutionalized inertia. Civil service personnel systems were established in state and local governments, in large part through personnel standards fostered by Maternal and Child Health (MCH) funding with the enactment of Title V of the Social Security Act in 1935. Although the initial intent was to provide added security for government workers, there has been long-standing discontent with the system and tension and conflict between government workers and elected officials ever since. Civil service employees generally lack the power to strike, unlike their private-sector counterparts who are organized into unions.

For many years, public health agencies operated under a command-and-control approach to management. If a problem was assigned to the public health agency, the agency sought to acquire the resources needed to deal with that problem. Resources were deployed directly from the agency; this approach worked well when the major problems called for environmental engineering solutions or communicable disease control expertise. As problems became more complex, however, encroaching on the territory of other health and human service agencies, command-and-control approaches became problematic. To resolve delicate turf issues, cooperating with other agencies and collaborative approaches began to supplement more directly-controlled strategies.

These added to the challenges of public agency managers, which also included promoting workers' efficiency and effectiveness. Management training has never been well supported in the public sector, certainly not to the extent that it has been in the private sector. As a result, public health agencies often are poorly managed; this generates tensions and conflicts between professional staff and administrators brought into an agency to maximize efficiency and effectiveness, as well as between the agency and its community collaborators. For example, there has been a declining proportion of LPHA heads with medical degrees. For larger health departments (especially those serving populations of 100,000 or more), this trend is partly explained by the employment of non-physician agency heads to manage the increasingly complex array of community and clinical services. Clinical professionals in health departments have not always adjusted well to these changes, and the result has sometimes been management and morale problems.

Public health agencies at the state and local levels often have boards to guide their efforts. More than four-fifths of LPHAs reported the presence of a local board of health in the 1996–1997 NACCHO profile.[7] During the past century, boards have assumed roles less involved with direct agency operations than when initially established. Agency leadership today has assumed much of the direction of professional staff, and boards have retained roles of approving regulations, advising/approving agency budgets, and often hiring the agency director. The role of many local boards of health has become unclear and largely advisory to the agency, prompting debate as to their role in the modern practice of public health. In response to concerns over past and current roles, the IOM report calls for public health councils, so that any historic baggage attached to boards of health will be minimized. Public health agencies often have a plethora of advisory boards and committees developed for specific programs or activities. Although the proliferation of these advisory bodies can be seen as unwieldy and sometimes conflicting with the roles of more formally established bodies, such as the board of health itself, these groups also serve to greatly expand participation and communication with professional constituencies. Superfluous from a management perspective, these are, nevertheless, often effective constituency-building activities. Boards of health and various forms of advisory committees provide a link between the agency and the community it serves. Agency and community interests are better served by fostering the utilization of these relationships than by limiting or controlling them.

Within public health agencies, leadership positions carry several different responsibilities. The leader manages the agency, interacts with the major stakeholders and constituency groups, and carries out some largely ceremonial functions. The specific duties of the agency are vested in its director through statutes or ordinances; these are the only legal powers of that leader. Within state and local public health agencies, there has been a steady move away from physician directors of agencies, although about half of all LPHAs continue to hire physicians as chief executive officers. An evolving literature on leadership is developing within the public health community. CDC has developed a national public health leadership institute, and nearly a dozen regional and state-based leadership development initiatives were in place in the year 2000.

Leadership development programs are often organized around concepts such as envisioning the future, inspiring others to act, and generally acting through others. Public health leaders used these skills a century ago to foster public perceptions of sound science in action in deploying culture tubes and laboratory diagnostic capabilities in the war against infectious disease risks.

However, leadership in public health involves more than individual leaders or individuals in leadership positions. Public health is intimately involved in leadership as an agent of social change by identifying health problems and risks and stimulating actions toward their elimination. Because the work of public health emphasizes both collective and individual leadership, the battery of leadership principles and practices is pertinent throughout public health organizations and systems. In many respects, the tools described in Chapter 5 (Assessment Protocol for Excellence in Public Health [APEXPH], Mobilizing for Action through Planning and Partnerships [MAPP], Healthy Communities, etc.) are tools of and for public health leadership.

Non-governmental organizations have played major roles in public health activities since 1900. As the national network of federal, state, and local public agencies expanded and government assumed more responsibility for health issues, it assimilated public health initiatives that were initiated and supported by nongovernmental organizations. The modern public health system represents the work of both government and nongovernmental organizations. The Rockefeller Sanitary Committee's Hookworm Eradication during 1910–1920 stimulated the development of LPHAs; other foundations sponsored health department development and medical education reform. The National Tuberculosis Association worked for tuberculosis (TB) prevention and treatment, the National Consumers League championed maternal and infant health initiatives in the 1920s, the American Red Cross supported nutrition programs during the Depression years of the 1930s, and, in the 1940s and 1950s, the March of Dimes led the national effort to develop a successful polio vaccine. More recently, Mothers Against Drunk Driving began in 1980 through the efforts of a group of women in California (after a young girl was killed by an intoxicated driver) and grew into a national campaign for stronger laws against drunk driving. Professional organizations and labor unions also worked to promote public health. The American Medical Association advocated better vital statistics and safer foods and drugs. The American

Dental Association endorsed water fluoridation, despite the economic consequences to its members. Labor organizations worked for safer workplaces in industry. Today, non-governmental organizations sponsor diverse public health research projects and programs, including family planning, human immunodeficiency virus (HIV) prevention, violence prevention, vaccine development, and heart disease and cancer prevention.

Coalitions and Consortia

An increasingly important aspect of organizational resources is the ability to work through collaborative links with other agencies and organizations. Often, these arrangements are described as coalitions or consortia, although other terms are frequently used, and distinctions are often blurred (Exhibit 6–4).[24] Coalitions can be formed for short-term efforts or established to address ongoing problems on a long-term basis. They are most likely to be successful when they include representation from all groups affected by the problem and making efforts to deal with that problem. In general, coalitions and consortia are formal partnerships involving two or more groups working together to achieve specific goals according to a common plan. The rationale for a consortia approach is that the goals are believed to be beyond the capacity of any one participating organization. Goals can take various forms, from communication among members, to public and professional education, to advocating and lobbying for particular policy changes. It is essential that coalition members be in agreement that the problem is best addressed through a coalition approach and that they be comfortable with the scope of activities planned. Building on mutual interests allows a coalition to place expectations and demands on its member organizations. Most important, coalitions must do things that are important for their members; they must help their members, as well as the group.

Exhibit 6–4 Characteristics of Collaborative Organizations

Organization	Characteristics
Advisory committees	Generally respond to organizations or programs by providing suggestions and technical assistance
Commissions	Usually consist of citizens appointed by official bodies
Consortia and Alliances	Tend to be semiofficial, membership organizations; typically have broad policy-oriented goals, and may span large geographic areas; usually consist of organizations and coalitions, as opposed to individuals
Networks	Are generally loosely-knit groups, formed primarily for the purpose of resource and information sharing
Task forces	Most often come together to accomplish a specific series of activities, often at the request of an overseeing body

Source: Reprinted from Contra Costa Country Health Services Department Prevention Program, *Developing Effective Coalitions: An Eight Step Guide,* 1994.

There are many advantages to working through coalitions and consortia. Collaborative efforts can function more efficiently than single organizations because work plans are shared among collaborating organizations rather than carried out by a single group. This serves to conserve limited resources and provides a pathway for reaching a larger part of the community. When organizations band together around specific goals, their efforts carry greater credibility than when only one or a few organizations are involved. Collaborative efforts are also excellent mechanisms for ensuring a broad range of inputs and perspectives into the policy development process and for facilitating communication and information across agencies and organizations. This has the added benefit of helping staff from one organization to view problems and possible solutions from a broader perspective than their usual vantage point. By building trust and personal relationships around one issue, collaborative approaches facilitate future collaborations around other issues.

There are no set rules for developing coalitions and consortia, but some general principles and approaches are useful after the decision is made to use a collaborative approach (Exhibit 6–5). That decision may come from a lead agency determining that a coalition would facilitate achievement of some goal or, in some instances, being required to establish one by a funding organization. On other occasions, an organization may be requested by community leaders or other agencies to organize a collaborative effort. Unmet community needs, scandals, and service breakdowns all serve to promote the development of coalitions, as do both informal and formal ties that exist among members.

Most coalitions have an agency or organization that leads the effort. Lead agencies must have both the credibility and the resources necessary for a coalition to succeed.

If it is determined that a coalition is the best mechanism to address a particular goal, the resources needed from the lead agency and other coalition members should be assessed to determine whether the coalition represents the best use of those resources to accomplish that goal. This requires examination

---

Exhibit 6–5 Key Steps for Coalitions and Other Collaborative Organizations

Step 1: Analyze the program's objectives and determine whether to form a coalition.
Step 2: Recruit the right people.
Step 3: Develop a set of preliminary objectives and activities.
Step 4: Convene the coalition.
Step 5: Anticipate the necessary resources.
Step 6: Define elements of a successful coalition structure.
Step 7: Maintain coalition vitality.
Step 8: Make improvements through evaluation.

Source: Reprinted from Contra Costa Country Health Services Department Prevention Program, *Developing Effective Coalitions: An Eight Step Guide,* 1994.

of objectives and implementation strategies that might facilitate achievement of the coalition's goals. A range of implementation strategies is available to coalitions, including making advocacy efforts to influence policy and legislation, changing organizational behavior, promoting networks, educating providers, educating the community, and increasing individual knowledge and skills. One or more implementation strategies should be adopted by the coalition on the basis of how well these fit with the community's strengths and weaknesses.

After the decision is made to develop a coalition, recruitment of the appropriate members is necessary to advance the process. Questions to be addressed include whether membership will consist of individuals or organizations and, if the latter, who should represent a particular organization on the coalition. In some cases, it is desirable to have agency leaders; in others, lower-level staff more familiar with the issues and programs may make better members. The size of the coalition also requires careful consideration. Once these issues are decided, preliminary objectives and work plans are developed, and the coalition is convened. At this point, the role of the lead agency in chairing or staffing the coalition should be determined, and resources needed to carry out the coalition's work plan should be identified and made available. Early decisions of the coalition should establish its expected life span, criteria for membership and decision-making, and expectations for participation at and between meetings. Constant vigilance is necessary to identify problems internal to the coalition's operation. These can include loss of interest and participation from some members, tension and conflict over power and leadership of the coalition, lack of community representativeness, and turnover of coalition members. Frequently, coalition members perceive threats to their organizational autonomy or come to disagree about service priorities or, more specifically, about which members will provide specific services. Careful assessment of a coalition's strengths and weaknesses (Exhibit 6–6), together with a commitment to make a good process even better, is often necessary to maintain the vitality and momentum of even the best coalition.

Many of these steps and issues appear to be straightforward and non-controversial until they are addressed within the context of an actual coalition experience. The discussion questions and exercises at the end of this chapter provide an opportunity to address these issues in the development of a state wide injury control coalition (also see Exhibit 6–7).

INFORMATION RESOURCES

In addition to human, organizational, and collaborative resources, information and access to information represent important elements of the public health infrastructure. The information resources that support public health practice include both the scientific basis of public health and the network of data and information needed to assess and address health problems. In large part, this knowledge base is outlined in the competencies for public health professionals presented in the discussion of the public health workforce. It includes elements from the public health sciences consisting of epidemiology, biostatistics, environmental health sciences, health administration, and behavioral sciences. This knowledge base contributes to the development of

Exhibit 6–6 Sample Questions for Partnership Self Assessment

Synergy	• Ability to identify new and creative ways to solve problems • Ability to include the views and priorities of the people affected by the partnership's work • Ability to develop goals that are widely understood and supported among partners • Ability to identify how different services and programs in the community relate to the problems the partnership is trying to address • Ability to respond to the needs and problems of the community • Ability to implement strategies that are most likely to work in the community • Ability to obtain support from individuals and organizations in the community that can either block the partnership's plans or help move them forward • Ability to carry out comprehensive activities that connect multiple services, programs, or systems • Ability to clearly communicate to people in the community how the partnership's actions will address problems that are important to them
Leadership	• Taking responsibility for the partnership • Inspiring or motivating people involved in the partnership • Empowering people involved in the partnership • Communicating the vision of the partnership • Working to develop a common language within the partnership • Fostering respect, trust, inclusiveness, and openness in the partnership • Creating an environment where differences of opinion can be voiced • Resolving conflict among partners • Combining the perspectives, resources, and skills of partners • Helping the partnership be creative and look at things differently • Recruiting diverse people and organizations into the partnership
Efficiency	• Using the partners' financial resources • Using the partners' in-kind resources (e.g., skills, expertise, information, data, connections, influence, space, equipment, goods) • Using the partners' time.
Administration and Management	• Coordinating communication among partners • Coordinating communication with people and organizations outside the partnership • Organizing partnership activities, including meetings and projects • Applying for and managing grants and funds • Preparing materials that inform partners and help them make timely decisions • Performing secretarial duties • Providing orientation to new partners as they join the partnership • Evaluating the progress and impact of the partnership • Minimizing the barriers to participation in the partnership's meetings and activities (e.g., by holding them at convenient places and times and by providing transportation and childcare)

continues

Exhibit 6–6 continued

Non-Financial Resources	• Skills and expertise (e.g., leadership, administration, evaluation, law, public policy, cultural competency, training, and community organizing) • Data and information (e.g., statistical data, information about community perceptions, values, resources, and politics) • Connections to target populations • Connections to political decision-makers, government agencies, other organizations/groups • Legitimacy and credibility • Influence and ability to bring people together for meetings and activities
Financial and Other Capital Resources	• Money • Space • Equipment and goods
Decision Making	• Comfort with the way decisions are made in the partnership • Support of decisions made by the partnership • Frequency of feeling left out of the decision-making process
Benefits of Participation	• Enhanced ability to address an important issue • Development of new skills • Heightened public profile • Increased utilization of your expertise or service • Acquisition of useful knowledge about services, programs, or people in the community • Enhanced ability to affect public policy • Development of valuable relationships • Enhanced ability to meet the needs of your constituency or clients • Ability to have a greater impact than you could have on your own • Ability to make a contribution to the community • Acquisition of additional financial support
Drawbacks of Participation	• Diversion of time and resources away from other priorities or obligations • Insufficient influence in partnership activities • Viewed negatively due to association with other partners or the partnership • Frustration or aggravation • Insufficient credit given to you for contributing to the accomplishments of the partnership • Conflict between your job and the partnership's work • Comparison of the benefits of participating in this partnership to the drawbacks
Satisfaction with Participation	• Satisfaction with the way the people and organizations in the partnership work together • Satisfaction with your influence in the partnership • Satisfaction with your role in the partnership • Satisfaction with the partnership's plans for achieving its goals • Satisfaction with the way the partnership is implementing its plans

Source: Adapted from Center for the Advancement of Collaborative Strategies in Health, 2002.

Exhibit 6–7 Coalition-Building Exercise Scenario

You are the Director of the Center for Health Promotion, one of the units of the Office of Community Health within the Lincoln State Department of Public Health (LDPH). Your office is within a few blocks of the state capitol building, which lies in the heart of the city of Jackson Springs, the capital of Lincoln.

Data indicate that the number of deaths in the state attributable to injury continues to be a problem. The fourth leading cause of death in terms of numbers of deaths, injury accounts for more years of potential life lost before age 65 than any other cause among Lincoln residents each year. Resources in state government are increasingly scarce. To maximize available resources, you convince your agency director that an Injury Coalition should be formed.

The Injury Coalition would be composed of organizational and individual representatives from throughout Lincoln with an interest in injury control and an influence on potentially affected groups of people. Ideally, this broad participation would not only bring diversity of perspective but would also ensure "buy-in" or commitment by involved organizations to project goals as these are developed. The role of the Injury Coalition would be to determine, on the basis of presentations of data concerning the burden of injury in Lincoln, which populations in the state are at greatest risk of death from injuries and how these groups might best be reached with preventive services. The Coalition would help develop a statewide injury control plan, set priorities in areas of greatest concern, and determine future interventions. The annual budget allocated to cover planning and other activities of the Injury Coalition is $100,000.

You and the state health department have had some experience setting up and working with coalitions on tobacco control and maternal and child issues in the past. Contact with legislators is not always easy in Lincoln, due to both political and geographic considerations.

Discussion Questions
(Note: for these questions, respond as if Lincoln were your home state!)
1. Why should an Injury Coalition be formed? What do you see as potential advantages and potential drawbacks of working with a coalition for this purpose?
2. How can you and the state health department build on prior successful involvement with coalitions?
3. What is the ideal size for such a coalition? What factors might help determine size?
4. Who might you invite to coalition meetings? How would you recruit members? What other facts should be considered when planning on coalition membership? Should members represent organizations or participate on the basis of individual leadership in their fields? Should they be agency heads?
5. Are there organizations that you would not like to have represented on the Injury Coalition?
6. Assuming that you decide on developing such a coalition, who should be in charge?
7. Would you choose LDPH staff to serve as coalition members? Why or why not? Should they be in charge of the coalition? Should they staff the coalition?
8. What powers and authorities should be given to the coalition? How might decision making within the coalition take place? What are the advantages and disadvantages of different styles of decision making?
9. What geographic factors particular to Lincoln need to be considered when planning coalition meetings?
10. What can you expect to be the coalition's major expenses? How might these be reduced?
11. How would you evaluate the coalition's effectiveness?

Source: Adapted from Translating Science into Practice, 1991, CDC Case Study.

Exhibit 6–8 Principles of Public Health Information

1. Recognize different types of data: encounter-based data on individuals as they encounter providers and universal data on populations from surveys and environmental monitoring systems.
2. Provide for integrated management to improve meeting of individual needs and to portray fully individual participation in multiple, categorical programs.
3. Maintain a service orientation to address the overriding concern of public health information systems.
4. Ensure flexibility so as to adapt to differences in data collection resources at the local level while accommodating data needs to support a broad range of public health programs and objectives.
5. Achieve system compatibility to allow data flow and functioning across systems in a fully compatible fashion.
6. Protect confidentiality to provide better service and to preserve privacy.

Source: Reprinted from JR Lumpkin, Six Principles of Public Health Information, *Journal of Public Health Management & Practice* 1995;1(1)40–42. © 1995, Lippincott, Williams & Wilkins.

competencies across a broad range of analytical, communication, policy development and planning, cultural, basic public health science, and management skills. Although this knowledge base is provided through graduate-level public health education, it can also be acquired through other educational, training, and experiential opportunities.

Information resources to carry out the activities of public health are increasingly abundant and accessible. Several important principles[25] that underlie the effective use of information sets in public health are highlighted in Exhibit 6–8. The need to ensure both flexibility and compatibility within information systems creates a tension that is not always readily resolved. In addition, two general categories of data sets are commonly encountered in public health practice. It is important to recognize their differences, although there is often great value in using both categories in efforts to identify and address health problems.

One category includes service- or encounter-based data, which are collected for a variety of purposes, such as reimbursement, eligibility, and evaluation of care. These data sets are common to programs that provide primary or episodic health care services, nutrition services for women, infants, and children (WIC), mental health and substance abuse treatment, and many other services. The information is collected for individual recipients of these services, which may include important clinical preventive services, such as immunizations or cancer screening. Aggregate data from these service encounters provide useful information on health needs and the health status of a population, including program coverage and penetration rates. However, the population is limited to those seeking services and may not be representative of the larger population.

Another category of data sets describes populations, rather than individuals. Examples include many of the federal surveys of health status and service utilization, as well as behavioral risk factor surveys of the population that collect information on population samples (composed of individual respondents) that are representative of the entire population. For these data sets, the population is described through the use of sampling techniques. Other data sets capture information on specific health events and outcomes for a defined population, such as cancer incidence registries and vital records systems. For these, data are collected on individuals and aggregated in comparison with a reference population, often derived from census information (e.g., the rate of newly diagnosed lung cancers among women aged 45–64 in a state). Data sets that describe risks or hazards common to a population, such as environmental monitoring data, represent yet another form of population-based data.

The limitations of encounter-based information systems are apparent when individuals participate in more than one service program. A prenatal care program may have its own information system; the WIC program serving the same person may have another system, and the lead screening program yet another. The communicable disease program may have separate systems for general communicable diseases, HIV infections, TB, and sexually transmitted diseases. Beyond these health information systems, an individual may also be receiving services from other agencies for mental health, substance abuse, spousal abuse, and Medicaid. The information systems are often problem-specific, but individuals generally have multiple problems. Integration of information systems across the entire spectrum of human services programs and needs is essential both to promote efficiency in programs and to characterize the health status and needs of individuals and populations.

Confidentiality issues can be especially difficult to address in information systems. State statutes for the collection, sharing, and confidentiality of health statistics should make it impossible for individuals to be identified unless they have consented. Disclosure of personal identifiers should be permitted only to a government entity or research project that had a written agreement to protect the confidentiality of the information or to a governmental entity for the purpose of conducting an audit, evaluation, or investigation of the agency.

Information and Analytic Techniques

The capacity of the public health system to use information more effectively expanded during the twentieth century. Advances occurred in both study design and periodic standardized health surveys. Methods of data collection evolved from simple measures of disease prevalence, such as field surveys, to complex studies of precise analyses, such as case-control studies, cohort studies, and randomized clinical trials. The first well-developed, longitudinal cohort study was conducted in 1947 among the 28,000 residents of Framingham, Massachusetts, many of whom volunteered to be followed over time to determine incidence of heart disease. The Framingham Heart Study has served as a model for other longitudinal cohort studies, advancing understanding of the multiple risk factors that contribute to disease. The age of modern clinical trials began in 1948 with a study of streptomycin therapy for TB; this study involved randomization, selection criteria, predetermined evaluation criteria, and ethical considerations. In 1950 the first convincing evidence of an association between lung cancer and tobacco use was provided in a case-control study, adding credibility to this important study design. Subsequently, high-powered statistical tests and analytic computer programs enabled multiple variables collected in large-scale studies to be measured and tools to be developed for mathematical modeling. Advances in epidemiology contributed to the elucidation of risk factors for heart disease and other chronic diseases and the development of effective interventions.

The first periodic standardized health surveys in the United States began in 1921. In 1935 the first national health survey was conducted among U.S. residents. In 1956 these efforts culminated in the National Health Survey, a population-based survey that evolved from focusing on chronic disease to estimating disease prevalence for major causes of death, measuring the burden of infectious diseases, assessing exposure to environmental toxicants, and measuring the population's vaccination coverage. Other population-based surveys, such as the Behavioral Risk Factor Surveillance System, Youth Risk Behavior Survey, and the National Survey of Family Growth, were developed to assess risk factors for chronic diseases and other conditions. Survey methods used in epidemiologic studies were enhanced by new approaches to sampling and interviewing developed by social scientists and statisticians.

Information and the Assessment Function of Public Health

Information drives the assessment function of public health in at least three ways. First, public health agencies commonly utilize surveillance data to monitor community health status and trends and to identify any new health risks or hazards. Second, once health needs and problems are identified, information is needed on the community's resources that are available to address those needs and problems and on the effectiveness of those resources. Third, information from assessments of health needs and current efforts must be tailored to the needs of decision and policy makers to facilitate more effective interventions.[26] Data sources for these three facets of the assessment function are presented in Exhibit 6–9. This exhibit demonstrates that information is a resource widely utilized throughout public health practice in applications involving surveillance, planning processes, selection of scientifically-based interventions, and health communications.

Exhibit 6–9 Data Sets and Activities Associated with the Three Facets of the Assessment Process

I. Monitor health status and risk factors
  A. Health status
    1. Mortality
      a. vital statistics
      b. coroner and medical examiner reports
      c. infant mortality reviews
    2. Morbidity, injuries, and disabling conditions
      a. notifiable diseases
      b. hospital discharge records
      c. disease registries (e.g., cancer, trauma)

continues

Exhibit 6–9 continued

        d. health interview surveys
        e. newborn screening
    B. Risk factors
      1. Known risk factors
        a. health risk appraisals
        b. behavioral risk factor surveys
        c. knowledge and attitude surveys
        d. health care utilization surveys
        e. laboratory tests
        f. environmental measures
        g. family histories
        h. physical exams
      2. Unknown risk factors (research agenda)
        a. community studies
        b. clinical trials
        c. basic science research (e.g., gene mapping)
II. Identify and evaluate resources
    A. Types of resources
      1. Health resources
        a. health facilities
        b. health professionals
        c. medicines and vaccines
        d. emergency medical transportation systems
      2. Other resources
        a. sanitation programs
        b. educational programs
        c. disaster response plans
        d. counseling services
    B. Evaluation of resources
      1. Availability of resources
        a. proximity
        b. accessibility
        c. affordability
        d. acceptability
        e. appropriateness
      2. Effectiveness of resources
        a. size of population in need
        b. proportion of the population reached by programs
        c. effectiveness of current programs
        d. cost to provide the program
        e. cost for each unit outcome
        f. cost to meet some proportion of the unmet need
        g. evaluation of alternative ways to meet need
III. Inform and advise managers, policy makers, and the public
    A. Summarize and data simply and straightforwardly
    B. Tailor the data to the audience
    C. Provide information that answers questions
    D. Educate those who ask the questions

Source: Reprinted from K. G. Keppel and M. A. Friedman, What is Assessment?, *Journal of Public Health Management & Practice,* 1995;1(2)1–7. © 1995, Lippincott, Williams & Wilkins.

Information and Surveillance

Public health surveillance activities monitor health status and risk factors in the population. Although surveillance data sets have become both more sophisticated and more accessible in recent years, the most important consideration for their establishment relates to why and how they will be used. The very first collection of health statistics dates back to the work of John Graunt in England in the mid-seventeenth century.

Health data in the United States have had the benefit of national enumerations of the population every 10 years, although the decennial census was established to ensure fair representation in the Congress, rather than to serve as a source of health or even demographic information on the population. National disease monitoring was first conducted in the United States in 1850 when the federal government first published mortality statistics based on death registrations. In the late nineteenth century, Congress authorized the collection of morbidity reports on cholera, smallpox, plague, and yellow fever for use in quarantine measures and provided funding to expand weekly reporting from states and municipal authorities. The first annual summary of notifiable diseases appeared in 1912 with reports of 10 diseases from 19 states, the District of Columbia, and Hawaii. By 1928 all states were reporting on 29 diseases. In 1950 state and territorial health officers authorized the Council of State and Territorial Epidemiologists (CSTE) to determine which diseases should be reported to the U.S. Public Health Service (PHS). The CDC assumed responsibility for collecting and publishing national data on notifiable diseases in 1961. As of 2003, 56 infectious diseases were notifiable at the national level (Exhibit 6–10).

Exhibit 6–10 Nationally Notifiable Infectious Diseases, United States, 2003

- Acquired Immunodeficiency Syndrome (AIDS)
- Anthrax
- Botulism
  - Botulism, foodborne
  - Botulism, infant
  - Botulism, other (wound & unspecified)
- Brucellosis
- Chancroid
- Chlamydia trachomatis, genital infections
- Cholera
- Coccidioidomycosis
- Cryptosporidiosis
- Cyclosporiasis
- Diphtheria
- Ehrlichiosis
  - Ehrlichiosis, human granulocytic
  - Ehrlichiosis, human monocytic
  - Ehrlichiosis, human, other or unspecified agent

continues

Exhibit 6–10 continued

- Encephalitis/meningitis, Arboviral
  - Encephalitis/meningitis, California serogroup viral
  - Encephalitis/meningitis, eastern equine
  - Encephalitis/meningitis, Powassan
  - Encephalitis/meningitis, St. Louis
  - Encephalitis/meningitis, western equine
  - Encephalitis/meningitis, West Nile
- Enterohemorrhagic Escherichia coli
  - Enterohemorrhagic Escherichia coli, O157:H7
  - Enterohemorrhagic Escherichia coli, shiga toxin positive, serogroup non-O157
  - Enterohemorrhagic Escherichia coli shiga toxin+ (not serogrouped)
- Giardiasis
- Gonorrhea
- Haemophilus influenzae, invasive disease
- Hansen disease (leprosy)
- Hantavirus pulmonary syndrome
- Hemolytic uremic syndrome, post diarrheal
- Hepatitis, viral, acute
  - Hepatitis A, acute
  - Hepatitis B, acute
  - Hepatitis B virus, perinatal infection
  - Hepatitis, C, acute
- Hepatitis, viral, chronic
  - Chronic Hepatitis B
  - Hepatitis C Virus Infection (past or present)
- HIV infection
  - HIV infection, *adult* (≥13 years)
  - HIV infection, *pediatric* (<13 years)
- Legionellosis
- Listeriosis
- Lyme disease
- Malaria
- Measles
- Meningococcal disease
- Mumps
- Pertussis
- Plague
- Poliomyelitis, paralytic
- Psittacosis
- Q Fever
- Rabies
  - Rabies, animal
  - Rabies, human
- Rocky Mountain spotted fever
- Rubella
- Rubella, congenital syndrome
- Salmonellosis
- Shigellosis

continues

Exhibit 6–10 continued

- Streptococcal disease, invasive, Group A
- Streptococcal toxic-shock syndrome
- Streptococcus pneumoniae, drug resistant, invasive disease
- Streptococcus pneumoniae, invasive in children <5 years
- Syphilis
  - Syphilis, primary
  - Syphilis, secondary
  - Syphilis, latent
  - Syphilis, early latent
  - Syphilis, late latent
  - Syphilis, latent unknown duration
  - Neurosyphilis
  - Syphilis, late, non-neurological
- Syphilis, congenital
  - Syphilitic Stillbirth
- Tetanus
- Toxic-shock syndrome
- Trichinosis
- Tuberculosis
- Tularemia
- Typhoid fever
- Varicella (morbidity)
- Varicella (deaths only)
- Yellow fever

Source: CDC, 2003.

Numerous sources of data are available for epidemiologic surveillance data.[27] These range from well-known data sets, such as birth and death records, to lesser-known sources, such as school and work absenteeism reports. Similar information is available for surveillance of environmental health risks.[28] Several important data sources are operated through CDC's National Center for Health Statistics, which maintains systems for:

- Vital Statistics (births, deaths, fetal deaths, induced abortions, marriages, divorces, follow-back surveys to gather additional information)
- National Health Interview Survey (amount, distribution, and effects of illness and disability, using a multistage probability sample)
- National Medical Care, Utilization and Expenditure Survey (use of and expenditures for medical services, done in 1980 but not repeated since)
- National Ambulatory Medical Care Survey (location, setting, and frequency of ambulatory care encounters)
- National Health and Nutrition Examination Survey (direct physical, physiologic, and biochemical data from national sample)
- National Hospital Discharge Survey (characteristics of patients, lengths of stay, diagnoses, procedures, patterns of patient use by type of hospital)

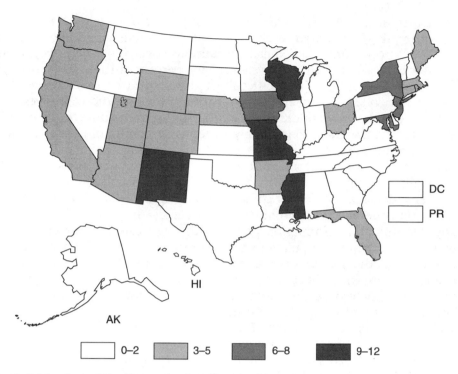

Figure 6–5 Number of Environmental Public Health Surveillance Systems, by Jurisdiction—United States, 1997

Surveillance is a multifaceted operation in that information is collected at a variety of levels. Surveillance information used in environmental public health applications illustrates this point. For any environmental agent that is considered to be a hazard, surveillance efforts can measure its effects at various steps in its chain of causation. For example, the agent's presence in the environment can be assessed, and its route of exposure can be measured through surveillance efforts that can be considered hazard surveillance. Beyond hazard surveillance, exposure surveillance can track actual exposures between the host and agent, the frequency in which the agent reaches its target tissue, and the early production of adverse effects. In addition, outcome surveillance can measure the actual adverse effects after these become clinically apparent.

Together, these three levels of surveillance activities provide a more complete picture of the problem and allow for a more rational strategy for its control and for evaluating whether control strategies are working.

There is wide variability in the capacity of state and local health agencies to maintain and utilize surveillance information. A CDC survey in 1997 identified 174 environmental public health surveillance systems from 51 jurisdictions[29] (see Figure 6–5). The mean number of systems per jurisdiction was three; the median was two. Of the 174, a total of 79 systems (45 percent) monitored lead exposure, with most systems monitoring childhood blood lead levels. The remaining 28 systems monitored non-occupational adult lead exposures. The environmental diseases least frequently monitored were heatstroke and hypothermia (four systems each). One state had surveillance systems for all 12 of the environmental public health conditions covered by the survey. One state did not have any surveillance systems. Nine percent of the surveillance systems collected data only, 27 percent collected data and conducted reviews, and 64 percent collected data and conducted both reviews and case investigations. Asthma was the only condition for which no systems conducted case investigations. LPHAs also vary considerably in terms of maintaining surveillance data on common public health problems. More than 80 percent maintain surveillance data on communicable diseases, but fewer than half track water quality, air quality, chronic diseases, behavioral risk factors, or injuries.

Most data sets are neither complete nor completely accurate. Each has problems and issues related to completeness, accuracy, and timeliness. For example, key denominator information provided through census enumerations under counts important subpopulations that are often at greater risk of adverse health effects. Even the data set often considered to be the most complete—birth and death records—includes some important data elements that are underreported or inaccurately recorded, including maternal behaviors, length of gestation, and congenital anomalies of newborn infants. Death records also suffer from variability in determining cause of death and, specifically, in identifying true underlying causes, such as tobacco or alcohol.

Vital records represent yet another example of an important federal health policy being operationalized through the states; there is no national mandate for uniform reporting of birth and deaths. Through a voluntary and cooperative effort with the states, a national model of these records is implemented by the states and localities, stimulated in part by federal grants for a national cooperative health statistics system.

Access to information and data for surveillance purposes has improved steadily with improved technology for electronic management and transfer. As of 2000, reports including a mix of text, tables, and figures were available from an increasing number of federal and state sources through a variety of electronic modes: telephone, fax, CD-ROM and diskettes, modem, and the Internet.[30] Increasingly, electronic systems are used in ongoing surveillance activities of federal, state, and local public health agencies. These include:

- National Electronic Telecommunications System for Surveillance (NETSS), which is used to collect, transmit, and analyze weekly reports of notifiable diseases from state and local health agencies; the system reports on a common set of diseases, using standard protocols for formatting and transmitting data, standard case definitions, a common record format, and designated individuals responsible for reporting from each agency
- HIV/AIDS Reporting System, which collects detailed demographic, risk, and clinical information on persons diagnosed with either AIDS or HIV infection; since 1985 CDC has provided state and local health agencies with standardized case report forms and microcomputer-based software for managing HIV and AIDS surveillance in their areas
- Public Health Laboratory Information System, which reports laboratory isolates to CDC to reduce the enormous paper burden in state laborato-

ries, to facilitate cluster identification, to provide states with better access to data, and to reduce the lag time between identification and reporting to CDC

- CDC WONDER, which is also used as a vehicle for transmission of surveillance files by a number of CDC surveillance systems

Surveillance systems are a major component of the public health preparedness activities that will be described in Chapter 8.

Information and Planning

Although there are various forms of planning, each relies heavily on information resources. In public health, planning information is widely employed for purposes of community health planning, agency strategic and operational planning, and program planning and management.

The community health planning role is new for many local governmental public health agencies. From the mid-1960s through the mid-1980s, community health planning was carried out through a national program of state and local planning agencies. The Comprehensive Health Planning Act of 1966 and the National Health Planning and Resource Development Act of 1974 established the framework for these structures and activities. At the state level, state health departments generally coordinated the development of state health plans, in part through the generation of local health plans. These local plans were developed by agencies known as health systems agencies (HSAs), whose role was to organize community participation in the development and implementation of the local plans. In large part, this form of planning focused on resources within the health system, assessing the availability of facilities, health manpower, and specific services. Where resources were lacking, plans were established to increase supply. Where resources were underutilized, plans sought to increase demand. As consumer majorities sat on planning boards at both the state and local levels, the focus was on resource planning, rather than needs-based planning.

Largely due to their focus on resources, inability to make change happen, and widespread provider resentment of consumer-dominated processes, political support for this effort waned, and the federal program was repealed. Very soon thereafter most of the local health planning agencies also disappeared, leaving a significant void. Local public health agencies, with a few exceptions, had not been very involved in community health planning and found it difficult to pick up the slack. LPHAs often lacked staff with the skills and expertise in community health planning: many information sources resided at levels of government outside their direct control, and they simply did not see it as part of their job description at a time when demands for serving the uninsured and the AIDS epidemic were at their doorsteps. These factors contributed to the need for the development of tools such as APEXPH, the Planned Approach to Community Health (PATCH), Model Standards, and the series of national Healthy People initiatives described in earlier chapters.

The framework of planning objectives in Healthy People 2000 encouraged states to develop more consistent state health plans. Most states used measures drawn directly from Healthy People 2000. However, this also meant that states replicated the lack of emphasis on mental health, substance abuse, environmental health, and occupational health issues that marked Healthy People 2000. In some states, these objectives were addressed in separate planning processes or not at all. States found that baseline data were generally available for state planning efforts modeled on Healthy People 2000, but they also found that such data were generally not available at the county or city level. Planning efforts relied heavily on vital records and, to a lesser extent, behavioral risk factor and notifiable disease data. Only infrequently were sources such as youth behavioral surveys, hospital discharge data, or morbidity data such as that provided in Table 6–3 used in state planning processes during the early 1990s. Stimulated by renewed interest in community-level health planning in the latter part of the decade, however, this situation has gradually improved.

APEXPH/MAPP and other community needs assessment processes call for a variety of mortality, morbidity, and risk factor information, as well as data and information on available resources to address priority health problems. Information describing the health status and needs of the local population is often available from federal and state sources but, more often, these sources must be supplemented with more locally-developed information. The lessons from earlier attempts at consumer-directed local health planning demonstrate that community health planning is as much a political process as it is an objective process based on statistical data. Diversity in values and perspectives within a community cannot be homogenized through the use of what some consider objective data. These past failures make it all the more difficult for local public health agencies seeking to reenter this minefield. Managerial planning improvements, however, have emerged, including planning-programming-budgeting systems, operations research, systems analysis, and program evaluation and review techniques.

Information resources also support the strategic and operational planning activities of an organization. Strategic planning seeks to identify external and internal trends that might influence the agency's ability to carry out its mission and role. Operational planning looks to maximize the use of available resources to achieve specific objectives that have been established for a specific period of time, generally one year.

Information and Scientifically Based Interventions

At the heart of public health interventions for improving the quality of life and reducing preventable mortality and morbidity are scientifically sound strategies and approaches. Although the scientific basis for public health interventions has always been highly valued, the formal application of rigorous assessments to the evidence for effectiveness is a relatively new undertaking for public health. Considerable progress has been made on this front during the 1990s; Chapter 7 presents principles, strategies, and tools that will drive public health interventions in the early twenty-first century. These build on public health achievements throughout the twentieth century, such as the efforts to assure safer and healthier foods, described in "Public Health Achievements in Twentieth-Century America: Safer and Healthier Foods."

Table 6–3 Injuries Associated with Selected Sports and Recreation Equipment Treated in Emergency Departments, 1994

Product Groupings	Estimated No. of Cases	All Ages	Age (yr)					Disposition	
			0–4	5–14	15–24	25–64	65+	Treated and Released	Hospitalized or DOA
ATVs, mopeds, minibikes, etc.	125,136	48.1	14.5	111.7	116.8	27.0	6.5	45.1	3.0
Baseball, softball	404,364	155.3	45.0	410.7	294.4	100.1	3.3	153.4	1.7
Basketball	716,114	275.1	13.4	584.0	955.3	111.6	3.2	272.9	1.8
Bicycles and accessories	604,455	232.2	247.8	908.2	243.2	87.5	28.2	223.3	8.6
Exercise and exercise equipment	155,231	59.6	45.2	68.8	134.6	49.6	16.6	58.5	1.0
Football	424,622	163.1	5.0	484.7	557.1	30.4	1.3	160.8	2.2
Hockey	81,885	31.5	5.4	85.1	81.9	14.4	0.3	30.9	0.5
Horseback riding	71,162	27.3	7.9	38.7	41.0	29.4	3.0	25.1	2.2
Lacrosse, rugby, misc. ball games	90,252	34.7	18.4	126.4	63.4	11.9	1.1	34.2	0.3
Playground equipment	266,810	102.5	386.1	468.7	16.4	5.9	1.6	99.5	2.9
Skateboards	25,486	9.8	7.3	37.5	24.0	1.0	—	9.7	0.1
Skating (excludes in-line)	146,082	56.1	15.6	226.8	57.3	27.1	2.6	54.8	1.3
In-line skating	75,994	29.2	2.3	115.6	40.4	12.9	0.7	28.3	0.8
Soccer	162,115	62.3	2.7	190.6	180.7	18.5	0.6	61.4	0.8
Swimming, pools, equipment	115,139	44.2	62.4	128.8	63.3	21.1	10.1	42.5	1.7
Track and field activities, equipment	18,774	7.2	—	24.3	24.2	0.5	1.0	7.1	0.1
Trampolines	52,892	20.3	27.7	93.5	20.6	3.6	0.1	19.8	0.5
Volleyball	97,525	37.5	2.0	52.4	111.4	27.7	0.6	37.2	0.2

DOA, dead on arrival.

Source: Reprinted from National Electronic Injury Surveillance System, U.S. Consumer Product Safety Commission.

Public Health Achievements in Twentieth-Century America:
Safer and Healthier Foods

The resources and relationships that comprise the infrastructure of the public health system include workforce, organizational, informational, and financial components. Coordinating these components to improve the safety of foods and provide population-wide protection from dental caries demonstrates how public health practice can be greater than the sum of its parts.

During the early twentieth century, contaminated food, milk, and water caused many food-borne infections, including typhoid fever, tuberculosis, botulism, and scarlet fever. In 1906 Upton Sinclair described in his novel, *The Jungle*, the unwholesome working environment in the Chicago meat-packing industry and the unsanitary conditions under which food was produced. Public awareness dramatically increased, leading to the passage of the Pure Food and Drug Act. Once the sources and characteristics of food-borne diseases were identified—long before vaccines or antibiotics—they could be controlled by hand washing, sanitation, refrigeration, pasteurization, and pesticide application. Healthier animal care, feeding, and processing also improved food supply safety. In 1900 the incidence of typhoid fever was approximately 100 per 100,000 population; by 1920 it had decreased to 33.8, and by 1950 to 1.7 (Figure 6–6). During the 1940s studies of autopsied muscle samples showed that 16 percent of persons in the United States had trichinellosis: 300–400 cases were diagnosed every year, and 10–20 deaths occurred. Since then the rate of infection has declined markedly; from 1991 through 1996, three deaths and an average of 38 cases per year were reported.

Perishable foods contain nutrients that pathogenic microorganisms require to reproduce. Bacteria such as Salmonella, Clostridium, and Staphylococcus species, can multiply quickly to sufficient numbers to cause illness. Prompt refrigeration slows bacterial growth and keeps food fresh and edible.

At the turn of the twentieth century, consumers kept food fresh by placing it on a block of ice or, in cold weather, burying it in the yard or storing it on a window sill outside. During the 1920s refrigerators with freezer compartments became available for household use. Another process that reduced the incidence of disease was invented by Louis Pasteur—pasteurization. Although the process was applied first in wine preservation, when milk producers adopted the process, pasteurization eliminated a substantial vector of food-borne disease. In 1924 the PHS created a document to assist Alabama in developing a statewide milk sanitation program. This document evolved into the Grade A Pasteurized Milk Ordinance, a voluntary agreement that established uniform sanitation standards for the interstate shipment of Grade A milk and now serves as the basis of milk safety laws in the 50 states and Puerto Rico.

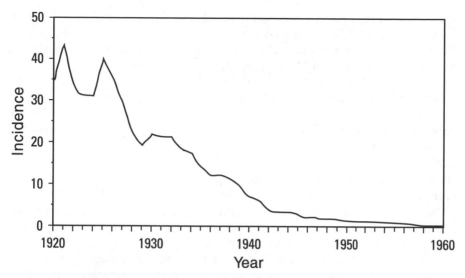

Figure 6–6 Incidence of Typhoid Fever, by Year—United States, 1920–1960. *Source:* Reprinted from Achievements in Public Health, United States, 1900–1999: Safer and Healthier Foods, *Morbidity and Mortality Weekly Report,* Vol. 48, No. 40, pp. 905–913, the Centers for Disease Control and Prevention, 1999.

Along with improved crop varieties, insecticides and herbicides have increased crop yields, decreased food costs, and enhanced the appearance of food. Without proper controls, however, the residues of some pesticides that remain on foods can create potential health risks. Before 1910 no legislation existed to ensure the safety of food and feed crops that were sprayed and dusted with pesticides. In 1910 the first pesticide legislation was designed to protect consumers from impure or improperly labeled products. During the 1950s and 1960s pesticide regulation evolved to require maximum allowable residue levels of pesticides on foods and to deny registrations for unsafe or ineffective products. During the 1970s, acting under these strengthened laws, the newly formed Environmental Protection Agency (EPA) removed DDT and several other highly persistent pesticides from the marketplace. In 1996 the Food Quality Protection Act set a stricter safety standard and required the review of older allowable residue levels to determine whether they were safe. In 1999 federal and state laws required that pesticides meet specific safety standards; the EPA reviews and registers each product before it can be used and sets levels and restrictions on each product intended for food or feed crops.

Newly recognized food-borne pathogens have emerged in the United States since the late 1970s; contributing factors include changes in agricultural practices and food processing operations and the globalization of the food supply. Seemingly healthy food animals can be reservoirs of human pathogens. During the 1980s, for example, an epidemic of egg-associated Salmonella enteritidis infection spread to an estimated 45 percent of the nation's egg-laying flocks, which resulted in a large increase in egg-associated food-borne illness within the United States. *Escherichia coli O157:H7*, which can cause severe infections and death in humans, produces no signs of illness in its nonhuman hosts. In 1993 a severe outbreak of *E. coli O157:H7* infections, attributed to consumption of undercooked ground beef, resulted in 501 cases of illness, 151 hospitalizations, and 3 deaths, and led to a restructuring of the meat inspection process. The most common food-borne infectious agent may be the calicivirus (a Norwalk-like virus), which can pass from the unwashed hands of an infected food handler to the meal of a consumer. Animal husbandry and meat production improvements that have contributed to reducing pathogens in the food supply include pathogen eradication campaigns, the Hazard Analysis and Critical Control Point (HACCP) programs, better animal feeding regulations, the use of uncontaminated water in food processing, more effective food preservatives, improved antimicrobial products for sanitizing food processing equipment and facilities, and adequate surveillance of food handling and preparation methods. HACCP programs also are mandatory for the seafood industry.

Improved surveillance, applied research, and outbreak investigations have elucidated the mechanisms of contamination that are leading to new control measures for food-borne pathogens. In meat-processing plants, the incidence of Salmonella and Campylobacter infections has decreased. However, in 1998, apparently unrelated cases of Listeria infections were linked when an epidemiologic investigation indicated that isolates from all cases shared the same genetic DNA fingerprint; approximately 100 cases and 22 deaths were traced to eating hot dogs and deli meats produced in a single manufacturing plant. In 1998 a multi-state outbreak of shigellosis was traced to imported parsley. During 1997–1998 in the United States, outbreaks of cyclosporiasis were associated with mesclunmix lettuce, basil/basil-containing products, and Guatemalan raspberries. These instances highlight the need for measures that prevent food contamination closer to its point of production, particularly if the food is eaten raw or is difficult to wash.

Nutritional sciences also were in their infancy at the start of the century. Unknown was the concept that minerals and vitamins were necessary to prevent diseases caused by dietary deficiencies. Recurring nutritional deficiency diseases, including rickets, scurvy, beri-beri, and pellagra were thought to be infectious diseases. By 1900 biochemists and physiologists had identified protein, fat, and carbohydrates as the basic nutrients in food. By 1916 new data had led to the discovery that food contained vitamins, and the lack of "vital amines" could cause disease. These scientific discoveries and the resulting public health policies, such as food fortification programs, led to substantial reductions in nutritional deficiency diseases during the first half of the century. The focus of nutrition programs shifted in the second half of the century from disease prevention to control of chronic conditions, such as cardiovascular disease and obesity.

Source: Adapted from Achievements in Public Health, United States, 1900–1999: Safer and Healthier Foods, *Morbidity and Mortality Weekly Report,* Vol. 48, No. 40, pp. 905–913, the Centers for Disease Control and Prevention, 1999.

FISCAL RESOURCES

The fiscal resources available for public health activities can be viewed as both inputs and outputs of the system. They are clearly inputs in that they represent an economic measure of the human, organizational, and informational resources described earlier, as well as the physical facilities, equipment, and other inputs that do not fit nicely into any of the other categories. However, the fiscal resources provided for public health programs also represent the perceived worthiness of these activities in comparison with other public policy goals. In this light, fiscal resources are a product of public health activities and an expression of their value in the eyes of society. In either interpretation, however, it is useful to quantify their extent.

It is no simple task to link financial expenditures to the essential public health services framework. The public sector provides many, but not all, of the population-based activities included among the essential public health services. Also, whereas some of the personal health services provided through public sector resources fall into the essential public health services framework, such as those linking people with needed services and assuring the provision of care when otherwise unavailable, others do not. In the public sector, many agencies other than official health agencies provide essential public health services; mental health, substance abuse, environmental protection, and other agencies contribute, as well. In addition, both some essential personal health services, including even some of the population-based essential services, are also provided outside the public sector. Although precise determinations are not possible, estimates using data derived from national health expenditure tracking systems and focused examinations allow for reasonable approximations.

Overall expenditures for health in the U.S. were $1.3 trillion in 2000, with about $44 billion (or 3.4 percent) identified as governmental public health expenditures for both population-based services and personal health care services provided directly by government. In effect, the $44 billion figure approximates governmental expenditures for the essential public health services, with $17 billion (1.3 percent of total health spending) supporting population-based public health activities. Expenditures in 2000 for essential public health services were $157 per capita, $61 of which supported population-based services. For comparison purposes, per capita spending for health purposes exceeded $4600 per person for each American in 2000.

These levels are consistent with results from a series of studies of public health expenditures in the mid-1990s,[31–33] including one that examined public health expenditures in 1994 across a variety of state and local governmental agencies in nine states. Median per capita expenditures for public health core functions (similar to the essential public health services framework) were $137 and median per capita expenditures for population-based services were $43 per capita in the nine-state study. Extrapolations to the entire U.S. for that year, together with the inclusion of federal expenditures that were not channeled through state or local governments, provided an estimate that about $38 billion was spent by the states on core functions and $15 billion on population-based services in 1994.

The nine-state study provides interesting information on spending patterns at the federal and state level, as well as insights into overall funding sources and expenditure patterns within the states in the mid-1990s.

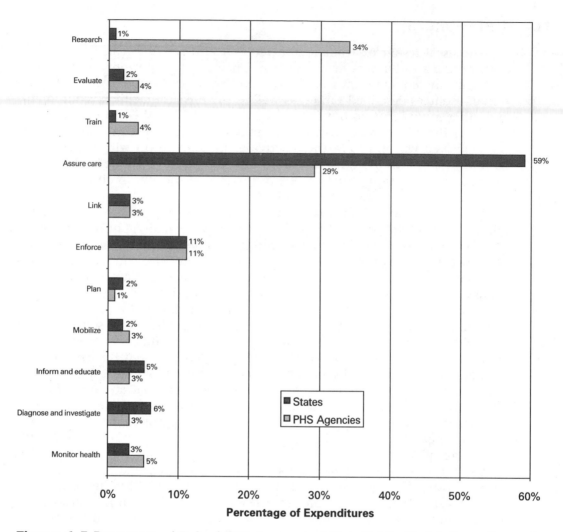

Figure 6–7 Percentage of Federal PHS Agency and State Public Health Expenditures for Essential Public Health Services by Essential Service. *Source:* Adapted with permission from Eilbert et al., *Measuring Expenditures for Essential Service,* © 1996, Public Health Foundation.

At the federal level, PHS expenditures for essential public health services differ from state/local expenditures for several essential services as illustrated in Figure 6–7. The federal agencies spend proportionately more on research, evaluation, training, and monitoring health status. State and local governments spend proportionately more on assuring care, informing and educating the public, and diagnosing and investigating health risks.

Additional findings from the study of state and local expenditures for public health core functions in nine states are presented in Table 6–4. Of the total expenditures by health, substance abuse, mental health, and environmental agencies in these nine states, 79 percent was expended on public

Table 6–4 Estimated Percentages of Public Health Expenditures for Essential Public Health Services, WIC, and Other Activities by Agency Type in Nine States

	Essential Public Health Services		Other Activities		Total
	Personal Health	*Population Health*	*WIC (food only)*	*Other*	
State Health Agencies	5.8	10.8	7.7	2.5	26.9
Local Health Departments	4.3	4.8		0.7	9.8
Mental Health Agencies	38.7	0.7		NA	39.4
Substance Abuse Agencies	5.5	2.4		0.6	8.5
Environmental Agencies	NA	5.5		9.9	15.4
Total	54.4	24.2	7.7	13.7	100.0

NA, not applicable.

Source: Reprinted with permission from Eilbert et al., *Measuring Expenditures for Essential Public Health Service,* © 1996, Public Health Foundation.

health core functions, with more than twice as much spent on personal health services as on population-based public health activities.

Expenditures for population-based services accounted for approximately one-fourth of the total resources available to the state and local health, environmental protection, mental health, and substance abuse agencies. About one-fourth of all expenditures for population-based activities involved enforcing laws and regulations related to protection of the environment, housing, food, water, and the workplace. State and local public health agencies accounted for about two-thirds of all population-based service expenditures and, together with environmental health agencies, expended about 90 percent of the total. For state and local public health agencies, 50–60 percent of the agencies' expenditures were for population-based services. For environmental health and substance abuse agencies, 30–40 percent supported population-based activities.

As illustrated in Figure 6–8, population-based expenditures were derived largely from federal and state funds, each accounting for about one-third of the total. State fees and local funds accounted for another third; Medicaid accounted for only 2 percent of the total expended by state and local governments. More than two-thirds of population-based service expenditures in the states were derived from nonfederal sources, reinforcing the observation that state and local governments bear the brunt of the burden for funding public health activities in the United States. Who currently pays the bills says much about the likelihood for expansion of public health efforts in the future. Tax bases of state and, especially, local governments and political opposition to tax increases of any kind do not augur well for increased state and local public health resources in the future.

The $44 billion figure for essential public health services and the $17 billion figure for population-based services understate public health expenditures because they do not include spending by nongovernmental public health agencies for core functions and essential public health services. It is estimated that nongovernmental organizations are responsible for performing

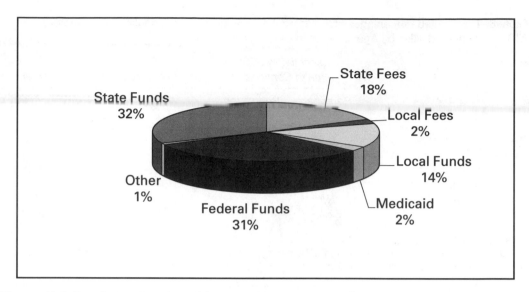

Figure 6–8 Population-Based Health Expenditures in Nine States by Source of Funds. *Source:* Reprinted from Eilbert et al., Public Health Expenditures: Developing Estimates for Improved Policy Making, *Journal of Public Health Management Practice,* Vol. 3, No. 3, p. 8, © 1997, Aspen Publishers, Inc.

about one-fourth to one-third of the total performance of essential public health services in the community.[34] The costs of these activities should also be considered in estimating total expenditures for public health. All factors considered, a reasonable estimate is that about $60–65 billion—or 5 percent of national health expenditures—supports activities related to public health core functions and essential services. About $20 billion funds population-based services, and the remaining $40 billion supports personal care. This amounts to about 20 cents per person per day for population-based services and 60 cents per day—the cost of a pack of gum—for the entire package of essential public health services.

HEALTHY PEOPLE 2010 INFRASTRUCTURE OBJECTIVES

Only one of the more than 500 national health objectives included in the Healthy People 1990 and Healthy People 2000 processes directly addressed the national public health system. That objective (from Healthy People 2000) called for 90 percent of the population to be served by an LPHA that was effectively carrying out public health's three core functions. The pursuit of this objective during the 1990s focused attention on the infrastructure capacity that must be in place for this target to be achieved. As a result, a more comprehensive panel of objectives related to the public health infrastructure was established for the Healthy People 2010 national health objectives. These infrastructure objectives address the human, organizational, informational, and financial aspects of the public health infrastructure described in this chapter. Exhibit 6–11 presents the final panel of infrastructure objectives included in Healthy People 2010.[35] Together these represent the national agenda for strengthening the public health infrastructure.

Exhibit 6–11   Healthy People 2010 Public Health Infrastructure Objectives

Data and Information Systems
- Increase the proportion of public health agencies that provide Internet and e-mail access for at least 75 percent of their employees and that teach employees in how to use the Internet and other electronic information systems to apply data and information to public health practice.
- Increase the proportion of public health agencies that have made information available to the public in the last year on the Leading Health Indicators, Health Status Indicators, and Priority Data Needs.
- Increase the proportion of all major national, state, and local health data systems that use geocoding to promote the development of geographic information system (GIS) at all levels.
- Increase the proportion of population-based Healthy People 2010 objectives for which national data are available for all population groups identified for the objective.
- Increase the proportion of Leading Health Indicators, Health Status Indicators, and Priority Data Needs for which data—especially for select populations—are available at the tribal, state, and local levels.
- Increase the proportion of Healthy People 2010 objectives that are tracked regularly at the national level.
- Increase the proportion of Healthy People 2010 objectives for which national data are released within one year of data collection.

Skilled Work Force
- Increase the proportion of public health agencies that incorporate specific competencies in the essential public health services into personal systems.
- Increase the proportion of schools for public health workers that integrate into their curricula specific content to develop competency in the essential public health services.
- Increase the proportion of public health agencies that provide continuing education to develop competency in essential public health services for their employees.

Effective Public Health Organizations
- Increase the proportion of public health agencies that meet national performance standards for essential public health services.
- Increase the proportion of tribes, states, and the District of Columbia that have a health improvement plan and increase the proportion of local jurisdictions that have a health improvement plan linked with their state plan.
- Increase the proportion of state and local public health agencies that provide or assure comprehensive laboratory services to support essential public health services.
- Increase the proportion of public health agencies that provide or assure comprehensive epidemiology services to support essential public health services.
- Increase the proportion of federal, state, and local jurisdictions that review and evaluate the extent to which their statutes, ordinances, and bylaws assure the delivery of essential public health services.

Resources
- Increase the proportion of federal, state, and local public health agencies that gather accurate data on public health expenditures, categorized by essential public health service.

Prevention Research
- Increase the proportion of public health agencies that conduct or collaborate on population-based prevention research.

Source: Reprinted from *Healthy People 2010: Understanding and Improving Health,* U.S. Department of Health and Human Services, Public Health Service, 2000.

CONCLUSION

Public health infrastructure includes the inputs and ingredients of the public health system that are blended together to carry out public health's core functions and essential public health services. Although these can be presented in various categories, several key elements are easily recognized. The first of these is the workforce of public health, an army of individuals committed to improving the public health, although relatively few have had other than on-the-job training for their roles. The diversity of this workforce in terms of educational and experiential backgrounds represents both a major strength and a potential weakness for efforts to focus and direct their collective efforts. Facilitating the contributions of the workforce are the organizations in which they work. These organizations exist at all levels of government, as well as in all corners of the community. The relationships between and among the agencies, organizations, institutions, and individuals committed to this work are more often informal and collaborative than formalized and centrally directed. Leadership within and across organizations to assess and address health issues and needs in the community is essential to initiate the community problem identification and problem-solving activities that can foster the changes necessary for improved health outcomes. The workforce, the organizations, and their leadership rely heavily on information for identifying problems, determining interventions, and tracking progress toward agreed-upon objectives. Together, these essential ingredients of the public system formulate the system's capacity to act in serving the public health. The public health infrastructure has evolved to provide the elements necessary for successful public health interventions: organized and systematic observations through morbidity and mortality surveillance, well-designed epidemiologic studies and other data to facilitate the decision-making process, and individuals and organizations to advocate for resources and to ensure that effective policies and programs were implemented and conducted properly. In the twenty-first century, public health is a complex partnership among federal agencies, state and local governments, nongovernmental organizations, academia, and community members. This infrastructure, and the essential public health services that it provides, represents a small portion of the national economy and only about 5 percent of all health-related expenditures, but its contribution to improved health status and its potential for realizing further gains and closing current gaps suggest that it is worth its weight in gold.

DISCUSSION QUESTIONS AND EXERCISES

1. Choose a recent (within the last three years) outbreak or other public health emergency situation that has drawn significant media attention. Describe how specific aspects of the public health infrastructure contributed to either the emergency situation or its solution. The MMWR contents for recent weeks would be a good place to look for recent outbreaks; various print and electronic media may also be useful sources of information.

2. What distinguishes a public health professional from a professional working for a public health organization?
3. Are public health professionals viewed as change agents in their communities today? Why or why not? Do you hold the same opinion for public health organizations? Why or why not?
4. What factors determine the optimum size for a coalition?
5. How have the roles of local boards of health changed over the past century? What would be the most useful roles for such boards in the future?
6. What factors limit our ability to use the extensive amount of data and information that is currently available? How can these obstacles be overcome?
7. Is health planning at the community level necessary? If so, who should be responsible? How can duplication and replication of community health planning be averted?
8. Examine the data provided in Table 6–3 and, in small groups, prioritize the various injuries to determine which should be the target of a statewide injury-reduction campaign focusing on sports and recreation equipment injuries. Which three should be targeted? Why?
9. Review the scenario described in Exhibit 6–7, and discuss the questions in small groups.
10. Describe how the various components of the public health infrastructure have contributed to the gains in food safety described in "Public Health Achievements in Twentieth-Century America: Safer and Healthier Foods." Which components were most important?

REFERENCES

1. Roper WL, Baker EL, Dyal WW, Nicola RM. Strengthening the public health system. *Public Health Rep.* 1992;107:609–615.
2. U.S. Department of Health and Human Services (DHHS). *Health United States, 2002.* Washington, DC: National Center for Health Statistics; 2002.
3. Health Resources and Services Administration (HRSA). The health professions workforce. *Health Workforce Newslink,* 1999.
4. Health Resources Services Administration, U.S. Department of Health and Human Services. *Public Health Enumeration 2000.* Washington, DC: Government Printing Office, December 2000.
5. Health Resources and Services Administration, U.S. Department of Health and Human Services. *Health Personnel in the United States: Eighth Report to Congress.* Washington, DC: U.S. Public Health Service (PHS); 1992.
6. U.S. Bureau of the Census. Federal, State, and Local Governments, Public Employment and Payroll Data. Available at *www.census.gov/govs/www/apes.html.*
7. National Association of County and City Health Officials. *Profile of Local Health Departments, 1996–1997 Dataset.* Washington, DC: NACCHO; 1997.
8. National Association of County and City Health Officials. Local Public Health Agency Infrastructure: A Chartbook, Washington, DC: NACCHO; 2001.

9. Gerzoff RB, Baker EL. The use of scaling techniques to analyze U.S. local health department staffing structures, 1992–1993. *Proceedings of the Section on Government Statistics and Section on Social Statistics of the American Statistical Association.* 1998;209–213.

10. Kennedy VC, Spears WD, Loe HD, Moore FI. Public health workforce information: A state-level study. *J Public Health Manage Pract.* 1999;5(3):10–19.

11. Kennedy VC. Who provides the essential public health services? A method and example. *J Public Health Manage Pract.* 1999;5(5):98–101.

12. Kennedy VC and Moore FI. A systems approach to public health workforce development. *J Public Health Manage Pract.* 2001;7(4):17–22.

13. Gerzoff RB, Richards TB. The education of local health department top executives. *J Public Health Manage Pract.* 1997;3(4):50–56.

14. Turnock BJ and Hutchison KD. *The Local Public Health Workforce: Size, Distribution, Composition, and Influence on Core Function Performance, Illinois 1998–1999.* Chicago IL; Illinois Center for Health Workforce Studies; 2000.

15. The Core Functions Steering Committee. *The Public Health Workforce: An Agenda for the 21st Century.* DHHS-PHS; 1997.

16. CDC Strategic Plan U.S. Department of Health and Human Services, Centers for Disease Control and Prevention, Public Health Practice Program Office. Strategic Plan for Public Health Workforce Development: Report from the Task Force on Public Health Workforce Development. Atlanta, GA: 1999.

17. Turnock BJ. Roadmap for Public Health Workforce Preparedness. *J Public Health Manage Pract.* 2003;9(6): 471–480.

18. Institute of Medicine. *The Future of Public Health.* Washington, DC: National Academy Press; 1988.

19. Sorenson AA, Bialek RG, eds. *The Public Health Faculty/Agency Forum.* Gainesville, FL: University of Florida Press; 1992.

20. Council on Linkages. Public Health Foundation, Council on Linkages Between Academia and Public Health Practice, Competencies Project, available at *www.trainingfinder.org/competencies.*

21. Gordon AK, Chung K, Handler A, et al. Final report on public health practice linkages between schools of public health and state health agencies: 1992–1996. *J Public Health Manage Pract.* 1999;5(3):25–34.

22. Pew Health Professions Commission. *Critical Challenges: Revitalizing the Health Professions for the Twenty-First Century.* San Francisco, CA: University of California, San Francisco, Center for Health Professions; 1995.

23. Institute of Medicine. *Who Will Keep the Public Healthy? Educating Public Health Professionals for the 21st Century.* Washington, DC: National Academy Press; 2003.

24. *Developing Effective Coalitions: An Eight Step Guide.* Martinez, CA: Contra Costa County Health Services Department; 1994.

25. Lumpkin JR. Six principles of public health information. *J Public Health Manage Pract.* 1995;1(1):40–42.

26. Keppel KG, Freedman MA. What is assessment? *J Public Health Manage Pract.* 1995;1(2):1–7.

27. Friis RH, Sellers TA. *Epidemiology for Public Health Practice.* Gaithersburg, MD: Aspen Publishers; 1996.

28. Thacker SB, Stroup DF, Parrish RG, Anderson HA. Surveillance in environmental public health: Issues, systems and sources. *Am J Public Health.* 1996;86:633–638.

29. CDC. Monitoring environmental disease—United States, 1997. *Morb Mortal Wkly Rep.* 1998;47(25):522–525.

30. Friede A, O'Carroll PW. CDC and ATSDR electronic information resources for health officers. *J Public Health Manage Pract.* 1996;2(3):10–24.

31. Eilbert KW, Barry M, Bialek R, Garufi M. *Measuring Expenditures for Essential Public Health Services.* Washington, DC: Public Health Foundation; 1996.

32. Eilbert KW, Barry M, Bialek R, et al. Public health expenditures: Developing estimates for improved policy making. *J Public Health Manage Pract.* 1997;3(3):1–9.

33. Barry M, Centra L, Pratt E, Brown CK, Giordano L. *Where Do the Dollars Go? Measuring Local Public Health Expenditures.* Washington, DC: Public Health Foundation; 1998.

34. Mays GP, Miller CA, Halverson PK, Baker EL, Stevens R, Vann JJ. Availability and perceived effectiveness of public health activities in the nation's most populous communities. *Am J Public Health.* 2003 (in press).

35. U.S. Department of Health and Human Services. *Healthy People 2010: Understanding and Improving Health.* Washington, DC: DHHS-PHS; 2000.

Chapter 7

Public Health Interventions

Public health practice affects everyone in the community in one way or another. Still, the image that the public most commonly associates with public health is the provision of medical—mostly treatment—care to low-income populations. Although this image is understandable, for public health professionals it is disconcerting.

There are several reasons why this image is prevalent. Many people equate public health with what public health agencies do, and public-sector agencies play an important safety-net role in serving individuals who otherwise lack access to care. This vital safety-net role often overshadows the population-based interventions of these agencies. In fact, the major share of public health resources supports personal care, as opposed to population-based interventions. Public perceptions as to the primary products of public health practice differ from those of most public health practitioners who believe that population-based interventions are the heart and soul of public health practice. However, public health professionals also know that public health is broader than what public health agencies do and that both the public and private sectors provide preventive as well as treatment interventions.

Preventive interventions that target individuals are considered clinical prevention; those that target populations are considered community prevention. Although population-based prevention is usually ascribed to public sector efforts, this should not imply that disease prevention and health promotion are offered only through the public sector or that future shifts in the level and proportion of these strategies offered by public and private providers are not possible. However, the public appears to understand and highly value personal care, both curative and preventive. Its understanding of population-based interventions is much less complete, although public opinion polls provide evidence that these interventions are also highly valued.

Just as people wish to be known as much for their aspirations as for their deeds, public health seeks to be identified with the wide variety of strategies that promote, protect, and maintain health. These strategies, in the form of various interventions, are often organized as programs. Programs represent identifiable products of the public health system's functioning. This chapter will examine various forms of public health interventions, as well as the key steps in their planning, development, and evaluation. Key questions addressed in this chapter include:

- What are the important interventions and programs of public health?
- What characteristics distinguish clinical preventive interventions from population-based interventions?
- How are public health interventions planned and evaluated?

INTERVENTIONS, PROGRAMS, AND SERVICES

The outcomes of the public health system result from carrying out the system's important processes. The important processes of public health, embodied in the essential public health services framework, affect outcomes both directly and indirectly. They directly affect outcomes by identifying important health problems and mobilizing efforts to address those problems. Interventions occur in a variety of forms, including statutes, regulations, policies, and programs intended to improve health status. Many interventions are organized into programs consisting of component processes that together seek to achieve specific outcomes. In this light, public health processes contribute to both the generation and operation of programs. As such, programs are understandable and useful constructs that link public health practice with specific outcomes.

Programs are collections of processes sharing the same objectives; lumping and splitting otherwise discrete programs can result in different formulations. For example, measles immunizations and measles surveillance can be considered as either separate programs or as components of a single program, depending on the formulation of their program objectives. A separate measles immunization program might have an objective to achieve a 90 percent immunization rate among two- to three-year-old children in a particular community. A separate measles surveillance program's objective might be to investigate newly reported cases of measles within 48 hours. Both of these could be considered as part of a more comprehensive measles prevention and control program whose objective might be stated as seeking a reduction in the incidence of measles by some percentage from the current rate.

Programs also provide an understandable framework for describing the scope and content of public health practice and for cataloging public health expenditures. Organizations generally develop budgets and track expenditures on a program-by-program basis. As a result, information on the economic dimensions of public health programs, similar to that presented in Chapters 4 and 6, is available at a variety of levels. Yet, public health practice is more than an aggregation of programs, and public health organizations are more than 40 different companies under one roof, as one health officer described his agency in the early 1990s before refocusing the agency from a program focus to one emphasizing public health's core functions.

Programs and their component processes are sometimes referred to as services if some benefit is bestowed on the individual or groups targeted for those interventions. Other processes of programs may be performed to support the provision of services. Some public health services, such as childhood immunizations, can be classified as clinical services if directly aimed at protecting or improving individual well-being. Others, such as the fluoridation of public water supplies, can be considered population-based services if directed toward a group of individuals or the entire population.

This connotation of services represents one aspect of what programs do, although programs are often known for the services that are provided through them. For example, immunization programs are commonly thought of as vaccinations given to individuals, although the actual shots given represent only one activity of that program. Public education, provider education, outreach, compliance determination, record keeping, and follow-up are also activities of immunization programs. Together, these make up a program whose best known services are vaccinations. The terms *programs* and *services* are often used interchangeably when public health activities are reported. The use of the term *services* (rather than processes) in the essential public health services framework further muddies the water because these are not services in the same way as the clinical preventive and population-based services described previously.

Data from the National Association of County and City Health Officials (NACCHO) profiles of local public health agencies (LPHAs) provide a general measure of the prevalence of public health programs.[1,2] Exhibit 7–1 summarizes information from NACCHO's 1999–2000 survey, using categories derived from the Public Health in America[3] document. Programs and services to prevent epidemics and spread of disease and to protect against environmental hazards are prevalent among LPHAs. Many are provided by more than 70 percent of the nation's LPHAs, including communicable disease control, immunizations for children and adults, tuberculosis (TB) testing, high blood pressure screening, food safety, lead screening, sewage disposal, private water supplies, and restaurant inspections.

Several programs to promote and encourage healthy behaviors are also prevalent, especially general health education; tobacco use prevention; and women, infants, and children (WIC) services. Injury prevention, disaster and emergency services, and activities to assure the quality and accessibility of health services are less consistently provided in the community through LPHA involvement. Among personal health programs, 77 percent of LPHAs link individuals to needed services in the community, while 40–70 percent of LPHAs provide early periodic screening, diagnosis, and treatment (EPSDT) for Medicaid-eligible children, as well as a variety of maternal and child health services in the form of maternal and prenatal care, family planning, and case management. For environmental health programs, 40–70 percent of LPHAs provide indoor air quality, vector control, laboratory, and environmental emergency response services. Fewer than half of the nation's LPHAs are involved in providing injury control, occupational health and safety, dental health, behavioral health, substance abuse, home health, or primary care services. More than 75 percent of LPHAs offer community assessment, community outreach and health education, and epidemiology and surveillance activities. Together, these profiles describe a constellation of local public health programs and services that are noteworthy for both their extensive scope and their local variability.

Exhibit 7–1 Percent of Local Health Departments Directly Providing, Contributing Resources to, or Contracting for Public Health Programs and Services in the Community

Prevent Epidemics & Spread of Disease		Sewage disposal	74%
Communicable disease control	94%	Private water supplies	72%
HIV/AIDS testing/counseling	64%	Vector	61%
STD testing/counseling	65%	Laboratory services	45%
Tuberculosis testing	88%	Solid waste management*	55%
Childhood immunizations	89%	Public water supplies*	63%
EPSDT	59%		
Influenza immunizations	91%	*Promotes & Encourages Healthy Behaviors*	
Hepatitis B immunizations	86%	Health education/risk reduction	87%
Cancer screening	58%	Tobacco prevention	68%
Diabetes screening	57%	Cardiovascular screening	50%
High blood pressure screening	81%	WIC	67%
		School health	46%
Prevents Injuries		Dental health	30%
Occupational health & safety	19%	Violence Prevention	22%
Injury control	37%		
		Assures Quality & Accessibility of Services	
Responds to Disasters/Assists Recovery		Linkage to needed care	77%
Environmental emergencies	61%	Primary care	18%
Hazardous substances*	57%	Prenatal care	41%
Behavioral & mental health*	26%	Maternal health	70%
		Obstetrical care*	31%
Cross-Cutting		Family planning	58%
Community assessment	79%	Case management	67%
Community outreach & education	90%	Health facilities licensing	38%
Epidemiology & surveillance	84%	Home health services	36%
		HIV treatment	25%
Protects Against Environmental Hazards		Substance abuse*	26%
Indoor air quality	44%	School-based clinics*	33%
Food safety	85%	TB treatment	71%
Restaurant inspections	80%	Homeless health services	10%
Lead screening & abatement	74%		

Source: Data from National Association of County and City Health Officials, *Local Public Health Agency Infrastructure: A Chartbook.* Washington, DC; NACCHO; 2001 except for * data from National Association of County and City Health Officials, Profile of Local Health Departments 1996–1997 Data Set. Washington, DC; NACCHO, 1997.

CATEGORIZING PROGRAMS AND SERVICES OF PUBLIC HEALTH

Aggregating programs into categories that focus on broad outcomes provides additional insights into the products of public health practice. External audiences who think of public health in terms of programs and services, rather than internal processes, readily understand this approach. The mega-outcome categories included in the Public Health in America statement (see Exhibit 1–5 and Exhibit 7–1) represent what public health does.[3] The six categories of programs provide a clear and comprehensive aggregation of the products of the public health system that seek to:

- prevent epidemics,
- protect the environment, workplaces, housing, food, and water,
- prevent injuries,
- promote healthy behaviors,
- respond to disasters, and
- ensure the quality, accessibility, and accountability of health services.

Each of these categories includes a mixture of preventive interventions targeted both to populations and to individuals. Preventing epidemics includes efforts such as disease surveillance, disease investigation, contact tracing, case management, prophylactic treatment, laboratory services, and immunizations. Environmental protection includes air and water quality monitoring and permitting; food, housing, and workplace safety standards enforcement; toxic waste permitting and hazardous conditions monitoring; environmental risk assessment services; toxicology evaluation services; laboratory services; and enforcement activities. Injury prevention includes injury surveillance, trauma network services, public education and awareness campaigns, child car seat loaner programs, and the like. Promoting healthy behaviors includes behavioral risk factor monitoring, fitness programs, comprehensive school health education, work site health promotion, community-wide risk reduction programs, media involvement, health education, parenting education, and information clearinghouses and other referral sources. Disaster response includes disaster planning, emergency medical system maintenance, trauma networks, disaster management drills, and emergency information system establishment. Assuring the quality, accessibility, and accountability of health services can include health professions licensing and certification, medical facilities licensing and certification, laboratory services quality assurance, hospital outcomes monitoring, personal services outcomes monitoring, personal services availability assessment, patient satisfaction assessment, cost-effectiveness studies, and automated and linked database management.

Using the framework presented in Chapter 3, these programs and services can also be described in terms of their intervention strategy, level of prevention, practice domain, and target population. Intervention strategies include health promotion, specific protection, early identification and treatment, disability limitation, and rehabilitation. By level of prevention, interventions can be classified as primary, secondary, or tertiary. By practice domain, interventions can be furnished by either public health or medical care practitioners. Interventions are also grouped by their target population, either individuals or populations.

As demonstrated in Exhibit 7–1, the activities available to carry out public health's core functions are extensive. Some are clinically-oriented preventive services for individuals; others are population-based programs and services. The clinical preventive services emphasize early case finding and other aspects of primary care, whereas population-based programs and services largely involve a variety of health promotion and specific protection services. There is considerable overlap between the two, especially for specific protection and early case-finding services.

Clinical Preventive Services

Clinical preventive services include screening tests, counseling interventions, immunizations, and prophylactic regimens for individuals of all age groups and risk categories. Although many of these interventions have been widely accepted and deployed by practitioners, there have been increasing concerns as to whether they truly improved clinical outcomes. Since the 1980s, both the Canadian Task Force on Preventive Health Care and the U.S. Preventive Services Task Force have reviewed information on the effectiveness of specific clinical preventive services.[4] At the heart of this examination are five key questions:[5]

- How important is the target condition?
- How important is the risk factor?
- How accurately can the risk factor or target population be identified?
- Is the preventive service effective?
- Do the benefits of implementation outweigh the costs?

Importance of the target condition is assessed using measures of frequency and severity. Incidence and prevalence are two key measures of frequency, whereas mortality, morbidity, and survival rates are useful measures of severity. Importance of a risk factor is determined by its frequency (incidence and prevalence) and measures of the magnitude of the relationship between the risk factor and the target condition, such as absolute and attributable risk. Absolute risk measures the incidence of the target condition in the population with the risk factor. Attributable risk measures the amount of the risk that is attributable to one particular risk factor.

Risk factor or target population accuracy depends on measures of sensitivity (the proportion of persons with a condition who correctly test positive), specificity (the proportion of persons without a condition who correctly test negative), and positive predictive value (proportion of positive test results that are correct). For screening tests, the criteria consider the accuracy and effectiveness of early detection. For counseling interventions, the criteria relate to the efficacy of risk reduction and the effectiveness of counseling. Efficacy of vaccines is the primary criterion for evaluating these interventions. For chemoprophylaxis, the criteria relate to efficacy, as well as to the effectiveness of counseling. Recommendations for clinical preventive services were first published in 1989 and revised in 1995 for the various age and risk status groups. The second *Task Force Guide to Clinical Preventive Services* was published in 1996 and became the basis for the 1998 *Clinicians Handbook of Preventive Services*[5] and the *Put Prevention into Practice* national implementation program. The third edition of these recommendations is an ongoing process involving reexamination of previous recommendations and consideration of new ones. In order to expedite their translation into practice, recommendations are now released soon after the task force concludes its examination of a specific clinical preventive service. A summary of the topics and clinical preventive services addressed by the task force through June 2003 is provided in Exhibit 7–2. It is important to note that these recommendations were not intended to serve as standards of care; rather, they were meant to be statements as to the quality of the evidence available to justify the use of practices as effective preventive interventions.

Exhibit 7–2 U.S. Preventive Services Task Force Recommendation Topic List, 2003

	Screening	Counseling	Immunizations	Chemoprevention
Abdominal Aortic Aneurysm	•			
Adolescent Idiopathic Scoliosis	•			
Adult Immunizations			•	
Aspirin for Primary Prevention of Cardiovascular Events				•
Aspirin Prophylaxis in Pregnancy				•
Asymptomatic Carotid Artery Stenosis	•			
Asymptomatic Coronary Artery Disease	•			
Bacterial Vaginosis in Pregnancy	•			
Breast Cancer	•			•
Bladder Cancer	•			
Cervical Cancer	•			
Child Developmental Delay	•			
Childhood Immunizations			•	
Chlamydial Infection	•			
Colorectal Cancer	•			
Congenital Hypothyroidism	•			
D (Rh) Incompatibility	•			
Dementia	•			
Dental and Periodontal Disease		•		
Depression	•			
Diabetes Mellitus	•			
Down Syndrome	•			
Drug Abuse	•			
Elevated Lead Levels in Childhood and Pregnancy	•			
Family Violence	•			
Genital Herpes Simplex	•			
Gestational Diabetes	•			
Glaucoma	•			
Gonorrhea	•			
Gynecologic Cancers		•		
Healthy Diet		•		
Hearing Impairment	•			
Hemoglobinopathies	•			
Hepatitis B Virus Infection	•			
Home Uterine Activity Monitoring	•			
Hormone Replacement Therapy				•
Household and Recreational Injuries		•		
Human Immunodeficiency Virus (HIV) Infection	•	•		
Hypertension	•			
Intrapartum Electronic Fetal Monitoring	•			
Iron Deficiency Anemia	•			
Lipid Disorders	•			
Low Back Pain		•		
Lung Cancer	•			
Motor Vehicle Injuries		•		

continues

Exhibit 7-2 continued

	Screening	Counseling	Immunizations	Chemoprevention
Neural Tube Defects	•			
Newborn Hearing: Screening	•			
Obesity	•			
Oral Cancer	•			
Osteoporosis	•			
Ovarian Cancer	•			
Pancreatic Cancer	•			
Peripheral Arterial Disease	•			
Phenylketonuria	•			
Physical Activity		•		
Postexposure Prophylaxis for Selected Infectious Diseases				•
Postmenopausal Hormone Replacement Therapy		•		•
Preeclampsia	•			
Problem Drinking	•			
Prostate Cancer	•			
Rubella	•			
Skin Cancer	•	•		
Suicide Risk	•			
Syphilis	•			
Testicular Cancer	•			
Thyroid Disease	•			
Thyroid Cancer	•			
Tobacco Use		•		
Tuberculous Infection	•			
Ultrasonography in Pregnancy	•			
Unintended Pregnancy		•		
Visual Impairment	•			
Vitamin Supplementation to Prevent Cancer and Coronary Heart Disease				•
Youth Violence		•		

Source: U.S. Preventive Services Task Force, 2003.

Assessments of the effectiveness of preventive services are made, in part, by examining the quality of the scientific evidence available for specific interventions. Evidence from properly designed randomized controlled trials is most heavily weighted in this process followed, in order, by evidence from controlled trials without randomization, well-designed cohort or case control studies (preferably multi-center studies), multiple time series or uncontrolled studies, and expert clinical opinion.

The effectiveness of immunizations has been well established through reductions of more than 99 percent for diseases that include poliomyelitis, rubella, diphtheria, and pertussis. Several screening tests have also contributed to reductions in disease mortality and morbidity. For example, hypertension screening has contributed to the 67 percent reduction in stroke mortality since 1968, and newborn screening for both congenital hypothyroidism and

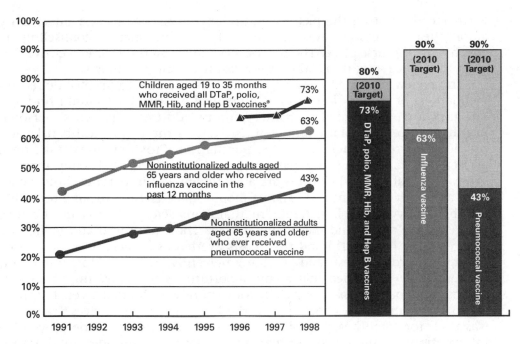

Figure 7–1 Immunization Coverage, United States, 1991–1998, and Year-2010 Targets. *Source:* Reprinted from *Healthy People 2010: Understanding and Improving Health,* U.S. Department of Health and Human Services, Public Health Service, 2000.

phenylketonuria and cervical cancer screening through Pap tests have greatly reduced the burden of these diseases. Chemoprophylaxis, especially for diseases such as tuberculosis, has also contributed to reductions in mortality and morbidity in recent decades. Despite the successes with these forms of clinical preventive services, the greatest potential lies in changing personal behaviors. In the clinical setting, counseling, often supported with screening tests, appears to be the clinical preventive service with the greatest potential.[4]

Complementing the scientific assessment of efficacy (answering the question "Does it work?"), the task force has increasingly focused on assessment of economic benefits and costs (answering the question "Is it worth it?"). These economic evaluations provide an additional dimension to the review of clinical preventive services that takes on greater importance in a world of finite resources, conflicting claims, and competing demands on decision-makers.

Notwithstanding the demonstrated effectiveness of many clinical preventive interventions, they remain underutilized, as demonstrated by the Healthy People 2010 targets for specific clinical preventive interventions included in Figure 7–1. Reasons for the failure to provide clinical preventive interventions often relate to reimbursement practices, provider education and practice patterns, and the pluralistic and fragmented health system in the United States. In addition to these factors, the proliferation of recommendations as to appropriate use of these interventions has created confusion and uncertainty among many health providers as to exactly what should be done and when.

Further complicating the picture are underlying suspicions and uncertainty among health providers as to whether interventions such as counseling are effective in the first place. The process developed by the U.S. Preventive Services Task Force sought to address these last two concerns directly.

The review of evidence leading to the age- and risk group-specific recommendations of the task force was accompanied by several important findings. The task force concluded that interventions addressing patients' personal health practices are vitally important in view of the major health risks and problems currently facing the U.S. population. Providers must take on a greater role in assisting their patients to reduce risks in their daily lives. In short, personal health behaviors are a legitimate and important clinical concern, and both clinicians and patients should share decision making regarding possible interventions. In determining that many screening tests are effective, the task force also found that many are not. These unproved and ineffective services must be avoided and their costs averted as clinicians become more selective in ordering tests and providing preventive services. Most important, the task force concluded that many opportunities for delivering preventive services were being missed, especially for persons with limited access to care.

Another important conclusion of the U.S. Preventive Services Task Force was that, for some health problems and risks, community-wide preventive interventions are more effective than clinical services. This does not diminish the role of clinical providers, however, because their standing in the community can do much to advance community interventions and link them more effectively with the provision of clinical services.

Additional insights into the scope and extent of public health interventions are provided through information on clinical preventive services. Until relatively recently, very little information on these services has been available. Through national surveys conducted by the Centers for Disease Control and Prevention's (CDC) National Center for Health Statistics (see Chapter 6), information on the general population has been generated. This information is less available at the local level, with just over one-half of local health agencies collecting information on clinical preventive services (Figure 7–2).

EVIDENCE-BASED COMMUNITY PREVENTIVE SERVICES

Scientifically sound strategies and approaches are essential for public health interventions to be successful in improving quality of life and reducing preventable mortality and morbidity. Public health practitioners have always highly valued the science base for public health practice, but only recently has the evidence for the effectiveness of community-based interventions been subjected to rigorous scrutiny. This effort is modeled on the work of the U.S. Preventive Services Task Force, which reviewed data and information related to the provision of clinical preventive services to assess what works and what does not. The clinical practice guidelines that emerged from that process have been widely accepted and have served to raise the standard of practice for clinical preventive services for specific age groups.

For preventive interventions, the job only begins with demonstrating efficacy: that an intervention works well under ideal circumstances. Although an

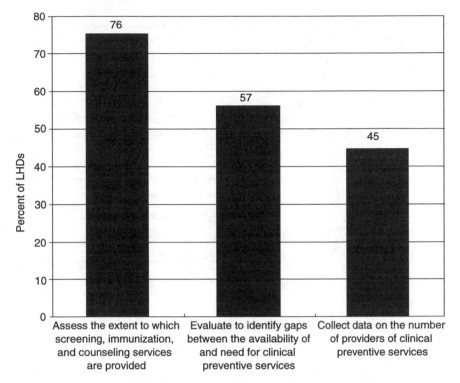

Figure 7–2 Local Health Department Activity in Assessing Clinical Preventive Services, 1992–1993. *Source:* Reprinted from National Association of County and City Health Officials and Centers for Disease Control and Prevention, *Profile of Local Health Departments, 1992–1993,* 1995, Washington, DC.

intervention may be efficacious, it may not work somewhere else because of the particular conditions and circumstances that exist there. Such an intervention would not be considered effective: that is, it would not have the impact intended. Many different social, ethical, legal, and distributional factors may limit effectiveness in a particular setting.[6] Figure 7–3 illustrates the life cycle of a preventive intervention, from its development through basic research to its eventual widespread intervention. In between, applied research activities and community demonstrations are necessary to provide a complete picture of its effectiveness in terms of its impact on outcomes, economic considerations, and safety.

Although these analyses have been applied to clinical preventive services for more than a decade, efforts to apply them to community prevention activities are of more recent vintage. In 1995 the first steps were taken toward the development of practice guidelines for public health, using similar principles.[7] An assessment of the feasibility of such an undertaking was completed through the Council on Linkages between Academia and Public Health Practice. The conclusions and recommendations of this assessment are presented in Exhibit 7–3; they indicate strong support for developing population-based practice guidelines. The primary purpose of guidelines for community preventive services is to

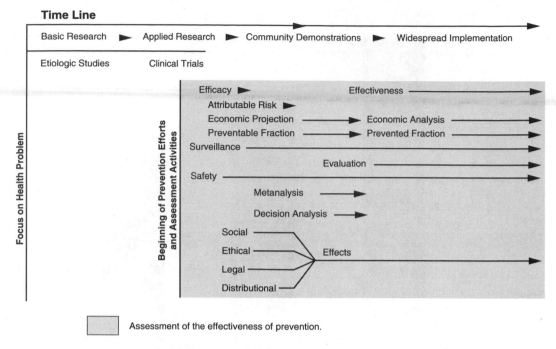

Figure 7–3 Natural History of the Development of an Effective Prevention Strategy and Temporal Relationship to the Types of Assessment Activities. *Source:* Reprinted from S. Teutsch, A Framework for Assessing the Effectiveness of Disease and Injury Prevention, *Morbidity and Mortality Weekly Report,* Vol. 41, p. RR-3, 1992, Centers for Disease Control and Prevention.

Exhibit 7–3 Practice Guidelines for Public Health: Recommendations for Assessment of Scientific Evidence, Feasibility, and Benefits

1. Public health practice guidelines are feasible, based on scientific evidence and other empirical information.
2. The potential benefits of public health practice guidelines are immediate and far-reaching.
3. Each set of guidelines should have a carefully circumscribed scope.
4. Guidelines should be flexible, rather than proscriptive.
5. Guidelines should be dynamic.
6. All major stakeholders should be involved as the guidelines are developed.
7. Critical questions are an efficient tool to structure the evidence-collection process.
8. A database search for scientific studies is a useful first step.
9. Additional sources of documentary evidence should be tapped and systematically evaluated.
10. Empiric evidence from state and local public health programs should be sought, evaluated, and incorporated into the guidelines.
11. Development of guidelines will stimulate needed research.
12. Guidelines should be pilot-tested before dissemination, then continuously evaluated.

Source: Reprinted from Council on Linkages Between Academia and Public Health Practice, *Practical Guidelines for Public Health: Assessment of Scientific Evidence, Feasibility and Benefits,* October 1995, Council on Linkages, U.S. Public Health Services.

provide public health practitioners, their community partners, and policy makers with information needed for informed decision making on the most effective public health strategies, policies, and programs for their communities. Where interventions are found to be effective, this process then examines their cost-effectiveness, benefits and harms, generalizability, and barriers to implementation. This information provides the basis for evidence-based recommendations on the use of specific community preventive interventions.

Population-based community prevention focuses on assessing and addressing common, as well as emergent, health problems and needs. It is both an investment strategy and a tool for protecting and enhancing community health status. Several forces have accelerated interest in a more evidence-based approach to community prevention that complements recent advances in evidence-based medicine and clinical preventive services in order to assess what works and what doesn't. The increasing chronic disease burden is one of those forces necessitating greater interest in preventive (reducing incidence and prevalence) strategies that focus on education and behavioral change rather than on new treatment modalities. Lessons learned in terms of environmental interventions and public policy changes in laws, regulations, and enforcement can be extended to new threats and other conditions. Changes in the health-care system are also needed in order to promote and target effective clinical preventive services to reach more of those who would benefit from such services.

The progress made after 1950 in identifying risk factors associated with chronic diseases and injuries is sometimes called the second epidemiologic revolution. With the importance of heart disease, stroke, cancer, diabetes, chronic lung diseases, and injuries as major contributors to morbidity and mortality, health promotion programs have grown in number and scope over the past two decades. Examples include injury risk reduction through use of seat belts, education to prevent tobacco use abatement, campaigns against drinking and driving, nutrition education (fat intake), fitness campaigns, smokeless tobacco use abatement, stress management, and programs promoting safe sex and abstinence. Risk or harm reduction strategies often seek to reduce, rather than totally eliminate, risk factors in a population by focusing on multiple strategies and by not considering the risk behavior from a moral or value-laden perspective.

Although viewed as important for health purposes, and increasingly emphasized by public and voluntary organizations, these services have not been widely embraced by providers and organizations in the private sector. To some extent, this has occurred because insurance plans have not covered these services and because they are not viewed as valued by the public. As a result, providers have not sought to advertise or otherwise promote them. Instead, disease-specific services emphasizing sophisticated, high-technology services, including screening tests, have been used to attract patients and market share.

The convergence of these considerations led to the development of the Task Force on Community Preventive Services and the establishment of the *Guide to Community Preventive Services*[8] (Community Guide). The Community Guide provides answers as to which strategies work to promote healthy lifestyles, prevent disease, and increase the number of people who receive appropriate preventive counseling and screening. The Community Guide provides decision makers with recommendations regarding population-based interventions to promote health and to prevent injury, disease, disability, and premature death. These recommendations target communities and health-care providers and focus on three general areas:

- Changing risk behaviors
  - Tobacco product use, prevention, and control
  - Alcohol abuse
  - Physical activity
  - Sexual behavior
- Reducing diseases, injuries, and impairments
  - Vaccine preventable diseases
  - Cancer
  - Diabetes
  - Mental health
  - Motor vehicle occupant injury
  - Oral health
  - Violence
- Addressing environmental and ecosystem challenges
  - Social environment

Systematic reviews are conducted for specific interventions within each health topic and organized as a chapter of the Community Guide. The assessment evaluates evidence of effectiveness and translates that into a recommendation or a finding of insufficient evidence. Importantly, a determination that evidence is insufficient does not mean that there is evidence of ineffectiveness. Exhibit 7–4 provides a summary of some of the task force's conclusions regarding community preventive services that work.

Community preventive services embody the two basic strategies for primary prevention (health promotion and specific prevention) and foster appropriate utilization of various tools for secondary prevention. These strategies are largely targeted to populations—the entire population or specific groups. These services constitute public health practice regardless of whether they are provided by public- or private-sector organizations and providers. It is not essential that all community preventive services be provided by the public sector, although some specific services can be organized and provided only through that route (e.g., fluoridation of water supplies).

It is likely that, as more communities become engaged in community-wide health improvement initiatives across the United States, there will be greater recognition of the need for community prevention services geared toward chronic diseases and a variety of behavioral health problems. During the twentieth century public health priorities have shifted away from communicable disease control, environmental hazards, and maternal and child health services toward chronic disease prevention, injuries, violence, mental health, and substance abuse as community health priorities. Recent evidence of this shift is reflected in the categories of community health priorities that were established as a result of all certified LPHAs in Illinois completing a community needs assessment process and community health plan (an adaptation of the Assessment Protocol for Excellence in Public Health, described in Chapter 5) in 1993/1994, followed by a second round of assessments in 1999/2000.[9] More

Exhibit 7–4 Guide to Community Preventive Services: What Works?

	Community Preventive Interventions that Work
Community Interventions	• Community water fluoridation • School-based dental sealant delivery programs • Community-wide education campaigns to increase physical activity • Early childhood development programs • Mass media campaigns to reduce tobacco use • Tobacco cessation telephone support systems
Education and Behavior Change	• Distribution and education programs for child safety seats • Individually-adapted behavior change programs to increase physical activity • School-based physical education • Publicly funded, center-based comprehensive early childhood development programs for children 3–5 years old
Environmental Interventions	• Create or enhance access to places for physical activity combined with informational outreach • Use of tenant-based rental assistance vouchers improves household safety by giving qualified families a choice in moving to neighborhoods that offer reduced exposure to violence
Healthcare System Interventions	• Diabetes disease management and case management programs • Tobacco cessation provider reminders and provider education • Reduce patients' out-of-pocket costs for vaccinations • Client and provider reminder systems for vaccinations • Standing orders for vaccinations
Legislation, Regulation, and Enforcement	• Sobriety checkpoints • Reduce legal blood alcohol levels (BAC) to <0.08% • Maintain legal drinking age at 21 years • Child safety seat laws • Safety belt laws • Increase the unit price of tobacco products • Smoking bans and restrictions

Source: Task Force on Community Preventive Services, 2003.

than 90 local health jurisdictions completed developed community health plans with thousands of community participants across the state. In each round more than 335 health priorities were identified in nine categories. As illustrated in Figure 7–4, there were changes in the leading categories for priorities during the 1990s, with more local health jurisdictions in 1999/2000 identifying priorities related to access to care, chronic diseases, and mental health and fewer identifying environmental hazards, communicable disease control, and maternal and child health as priorities than in 1993/1994.

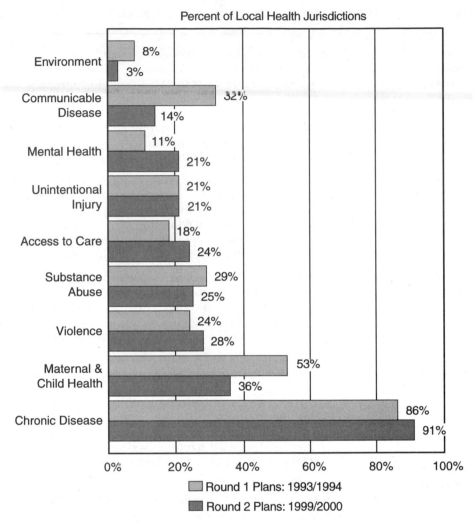

Figure 7–4 Categories of Health Problems Identified as Priority Community Health Problems through Community Needs Assessments, Illinois, 1993/1994 and 1999/2000. *Source:* Illinois Department of Public Health, IPLAN Objective Summary, 2002.

Mental health, substance abuse, violence, and injuries were more frequently identified as priorities than communicable disease control or environmental hazards in the 1999/2000 community health assessments.

Evidence-based public health practice presents formidable challenges for several important reasons. Frequently relying on cross-sectional and quasi-experimental designs that lack a true comparison or control group, the quality of evidence for public health interventions is often limited, in comparison with the evidence for medical interventions. In addition, there is a longer time period between intervention and outcome for many public health activities. Still, there is a variety of tools available to public health practitioners to assist in

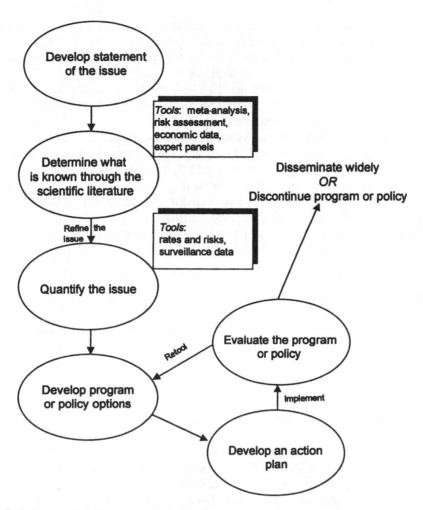

Figure 7–5 A Sequential Framework for Enhancing Evidence-Based Public Health. *Source:* Reprinted from Brownson et at., Evidence-Based Decision Making in Public Health, *Journal of Public Health Management and Practice,* 1999;5(5):86–97 © 1999, Lippincott, Williams & Wilkins.

determining when public health action is warranted, including meta-analysis, risk assessment, economic evaluation, public health surveillance, and expert panels and consensus conferences.[10,11] Basic steps useful for enhancing evidence-based public-health practice are illustrated in Figure 7–5; they include:

- developing an initial, concise, operation statement of the issue
- determining what is known through the scientific literature
- quantifying the issue
- developing program or policy options
- developing an action plan for the program or policy
- evaluating the program or policy[10]

It is clear that the needs of science and public policy differ in terms of their standards of evidence. Scientists would prefer that many true hypotheses go unproven rather than to "prove" one false hypothesis. Public health professionals, however, often cannot wait until definitive evidence is available. Evidence-based practice does not demand that judgment be suspended until all of the evidence is in or that only "gold standard" evidence is acceptable. For decades the tobacco industry dismissed evidence of the causal link between tobacco use and lung cancer as inconclusive because it was based largely on observational studies. This objection resonated with research scientists but did not deter public health activists from planning and implementing anti-tobacco interventions. A similar scenario existed with deploying both population-based and individual-oriented preventive interventions in reducing dental caries through fluoridation of public water supplies during the second half of the twentieth century (see "Public Health Achievements in Twentieth-Century America: Fluoridation of Drinking Water to Prevent Dental Caries").

Example

Public Health Achievements in Twentieth-Century America: Fluoridation of Drinking Water to Prevent Dental Caries

Fluoridation of public water supplies is a simple but extremely effective community-based intervention. Its story is one of the great accomplishments of public heath in twentieth-century America.

At the beginning of the twentieth century, extensive dental caries was common in the United States and in most developed countries. No effective measures existed for preventing this disease, and the most frequent treatment was tooth extraction. Failure to meet the minimum standard of having six opposing teeth was a leading cause of rejection from military service in both world wars. Pioneering oral epidemiologists developed an index to measure the prevalence of dental caries using the number of decayed, missing, or filled teeth (DMFT) or decayed, missing, or filled tooth surfaces (DMFS), rather than merely presence of dental caries, in part because nearly all persons in most age groups in the United States had evidence of the disease. Application of the DMFT index in epidemiologic surveys throughout the United States in the 1930s and 1940s allowed quantitative distinctions in dental caries experience among communities—an innovation that proved critical in identifying a preventive agent and evaluating its effects.

Soon after establishing his dental practice in Colorado Springs, Colorado, in 1901, Dr. Frederick S. McKay noted an unusual permanent stain or "mottled enamel" (termed *Colorado brown stain* by area residents) on the teeth of many of his patients. After years of personal field investigations, McKay concluded that an agent in the public water supply probably was responsible for mottled enamel. McKay also observed that teeth affected by this condition seemed less susceptible to dental caries. In 1930 a chemist with Aluminum Company of America, an aluminum manufacturing company that had bauxite mines in the town, used a newly available method of spectrographic analysis that identified high concentrations of fluoride (13.7 parts per million [ppm]) in the water of the abandoned well. Fluoride, the ion of the element fluorine, almost universally is found in soil and water, but generally in very low concentrations (less than 1.0 ppm). On hearing of the new analytic method, McKay sent water samples to Churchill (the chemist) from areas where mottled enamel was endemic; these samples contained high levels of fluoride (2.0-12.0 ppm).

The effectiveness of community water fluoridation in preventing dental caries prompted rapid adoption of this public health measure in cities throughout the United States. As a result, dental caries declined precipitously during the second half of the twentieth century. For example, the mean DMFT among persons aged 12 years in the United States declined 68 percent, from 4.0 in 1966–1970 to 1.3 in 1988–1994 (Figure 7–6). The American Dental Association, the American Medical Association, the World Health Organization, and other professional and scientific organizations quickly endorsed water fluoridation. Knowledge about the benefits of water fluoridation led to the development of other modalities for delivery of fluoride, such as toothpastes, gels, mouth rinses, tablets, and drops. Several countries in Europe and Latin America have added fluoride to table salt.

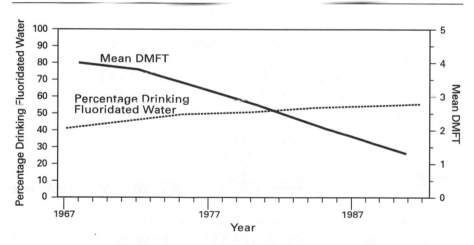

Figure 7–6 Percentage of population residing in areas with fluoridated community water system and mean number of decayed, missing (because of caries), or filled permanent teeth (DMFT) among children aged 12 years, United States, 1967–1992. *Source:* Reprinted from Achievements in Public Health, United States, 1900–1999: Fluoridation of Drinking Water to Prevent Dental Caries, *Morbidity and Mortality Weekly Report,* Vol. 48, No. 41, pp. 933–940, the Centers for Disease Control and Prevention, 1999.

Early studies reported that caries reduction attributable to fluoridation ranged from 50 percent to 70 percent, but by the mid-1980s, the mean DMFS scores in the permanent dentition of children who lived in communities with fluoridated water were only 18 percent lower than among those living in communities without fluoridated water. A review of studies on the effectiveness of water fluoridation conducted in the United States during 1979–1989 found that caries reduction was 8–37 percent among adolescents (mean: 26.5 percent).

Since the early days of community water fluoridation, the prevalence of dental caries has declined in communities both with and without fluoridated water in the United States. This trend has been attributed largely to the diffusion of fluoridated water to areas without fluoridated water through bottling and processing of foods and beverages in areas with fluoridated water and widespread use of fluoride toothpaste. Fluoride toothpaste is efficacious in preventing dental caries, but its effectiveness depends on frequency of use by persons or their caregivers. In contrast, water fluoridation reaches all residents of communities and generally is not dependent on individual behavior.

Although early studies focused mostly on children, water fluoridation also is effective in preventing dental caries among adults. Fluoridation reduces enamel caries in adults by 20–40 percent and prevents caries on the exposed root surfaces of teeth, a condition that particularly affects older adults.

Water fluoridation is especially beneficial for communities of low socioeconomic status. These communities have a disproportionate burden of dental caries and have less access than higher-income communities to dental-care services and other sources of fluoride. Water fluoridation may help to reduce such dental health disparities.

By the end of 1992, 10,567 public water systems serving 135 million persons in 8,573 U.S. communities had instituted water fluoridation. Approximately 70 percent of all U.S. cities with populations of greater than 100,000 used fluoridated water. In addition, 3,784 public water systems serving 10 million persons in 1,924 communities had natural fluoride levels greater than or equal to 0.7 ppm. In total, 144 million persons in the United States (56 percent of the population) were receiving fluoridated water in 1992, including 62 percent of those served by public water systems. However, approximately 42,000 public water systems and 153 U.S. cities with populations greater than or equal to 50,000 have not instituted fluoridation.

Water fluoridation costs range from a mean of 31 cents per person per year in U.S. communities of greater than 50,000 persons to a mean of $2.12 per person in communities of less than 10,000 (1988 dollars). Compared with other methods of community-based dental caries prevention, water fluoridation is the most cost-effective for most areas of the United States in terms of cost per saved tooth surface.

Water fluoridation reduces direct health-care expenditures through primary prevention of dental caries and avoidance of restorative care. Per capita cost savings from one year of fluoridation may range from negligible amounts among very small communities with very low incidence of caries to $53 among large communities with a high incidence of disease. One economic analysis estimated that prevention of dental caries, largely attributed to fluoridation and fluoride-containing products, saved $39 billion (1990 dollars) in dental-care expenditures in the United States during 1979–1989.

Early investigations into the physiologic effects of fluoride in drinking water predated the first community field trials. Since 1950 opponents of water fluoridation have claimed that it increased the risk for cancer, Down syndrome, heart disease, osteoporosis and bone fracture, acquired immunodeficiency syndrome, low intelligence, Alzheimer disease, allergic reactions, and other health conditions. The safety and effectiveness of water fluoridation have been reevaluated frequently, and no credible evidence supports an association between fluoridation and any of these conditions.

Source: Adapted from Achievements in Public Health, United States, 1900–1999: Fluoridation of Drinking Water to Prevent Dental Caries, *Morbidity and Mortality Weekly Report,* Vol. 48, No. 41, pp. 933–940, the Centers for Disease Control and Prevention, 1999.

PROGRAM MANAGEMENT IN PUBLIC HEALTH

Program management in public health includes the myriad activities involved with the development, implementation, and evaluation of interventions addressing public health problems. Effective program management is an organized response requiring a carefully designed problem statement, the availability of an appropriate intervention, and the capacity to deliver that intervention in a specific setting. Each of these is an essential component of an organized response. The task is to bring these elements together and direct them toward the solution of problems. Public health program management seeks to organize and direct public health workers, scientifically sound interventions, and appropriate strategies toward specific health problems.[12] The ultimate aim is to eliminate or reduce these problems to the maximum extent possible (effectiveness) and to achieve these results with the minimum resources necessary (efficiency). Effectiveness and efficiency are the primary criteria by which programs are judged or evaluated.

Management revolves around resource allocation and utilization. The resources of public health as described in Chapter 6 include the human, organizational, informational, fiscal, and other supportive resources. To utilize these resources both effectively and efficiently, there must be a process that carefully examines the problem for the pathways most likely to yield successful results. There are two cardinal sins of program management: (1) failing to achieve program objectives when adequate resources are available and (2) utilizing more resources than are necessary to achieve a program's objectives. The first situation is more commonly viewed as poor management than the second, although from a management point of view, each results in resources being wasted. When program management is improperly or only partially applied, either resources and technology are underutilized—and problems are not fully addressed—or resources and technology are inefficiently utilized—resulting in excess resource consumption and opportunity costs.

Program management calls for the development of a program hypothesis. This is best understood when programs are considered at the level of their basic elements, namely, the specific activities or tasks that are undertaken. The program hypothesis in its simplest form is that if the designated activities are successfully undertaken, the program's goals and objectives will be successfully addressed. For health programs, we expect that these activities will change characteristics of individuals or populations such that factors contributing to the level of the health problem will improve. With improvements in these various factors affecting the health problem, we expect that the level of the health problem itself will also be improved. Depending on how many intervening levels of factors there might be, we expect that improvement at one level will result in improvements in higher levels. These terms will be defined and clarified below; the major point here is that rational programs directly address the chain of causation that creates the health problem being targeted by the program.

The management cycle is often described as consisting of three phases: (1) planning (deciding what to do and how to do it), (2) implementation (acting to accomplish what has been planned), and (3) evaluation (comparing the results of what was accomplished with what was intended).[12] Very often, planning, implementation, and evaluation have been viewed as linear processes. First we plan. Then we implement. Finally, we evaluate what has occurred. In this linear model, we stop planning when we begin implementing, and we do not evaluate until after we have implemented our program. This approach views planning and evaluation as discrete, independent functions carried out at different points in the life span of a program. There are few fallacies more dangerous to sound management than this one! It is critical that planning and evaluation be viewed as interrelated and interdependent processes working together at varying levels of emphasis throughout the life of a program. Rather than a linear process, program management should be viewed as a cyclical process in which one step logically leads to the next, and feedback obtained at all steps is used to revise the directions established in preceding steps.

Program management centers on the development of objectives. Unfortunately, objectives are all too often viewed as the products of planners alone. Program management in public health and other areas is simply too important for objectives to be left to the planners! Objectives are more than abstract targets for achievement. Although they are often characterized as the blueprint of a program, they actually serve more as a roadmap than as a blueprint. Objectives point the program toward a specific destination and, at the same time, set its speed and its mile markers. Objectives guide program administration and establish the framework and strategy for program evaluation. Rather than serving primarily as tools for program planning, they guide all aspects of program planning, administration, and evaluation.

Linking Planning and Evaluation

A practical definition of planning views it as the application of rational decision making to the commitment of future resources. Planning is as much an art as it is a science. Planners do not have any special abilities to predict or foresee the future, and planning does not result in certainty as to what will happen. Rational planning serves to reduce, but not entirely eliminate, risk. The management purpose behind planning must be kept in mind; it is to make the most efficient use of resources. As a result, planning should not be judged solely by the accuracy of its predictions or even by whether planning targets, such as objectives, are met. Instead, planning should be judged on the basis of whether it helps an organization to achieve the best possible results in a changing environment. It is rare for programs to be carried out exactly as they were designed. Change occurs constantly among the external and internal factors that affect both the problem and programs designed to address the problem. Ongoing planning serves to recognize changes and modify implementation strategies accordingly. The ability of a program to evaluate itself continuously determines how quickly and effectively it can respond to changing conditions.

The key to the process of evaluation is the ability to ask the right questions. All too often, little thought is given to an evaluation strategy until the program is already in place and decision makers or funders begin to ask for evidence of its benefit. In short, evaluation is an afterthought. As a result, programs scurry around, asking the question, "What are we doing that we can measure?" Unfortunately, often very little can be done at this point. Evaluation strategies should be developed and agreed upon before programs are implemented, and they should be based on asking the quite different question, "What do we need to measure to know what we are doing?" We will return to these issues in greater detail as we discuss planning and evaluation in subsequent sections of this chapter. The point here is that these are not to be considered as bookends for program implementation; rather, they should be carried out concurrently and continuously. When this is done, planning and evaluation contribute substantially to a rational decision-making system in which managers are more likely to ask the right questions and direct resources toward the most promising intervention activities.

Key Questions for Managers

There are five key questions that guide the program management process:[12]

1. Where are we?
2. Where do we want to be?
3. Should we do something?
4. What should we do?
5. How do we know that we are getting there?

These questions provide managers with much of the essential information needed to make better decisions. They focus attention on the essential components of any decision process: the starting point, the ending point, and the intermediate measurements. The logic and rational nature of this process can be tracked through decision models, such as those developed by CDC for public health program managers. In Exhibit 7–5, the five questions serve as a roadmap of the program manager's major duties and tasks.

Even with a road map, journeys require a destination or goal. For public health programs, goals are generalized statements expressing a program's intended effect on one or more health problems. Goals are often described as timeless statements of overall aspirations; these generally serve to establish boundaries for the program's operational activities, but they also serve as the philosophic justification for a program's existence. It is unusual for program managers to be involved in the establishment of goals. Higher authorities, such as boards, legislative bodies, or even funding sources, usually establish these. Despite being somewhat abstract and externally developed, goals serve a valuable purpose for public health programs. Goals need to be clearly stated, and they need to be understood by all program staff, if only to serve as a common bond and continuous reminder of the program's aspirations.

Exhibit 7–5 Key Questions for Managers of Public Health Programs

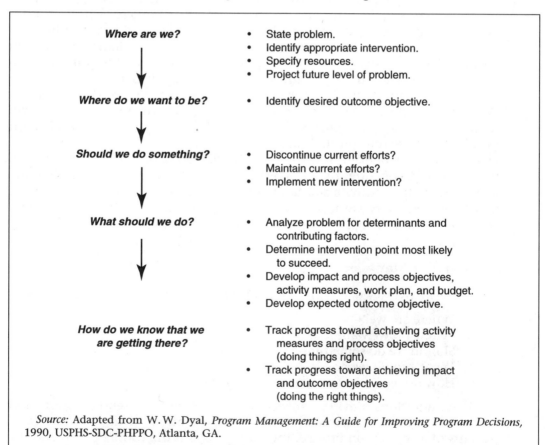

Where are we?
- State problem.
- Identify appropriate intervention.
- Specify resources.
- Project future level of problem.

Where do we want to be?
- Identify desired outcome objective.

Should we do something?
- Discontinue current efforts?
- Maintain current efforts?
- Implement new intervention?

What should we do?
- Analyze problem for determinants and contributing factors.
- Determine intervention point most likely to succeed.
- Develop impact and process objectives, activity measures, work plan, and budget.
- Develop expected outcome objective.

How do we know that we are getting there?
- Track progress toward achieving activity measures and process objectives (doing things right).
- Track progress toward achieving impact and outcome objectives (doing the right things).

Source: Adapted from W. W. Dyal, *Program Management: A Guide for Improving Program Decisions,* 1990, USPHS-SDC-PHPPO, Atlanta, GA.

Where Are We?

The essence of decision making at any level is deciding either to do some-thing or to do nothing. A rational decision to do or not do something calls for a thorough assessment of the current situation, or an asking of the question, "Where are we?" Determining the current status of things assists the manager in several ways. It provides information that can be later used to decide whether action should be taken; it also serves to describe the dimensions of a potential problem in terms of which groups might be more affected, and it establishes a baseline for comparisons over time.

In examining where things stand, it is important to assess in detail the problem, the interventions capable of addressing the problem, and the resources available to deploy those interventions. Although these three ele-ments need to be considered together in determining the current situation, the availability of an effective intervention is absolutely essential from the pro-gram management perspective. Without a potentially effective intervention, it makes little sense to plan and implement a program. The availability of an effective intervention refers to the current level of sophistication of the knowl-edge and techniques for its coordinated application. It is the science and knowledge base for developing and justifying a technical approach for accom-plishing a goal. The specific intervention approach could be drawn from any of the categories of health interventions strategies described in Chapter 3 (health promotion, specific protection, early case finding and treatment, disability lim-itation, and rehabilitation). As a result, the intervention could be based on medical sciences, physical sciences, or social sciences. Sometimes referred to as the state of the art, this knowledge or technical information convinces pro-gram managers that a particular health problem can be addressed.

In addition to the capability to intervene, there are two other considera-tions in assessing where things currently stand. These are the level of a health problem and the capacity or resources to intervene. A health problem is defined here as a situation or condition of people (expressed in health out-come terms, such as mortality, morbidity, or disability) that is considered undesirable and is likely to exist in the future unless additional interventions are implemented. The heart of any intervention strategy lies in the definition of the problem. The development of objectives and intervention strategies flows naturally from a careful and precise statement of the problem. Problem statements come in all formats and lengths, and they vary significantly in their complexity. Still, all good problem statements present a clear, concise, and accurate description of the condition to be controlled or prevented. The more carefully that a problem is stated, the more likely it is that it can be accurately measured.

Planning processes look to the future. Above all, planning is concerned with future resource allocation; therefore, decisions will need to address the anticipated future level of problems, rather than their current levels. It makes little sense to throw additional resources at a problem if that problem's level is declining and the level of the problem in the future may not be deemed unac-ceptable. This would constitute at least a partial waste of resources, something that is to be avoided with good management practices. Even a decreasing level of a problem may merit additional resource allocation if that level is judged to be unacceptable or if additional resources might accelerate the decrease.

Looking to both the past and the future is necessary to describe a problem adequately because its trends are an important aspect of its description. Tracking problems over time also helps to project their future levels through trend analysis techniques. Often, however, tracking the level of a problem provides only an incomplete picture of changes over time. It is also important to track changes and trends in the problem's major determinants. For example, changes in low birthweight (a major determinant of infant mortality) should be examined alongside infant mortality rates, and changes in tobacco use should be tracked alongside lung cancer rates. Projecting future levels of a problem on the basis of trends in the problem and its determinants is fraught with uncertainty and is imprecise at best. Nonetheless, it is both useful and rational in informing decisions that will allocate resources to achieve specific results.

In addition to trends and projections of levels, the process of problem specification calls for assessment of the size, scope, and distribution of a problem, beginning with a clear definition of the problem in terms of its nature and etiology, its magnitude and extent in terms of its incidence and prevalence, its affected populations in terms of specific populations at risk (by age, sex, race, occupation, or other risk factors), and its time and place of occurrence. In some respects, this reads like the major components of a news story in terms of who, what, when, where, and how much.

Just as problems need to be carefully specified in determining where we are, resources also need to be assessed for their trends over time in terms of financial resources, as well as human resources (number, types, skills), organizational resources, information resources, facilities, equipment, and other materials. Tracking both the problem and the resources over time allows for reasonable predictions to be made as to the effects (if any) of resources on the problem and what might be expected at various future resource levels. This information facilitates the development of realistic outcomes.

Where Do We Want To Be?

Determining where you are allows for a comparison with where you want to be. In answering this question, one makes an effort to identify the level at which a problem will be considered acceptable at some point in the future. This is the level at which a current problem will no longer be considered a problem, and it is very much dependent on how carefully and comprehensively the problem has been described. If a problem is well defined in terms of what, how much, who, when, and where, priorities can be established so that resources can be most efficiently utilized to achieve program results. Specific measurable objectives can also be established on the basis of these components of the problem description. The term *desired outcome objective* refers to the level to which a health problem should be reduced and/or maintained within a specified time period. It is meant to be of long term (generally two or more years), realistic (achievable through the intervention strategies proposed), and measurable. Outcome objectives are designed to measure directly the level of the health problem; they include a statement of how much and when the program should affect the health problem. An outcome objective is a quantitative measurement of the health problem at some future date and is something that the manager believes the program can and should accomplish. To establish meaningful outcome objectives, the three key ingredients are the availability of effective interventions, the resources and capacity to implement these interventions, and projections for the future level of the health problem. By assessing the past and current relationships among capability, capacity, and outcomes, one can project realistic and measurable outcome objectives for various levels of program activity.

Should We Do Something?

The purpose of asking the first two questions ("Where are we?" and "Where do we want to be?") is to force a decision as to whether something additional needs to be done. When where you are (and are likely to be) differs from where you would like to be, change is indicated. Change can take one of two forms, doing more or doing less. As a result, there are three options in terms of resource allocation and deployment: reduce (or even eliminate) current efforts, maintain current efforts, or implement a new intervention.

Discontinuing current efforts may be called for if the health problem has already reached or is projected to reach desirable levels, such that further resource allocation is unnecessary. From a manager's point of view, this represents an opportunity to save or redirect resources, rather than to waste them.

A second option is to continue to provide the same level of resources if that level will achieve the desired outcome level by the target achievement date. The decision for a maintenance level should never become automatic; an active, analytical decision-making process should precede it. If the expected level of the problem falls within the acceptable range and resources are available, maintenance of the current level of effort is appropriate.

Interventions are called for when the projected level of the problem exceeds the desired outcome objective and when the capability and capacity to intervene are available. With the availability of technology and resources, the trick is to determine the best implementation strategy that will utilize these to achieve the desired outcome. How a program gets from where it is to where it wants to be requires that decisions be made as to which specific strategies and activities are to be used. There are generally at least several strategies for affecting the level or extent of a health problem. The decisions to be made are based on which options are likely to be most successful and how much of the program's resources should be devoted to each strategy. A program's intervention strategy determines how a program's resources are to be deployed to achieve the desired outcome objective. The logic behind this is simple: If the strategies and activities are carried out as planned, the problem will be reduced to the expected level on schedule. Many uncertainties and unforeseen circumstances can prevent an intervention strategy from succeeding as planned. These can be viewed as analogous to the difference between efficacy (Will it work?) and effectiveness (Will it work here?). In any event, an intervention strategy is as much a hypothesis as it is a plan. It remains to be proven, and the likelihood of unforeseen problems and obstacles increases when the problem is inadequately defined and analyzed.

Exhibit 7–6 Levels of Program Management and Planning

Goal	*Defined Operational and Philosophical Parameters*
• Outcome objective	• Projected future level of the health problem
• Impact objective	• Projected future level of a direct determinant
• Process objective	• Projected future level of a contributing factor
• Activities	• Actual tasks performed by program personnel

Source: Adapted from W. W. Dyal, *Program Management: A Guide for Improving Program Decisions,* 1990, USPHS-CDC-PHPPO, Atlanta, GA.

What Should We Do?

When the problem has been clearly and concisely stated, when the capability to intervene exists, and when the capacity to deploy the interventions is on hand, an intervention strategy can succeed. Success will further depend on how thoroughly the problem has been analyzed so that its major determinants and their contributing factors are identified. This analysis provides information as to which approaches are most likely to be effective and allows for matching of program resources with activities that will address key contributing factors.

Consistent with the health problems analysis model described in Chapter 2, measures of health problems should be stated in terms of health outcomes, such as mortality, morbidity, incidence, and prevalence. Determinants are risk factors that, on the basis of scientific evidence or theory, are thought to directly influence the level of a specific health problem. Contributing factors are those factors that directly or indirectly influence the level of determinants. Analysis should continue until all pertinent direct determinants and their associated contributing factors have been identified. The direct determinants are then examined to determine which offer the greatest chance of success in achieving the desired outcome. For some determinants, there are either no or only partly effective interventions. Those that offer the best chances for success are selected as points of intervention.

In addition to the expected outcome objective, other levels of objectives guide the intervention process. The outcome objective relates to the level of the health problem. Similarly, some objectives relate to determinants, and still others relate to the contributing factors (Exhibit 7–6 and Table 7–1).

Impact objectives address the level to which a direct determinant is to be reduced within a specified time period. They are generally intermediate (1–5 years) in terms of time, and they are both realistic and measurable. An impact objective measures a determinant and states how much and when the program will affect the determinant. It is the quantitative measurement of the determinant at some future date.

Just as impact objectives measure determinants, process objectives measure contributing factors. For a program to function as planned, achieving process objectives will lead to achieving impact objectives, which, in turn, will result in achieving of the outcome objective. Process objectives are shorter

Table 7–1 Characteristics of Program Objectives

Term	Time Period	Description	Measurement
Outcome objective	Usually long-term	Related to health problem	Degree of accomplishment; addresses doing the right things
Impact objective	Intermediate	Related to direct determinants and risk factors	Degree of accomplishment; addresses doing the right things
Process objective	Short-term	Related to contributing factors	Degree of accomplishment; addresses doing things right
Activities	Usually short-term	Describes the use of program resources	Accomplishment (yes/no); addresses doing things right

Source: Adapted from W.W. Dyal, *Program Management: A Guide for Improving Program Decisions,* 1990, USPHS-CDC-PHPPO, Atlanta, GA.

term than outcome or impact objectives. They are of short term (usually one year), realistic, and measurable.

The establishment of process objectives initiates two activities, one focusing on developing a workplan for the activities necessary to address the process objectives and one revisiting the outcome objective. The former activity is seldom overlooked because it is essential in order to complete the program planning process. The latter activity, however, is often forgotten, resulting in programs operating with outcome objectives that cannot be achieved. The rationale for revisiting the outcome objective is that the intervention strategy selected, together with its process objectives and activity measures, is likely to be only partially successful in reducing the outcome objective to the desired level. Programs are seldom able to achieve the entire improvement called for in the desired outcome objective. As a result, an expected outcome objective is established by reassessing the probability of achieving the desired outcome objective within the estimated time frame for the program. The expected outcome objective represents an estimate of an important future event that can and should be accomplished through the program's efforts and within the resources available.

Completing the program-planning process requires the establishment of a workplan with specific activities and tasks that carry out the program's process objectives. Program resources are attached to these activities, and tasks and activity measures are used to track progress. Activity measures are generally very short term (often expressed in weeks or months), but are also realistic and measurable. The program budget is expended in carrying out these activities and tasks. These work statements are short term (less than one year), realistic, and measurable, and they describe what is to be done, by whom, when, and where. A budget is very much an operational plan for financial expenditures to support the actions agreed upon in the program plan.

As noted previously, the program plan is based on a set of theoretical linkages or assumptions involving the problem and its determinants, contributing factors, activities, and resources. Program resources are deployed through specific activities that serve to modify contributing factors, resulting in achievement of process objectives. Achievement of the process objectives affects the determinants, resulting in the achievement of impact objectives. Achievement of the impact objectives reduces the level of the health problem, resulting in the achievement of the expected outcome objective.

How Do We Know That We Are Getting There?

To answer the last question, "How do we know that we are getting there?" one examines the effectiveness of program design and implementation. Key to any evaluation strategy is the establishment of measurable checkpoints, or milestones, in both time and direction. These assist the manager in determining whether the program is moving in the right direction and whether it will arrive at its destination on time. Both the strategy and the importance of continuously assessing the effectiveness of a program are summed up in the well-known observation that it is more important to be doing the right things than it is to be doing things right. Evaluation focuses on both.

Evaluation was previously characterized as asking the right questions. With a well-analyzed problem statement and the selection of an appropriate intervention strategy, asking the right questions should be straightforward. The key questions are as simple as: "Was the outcome objective achieved?" "Were the impact objectives achieved?" "Were process objectives achieved?" "Were program activities performed as planned?" Evaluation within this framework calls for measuring the actual results and comparing them with the intended results. Information on intended results is derived from the program plan whereas data and information on the actual result must be provided by the program's information system. Goals, objectives, activities, and other standards establish the level of the intended result for comparison.

The intervention strategy represents a causal hypothesis that must be continuously reassessed because circumstances and conditions may change in ways that affect the initial assumptions and linkages. Evaluation is essential before decisions are made as to whether efforts should be expanded, reduced, or even maintained. In 1999 the CDC developed guidelines for public health professionals to use in program evaluations.[13] These guidelines focus less on the technical aspects of program evaluation than on six essential elements and four broad standards for program evaluations. The six steps include:

1. Identify stakeholders, including program implementers, those served or affected, and those who will use the results of the program evaluation.
2. Describe the program, including a clear description of need, expectations for the program, the logic model behind the program, resources

Table 7–2 Centers for Disease Control and Prevention Evaluation Steps and Relevant Standards

	Utility	Feasibility	Propriety	Accuracy
1. Identify stakeholders	✓		✓	
2. Describe program			✓	✓
3. Focus evaluation design		✓	✓	✓
4. Gather credible evidence	✓			✓
5. Justify conclusions	✓			✓
6. Ensure use, share lessons learned	✓		✓	✓

Source: Adapted from Framework for Program Evaluation in Public Health, *Morbidity and Mortality Weekly Report,* Vol. 48, pp. RR-11, the Centers for Disease Control and Prevention, 1999.

    to be used, activities to be implemented, and its stage of development and how it fits into the larger organizational and community context.

3. Focus the evaluation design, including a clearly stated purpose for the evaluation (its uses and users), as well as its specific evaluation questions and methods.
4. Gather credible evidence, including indicators that translate the general concepts of the program into specific measures; consider important sources of evidence, collect only what is needed, and use accepted data gathering and management techniques.
5. Justify conclusions, including analysis, synthesis, interpretation, and recommendations consistent with values of stakeholders.
6. Ensure use of and share lessons learned, including preparation for addressing both positive and negative findings and adequate mechanisms for feedback, follow-up, and dissemination with stakeholders.

The broad evaluation standards help determine whether an evaluation is well-designed and working to its full potential. They are very much interrelated to the essential steps in the evaluation, as illustrated in Table 7–2. The standards address four key questions:

1. Is the evaluation useful? (Utility)
2. Is the evaluation practical? (Feasibility)
3. Is the evaluation ethical? (Propriety)
4. Is the evaluation correct? (Accuracy)

There are several dimensions for evaluating preventive interventions. These include a program's reach (proportion of the target population that participated in the intervention), efficacy (success rate if implemented as intended), adoption (proportion of all potential settings that will adopt this intervention), implementation (extent to which the intervention is implemented as intended in the real world), and maintenance (extent to which a program is sustained over time).[14] Failure to assess impact in all five dimensions can contribute to inefficient use of resources, suboptimal influence on health outcomes, and limited research opportunities.

Effectiveness represents the ability to produce an intended result and achieve expected outcomes. When a program fails to achieve its expected outcomes, the cause of that failure must be identified. Programs may not be effective for several reasons that relate to the various levels of the program's objectives and activities: its outcome objectives, its impact objectives, its process objectives, and its activity measures.

In reverse order, activity measures may not be achieved if resources are lacking or if personnel fail to carry out their tasks. This results in activity measures not being met. If the activity measures are closely linked to their associated process measures, these also will not be met. Failure to address a program's activity measures and process objectives successfully means that a program is not doing things right. Successfully carrying out activity measures and achieving process objectives, on the other hand, means that a program is doing things right. Even when a program is doing things right, however, it may not be doing the right things. Doing the right things means that program outcome and impact objectives are achieved. Four combinations of program effectiveness can occur:

1. Programs can be doing the right things and doing things right. These are well-designed and well-managed programs that merit emulation.
2. Programs can be doing the right things, even though things are not being done right. The linkage between the program's process objectives and activity measures and the program's outcome and impact objectives has been poorly identified. These programs are neither well-designed nor well-managed. It is not possible to link program activities and resources to the outcomes achieved.
3. Programs can be neither doing the right things nor doing things right. These programs are poorly designed and executed on all accounts.
4. Programs can be doing things right but not doing the right things. Here, activity measures and process objectives are achieved, but impact and outcome objectives are not. Although the program staff may be satisfied with its performance, the program as a whole cannot be satisfactory. This situation occurs when a problem is inadequately analyzed. It can be argued that these programs, though poorly designed, are at least partly well-managed.

As suggested in these alternatives, programs can suffer from invalid assumptions or incomplete strategies linking process objectives to impact objectives or linking impact objectives to an expected outcome objective. Pinpointing the location of a program's weaknesses in design or implementation calls for continuously assessing the validity, reliability, and completeness of the intervention strategy.

"Doing things right" refers to the performance of activities and the achievement of process objectives. It is measured through process evaluation. Process objectives can be unmet for two reasons: (1) lack of resources, which calls for reassessing the impact and process objectives in order to align them with the available resources (lower expectations or locate additional resources), or (2) lack of performance, which calls for reassessing the program personnel

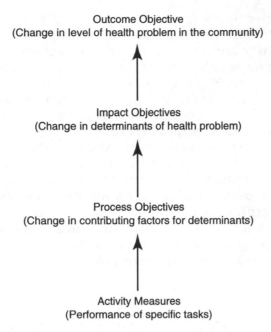

Outcome Objective
(Change in level of health problem in the community)

Impact Objectives
(Change in determinants of health problem)

Process Objectives
(Change in contributing factors for determinants)

Activity Measures
(Performance of specific tasks)

Figure 7–7 Multilevel Program Evaluation. *Source:* Adapted from W. W. Dyal, *Program Management: A Guide for Improving Program Decisions,* 1990, USPHS-CDC-PHPPO, Atlanta, GA.

in terms of motivation, skills, and knowledge (hire, fire, train, or motivate). If process objectives are being met, the program is doing things right.

"Doing the right things" refers to the achievement of impact and outcome objectives and measures the program's effectiveness. If the impact objectives are not being achieved, but the process objectives are, the manager must reexamine the assumed relationship between contributing factors and the determinants, revise the intervention strategy, and develop a new work plan. If the expected outcome objective is not being achieved, but the impact objective is, the manager must reexamine the assumed linkage between the determinants and the health problem, revise the intervention strategy, and develop a new work plan. If a program is doing things right (activities and process objectives), but is not achieving its projected impact or outcome, the only conclusion is that the program is not doing the right things. If the expected outcome objective is being achieved, the manager must reassess the need for the program and begin the management cycle again.

The three-level objective and evaluation procedure (process, impact, and outcome) facilitates locating the source of problems when a program does not achieve its expected outcome[12] (Figure 7–7). Many programs start off with a focus on achieving outcomes, but rapidly shift to a focus on accomplishing their activities and process measures. This is an example of outcome displacement in that outcomes are displaced as the driving force of programs by lower-level activities. Because every program needs to succeed, a program defines its success by doing things right, even if those things do not lead to the outcomes that the program was designed to produce. If a program cannot succeed in terms of outcome, it will shift its objectives to those it can achieve. Activities and processes then become the program's purpose and are accepted as surrogates for achieving the program's objectives. An analogous situation is apparent in the larger health system, where health outcomes have been displaced as objectives by processes such as access to medical care or the perceived quality of specific medical services.

This simple program management system works well in public health for many reasons. It is rational, flexible, and adaptable to most programs and allows for easily understood comparisons between programs. In addition, it fosters communications within an organization and serves to prevent outcome displacement. Most important, it provides a roadmap and mile markers for managers so that they can maintain a steady course along the road to achieving the program's stated outcome objectives. Exhibit 7–7 provides an opportunity to work through this framework.

CONCLUSION

The question, "What have you done for me recently?" conveys the expectation for services that permeates society. Interventions and the programs that orchestrate their implementation have become the hallmark of public health. Most people define public health in terms of the interventions that they most frequently encounter. Because personal health services represent such a large share of public health expenditures and because many of public health's population-based services are neither as visible nor as direct as clinical services, a common perception is that public health mainly provides clinical services for those without access to other providers.

There are a number of ways to categorize or classify the interventions and programs that result from collective efforts to identify and address health needs and risks in the community. One approach separates population-based community preventive from clinical preventive interventions. This approach is largely based on the different emphases of public health and medical practitioners. The interfaces between the two modes of practice are extensive and increasing.

Organizing and orchestrating these interventions are accomplished through program management methods that begin with and revolve around careful definition of health problems. Analysis of carefully defined health problems allows for the establishment of three levels of objectives for the problem, as well as its determinants and contributing factors. Outcome, impact, and process objectives, together with the specific tasks necessary to carry out the process objectives, constitute a framework for tracking progress and modifying program strategies and activities. This program management system helps programs to keep their "eyes on the prize," rather than allowing them to shift their emphases from their intended outcomes to their day-to-day tasks.

Exhibit 7–7 Exercise in Designing a Program Intervention

You have just completed a priority-setting process for a statewide injury control initiative. To that end, your governor has just ensured an appropriation of $1,000,000 for the next state fiscal year to begin an Injury prevention/control program for Injury Problem X. The overall goal is to reduce mortality due to Injury X in your state. All of the available resources are to be directed toward this goal. (Note that Injury X can be any of the following injury problems: homicide, suicide, family violence, gang violence, motor vehicle injuries, unintentional firearm injuries, occupational injuries, burns, falls, drowning.)

Assemble the information that you will need, and undertake the planning process with your statewide injury control coalition. Each coalition will do the following:

State the health problem and the desired outcome objective. This will call for
- describing the current state of the art for prevention/control of Injury X
- developing a carefully designed problem statement that includes the magnitude and extent of the problem, the population at risk, and pertinent trends
- discussing the resources available to address the problem and any additional resources that might be needed.
- developing a desired outcome objective for the health problem

Develop an intervention strategy by
- analyzing your injury problem in terms of the factors most amenable to intervention
- identifying the two most important determinants and, for each, two major contributing factors (upon completion, this logic model should describe selected paths through which an intervention can affect Injury X mortality)
- writing one or more desired outcome objectives
- developing an intervention strategy that would address one of the paths for the health problem. To do this, select a determinant and its associated contributing factors for which impact and process objectives are to be developed. Consider the state of the art and available resources in developing these objectives
- examining the projected impact and process objectives to develop an expected outcome objective if their accomplishment will not result in achieving the desired outcome objective

Develop a work plan by specifying the actual tasks or activities necessary to accomplish all process objective through the use of program personnel, such that
- tasks are in logical sequence and will lead to achievement of the process objectives
- program personnel (by job titles) responsible for each task are identified
- all necessary deadlines are specified
- the available budget is not exceeded

Develop an evaluation plan for the program that will provide evidence that the program really works in the setting in which it is being implemented by
- describing how each of the following will be assessed: activities, process objectives, impact objectives, and outcome objective. For each evaluation process, include information on items to be measured or counted, sources of information, flow or transfer of information, timeliness of data, how data and information will be analyzed, content of reports, and to whom and how often reports are to be made.

Assuming that you achieve all of your process objectives and that your outcome objective is 80 percent achieved, what actions would be appropriate? At 40 percent?

Source: Adapted from *Translating Science Into Practice,* 1991, CDC Case Study.

DISCUSSION QUESTIONS AND EXERCISES

1. How are planning and evaluation related to program implementation?
2. What are outcome, impact, and process objectives, and how do they contribute to program evaluation?
3. Identify a health problem related to oral health ("Public Health Achievements in Twentieth-Century America: Fluoridation of Drinking Water to Prevent Dental Caries") and an intervention that can reduce the level of that problem. Provide examples of possible outcome, impact, and process objectives for that intervention.
4. If your program is meeting its activity and process measures, but not affecting impact and outcome objectives, what should you do?
5. If a program is not meeting its activity and process objectives, what should be done?
6. Why is the definition of a health problem so important to program management?
7. What is the principle of "outcome displacement," and how does it affect programs and bureaucracies?
8. What is the difference between doing the right things and doing things right in public health?
9. Complete the development of an intervention for one of the injury problems identified in Exhibit 7–7.
10. If more extensively utilized, which of the community preventive services identified as effective in Exhibit 7–4 will be most effective in addressing health problems related to oral health ("Public Health Achievements in Twentieth-Century America: Fluoridation of Drinking Water to Prevent Dental Caries")?

REFERENCES

1. National Association of County and City Health Officials. *Local Public Health Agency Infrastructure: A Chartbook.* Washington, DC: NACCHO; 2001.
2. National Association of County and City Health Officials. *Local Health Department Profile 1996–1997 Data Set.* Washington, DC: NACCHO; 1997.
3. Public Health Functions Steering Committee. *Public Health in America.* Washington, DC: U.S. Public Health Service (PHS); 1994.
4. U.S. Preventive Services Task Force. *Guide to Clinical Preventive Services. 2nd ed.* Washington, DC: U.S. Department of Health and Human Services; 1995.
5. U.S. Public Health Service. *Clinician's Handbook of Preventive Services.* Germantown, MD: International Medical Publishers; 1998.
6. Teutsch S. A framework for assessing the effectiveness of disease and injury prevention. *Morb Mortal Wkly Rep.* 1992;41:RR-3.
7. *Practice Guidelines for Public Health: Assessment of Scientific Evidence, Feasibility and Benefits.* Baltimore: Council on Linkages between Academia and Public Health Practice; 1995.
8. Task Force on Community Preventive Services. Guide to Community Preventive Services. Available at *http://www.thecommunityguide.org.*

9. Illinois Dept of Public Health (IDPH). *Challenge and Opportunity: Public Health in an Era of Change.* Springfield, IL: IDPH; 1996.

10. Brownson RC, Gurney JG, Land GH. Evidence-based decision making in public health. *J Public Health Manage Pract.* 1999;5(5):86–97.

11. Brownson RC, Baker EA, Leet TL, Gillespe KN. *Evidence-Based Public Health.* New York NY: Oxford University Press, 2002.

12. Dyal WW. *Program Management: A Guide for Improving Program Decisions.* Atlanta, GA: PHS; 1990.

13. CDC. Framework for program evaluation in public health. *Morb Mortal Wkly Rep.* 1999;48:RR-11.

14. Glasgow RE, Vogt TM, Boles SM. Evaluating the public health impact of health promotion interventions: The RE-AIM framework. *Am J Public Health.* 1999;89:1322–1327.

Public Health Emergency Preparedness and Response

Public health crossed the threshold of a new century as an admittedly important but poorly understood contributor to the American way of life. Despite its contributions to population health status and quality of life throughout the twentieth century, the visibility and economic valuation of public health activities remained low. This situation changed rapidly after the terrorist attacks on the World Trade Center and Pentagon on September 11, 2001 and the bioterrorism events spreading anthrax through the U.S. postal system the following month. The nation responded quickly in the aftermath of these events, elevating international terrorism, bioterrorism preparedness, and emergency response to the top of the national agenda. Within months more than $2 billion was made available to federal, state, and local public health agencies for emergency preparedness and response activities, with additional funding allocated the following year. This explosion of attention, resources, and expectations typifies the history of public health in America, a dramatic health-related event focusing its spotlight on a largely neglected public health infrastructure followed by rapid infusion of resources to resuscitate the system.

This chapter describes the early years of efforts to enhance public health emergency preparedness, as well as some of the successes, failures, and lessons encountered along the way. The intent is to initiate an examination of whether public health preparedness will become one of the Public Health Achievements in Twenty-first Century America. In the process, this chapter will focus on several key questions:

- What is public health preparedness?
- What are the key components of preparedness?
- Is the public health system currently prepared?
- What can be done to become better prepared?

PUBLIC HEALTH ROLES IN EMERGENCY PREPAREDNESS AND RESPONSE

Previous chapters, especially Chapters 1 and 5, introduce and describe a framework for modern public health responses that is organized around six major functions:[1]

- preventing epidemics and the spread of disease
- protecting against environmental hazards

- preventing injuries
- promoting and encouraging healthy behaviors
- responding to disasters and assisting communities in recovery, and
- assuring the quality and accessibility of health services

Although only one of those functions explicitly refers to public health's role in responding to emergencies, all six drive the public health approach to emergency preparedness and response. Public health emergency preparedness and response efforts seek to prevent epidemics and the spread of disease, protect against environmental hazards, prevent injuries, promote healthy behaviors, and assure the quality and accessibility of health services. Each of these is expected by the public and each is evident in effective preparedness and response related to public health emergencies. Together they make preparedness and response a special and particularly critical component of modern public health practice.

For public health emergencies, preparedness and response are inextricably linked.[2] Preparedness is based on lessons learned from both actual and simulated response situations. Effective response is all but impossible without extensive planning and thoughtful preparation. Public health roles in health-related emergencies illustrate both facets.

Public Health Surveillance

Many public health emergencies are readily apparent, but others may not manifest themselves immediately. Effective preparedness and response rely on monitoring disease patterns, investigating individual case reports, and using epidemiological and laboratory analyses to target public health intervention strategies. For example, foodborne illness outbreaks may involve individuals who remain in the same location after being exposed making it easier to identify a common exposure pattern when these individuals seek medical care. Alternatively, an exposure at a convention or family reunion is more difficult to detect because individuals may present for medical care far from the location of exposure. Whether within the same community or in distant locations, it is often difficult for individual medical practitioners to recognize that an outbreak or widespread epidemic is occurring. Prompt recognition and reporting of cases to health authorities is a critical link in the public health chain of protection. A relatively new component of public health surveillance involves bio-surveillance, the early detection of abnormal disease patterns and non-traditional early disease indicators such as pharmaceutical sales, school and work absenteeism, and animal disease events.

Epidemiologic Investigation and Analysis

Once reported, public health agencies can uncover unusual patterns that help identify outbreaks and continuing risks. Public health professionals may use sophisticated analytic tools, such as pattern recognition software and geographic information systems, to determine patterns in disease cases. These surveillance activities help to ensure that disease outbreaks are identified quickly and that appropriate response actions, such as the issuance of health alerts for area providers and communication with response partners, are initiated. Many current disease surveillance systems act in a passive manner (that is, they rely on providers to initiate disease reports); however, public health agencies are increasingly using active surveillance activities, such as when public health workers proactively seek information from providers and other sources to monitor disease trends. In the event of an actual or threatened public health emergency, active surveillance activities are deployed and/or expanded.

Surveillance activities trigger more extensive and focused epidemiological investigations in order to determine the identity, source, and modes of transmission of disease agents. Epidemiological investigations seek to determine what is causing the disease, how the disease is spreading, and who is at risk. Answers to these questions inform efforts to mount rapid and effective interventions. Methods of obtaining epidemiological information, often characterized as disease detective activities, include contacting patients, obtaining detailed information on location and types of possible exposures, and examining both clinical specimens (such as blood and urine) and environmental samplings (such as food, water, air, and soil). Epidemiological investigations require trained personnel and, in many cases, are quite human resource-intensive in terms of the quantity and quality of manpower needed. Laboratory capacity to support these investigations is critical.

Laboratory Investigation and Analysis

In many situations, laboratories provide the definitive identification of causative agents, both biological and chemical, and through various fingerprinting activities link cases to a common source. Capabilities to identify rare or unusual diseases are often not present in every community, necessitating linkages with higher level laboratories. Specimens may be sent for analysis and confirmation to a regional or state public health laboratory or possibly even to a Centers for Disease Control and Prevention (CDC) reference laboratory. Some specialized capabilities found at these higher level laboratories include serotyping to determine the antigenic profile of a microorganism and DNA fingerprinting to not only identify the type of microorganism causing an infectious disease, but to also pinpoint the particular strain of bacterium or virus involved. In this way, public health authorities can determine if reported disease cases are part of the same outbreak, and therefore linked to a common source. Public health laboratories must rely on specialized protective laboratory equipment and facilities due to the dangerous agents with which they work. Some agents, such as smallpox, require special biocontainment equipment and procedures; laboratories are rated in terms of the level of safety they can provide.

Intervention

The primary reason for collecting, analyzing, and sharing information on disease is to control that disease. Expending resources for surveillance and analysis makes little sense if actions do not follow. Interventions that protect individuals from risks associated with environmental hazards are many, including setting standards for health and safety, inspecting food production and importation facilities, monitoring environmental conditions, abating conditions that foster infectious disease (for example, insect and animal control), and enforcing private-sector compliance with established standards. Disease and injury risks associated with these biological and chemical hazards, whether naturally occurring or initiated by man, are reduced through rigorous monitoring and enforcement activities. Public health agencies also play a substantial role in remediation of environmental hazards by decontaminating sites and facilities after they are identified. The extent of remediation necessary can vary greatly, just as the nature and extent of the contamination varies with different disease agents and their ability to remain viable outside a human host or animal/insect vector.

Risk Communication

Epidemiological and laboratory investigations drive the initiation of actions intended to limit the spread of disease and to prevent additional cases in the community. The range of possible actions can be quite broad, including restraining the activities of individuals through isolation and quarantine and imposing temporary or permanent barriers around sources of contamination (for example, sealing buildings, closing restaurants, and cutting off water supplies). In severe and unusual circumstances, special emergency powers may be put into effect limiting human and animal travel and/or restricting certain types of business activity. In these situations, the importance of effective public education and information activities to communicate risk to the public cannot be overstated. Commonly encountered examples include notices to boil drinking water when contaminated water supplies are suspected and product recalls and food safety advisories for potentially contaminated food products. The dissemination of information on mail handling practices during the anthrax attacks in late 2001 served both public education and risk communication purposes.

Promoting and encouraging healthy behaviors during public health emergencies represents another public health intervention strategy. It is not uncommon in the event of a natural disaster or terrorist attack for the most devastating effects to take the form of social disruption and infrastructure damage. The psychological effects of fear and terror, together with disruption of infrastructure components such as electricity, water, and safe housing, may create more casualties than any initial terrorist's biological or chemical assault. Such conditions can also foster toxicity and infectious disease threats, such as occurred with the mass evacuation of the area around the World Trade Center leading to the abandonment of food supplies in surrounding homes and restaurants. Public health officials in New York City took steps to secure these premises to avoid the proliferation of rodents and other pests that otherwise could have resulted in secondary health threats.

Preparedness Planning

Organizing responses to emergencies is another public health role that assures the availability and accessibility of medical and mental health services. Preparedness and planning cannot eliminate all biological, chemical, radiation, and mass casualty threats. But coordinated, community-wide planning for emergency medical and public health responses assures that emergency medical services and medical treatment services are deployed in a rapid and effective manner. Such planning foresees the need for public health measures to be activated in order to assure the safety of responders and to prevent secondary effects due to further disease transmission and injury risk. Planning for these coordinated responses includes monitoring available response resources, establishing action protocols, simulating emergency events to improve readiness, training public and private-sector personnel, assessing communication capabilities, supplies, and resources, and maintaining relationships with partner organizations to improve coordination.

Community-Wide Response

Public health agencies play an important, but not exclusive, role in community-wide responses to emergencies (Figure 8–1). In many response situations private sector medical care providers deliver the bulk of the triage and treatment services needed when a mass casualty emergency occurs. Although less involved with direct care, public health agencies play key roles in coordinating and overseeing the delivery of services as well as communicating with providers, the media, and the public. Supervision of decontamination and triage often falls to public health authorities. Countermeasures such as antibiotics, antitoxins, and chemical antidotes, as well as prophylactic medications and vaccines must be obtained, deployed, and delivered. Public health plays an active role in situations necessitating deployment of Strategic National Stockpile pharmaceuticals, supplies, and equipment. In some situations, public health professionals also provide direct medical care. Public health also contributes through mobilization of regional and national assets and resources when local resources are overwhelmed. Some emergency situations, such as the anthrax attacks of 2001, prompted public fear and overreactions resulting in mountains of unknown powdery substances being tested and thousands of individuals unnecessarily initiating prophylactic antibiotic treatments. That situation and others over recent years argue that the worried well can stress response systems even more than those actually affected.

Unique Aspects of Bioterrorism Emergencies

Across the spectrum of possible public health emergency scenarios, bioterrorism threats represent a particularly challenging form of public health emergency. Bioterrorism is the threatened or intentional release of biological agents (viruses, bacteria, or their toxins) for the purpose of influencing the

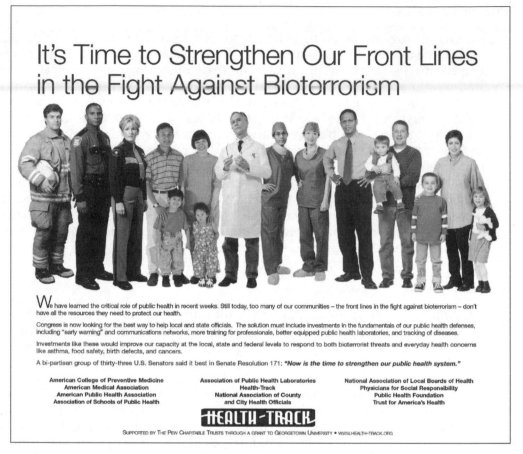

Figure 8–1 News Media Ad in Early 2002 Promoting Public Health Infrastructure as a Front Line of Defense against Bioterrorism. *Source:* Health Track Coalition, 2002.

conduct of government or intimidating or coercing a civilian population to further political or social objectives. These agents (see Exhibits 8–1 and 8–2) can be released by way of the air (as aerosols) food, water, or insects. Biological, chemical, radiation, and mass casualty threats that are intentionally inflicted differ from naturally occurring disease and injury threats in a number of important aspects. Central to these differences, bioterrorism is a criminal act requiring its prevention and response to include criminal justice, military, and intelligence agencies that are not likely to be familiar with naturally occurring disease outbreaks. Law enforcement agencies, including the Federal Bureau of Investigation, have lead responsibility for responding to a bioterrorism attack. In addition, bioterrorism attacks may involve disease agents that occur infrequently in nature and with which neither public health officials nor clinicians have had much experience. It is increasingly possible to genetically engineer chimeras to create, for example, microorganisms that blend the pathogenic qualities of multiple disease agents. Since such organisms do not

Exhibit 8–1 Biological Agents with Bioterrorism Potential

Category A
- Variola major (smallpox)
- Bacillus anthracis (anthrax)
- Yersinia pestis (plague)
- Clostridium botulinum (botulism)
- Francisella tularensis (tularemia)
- Filoviruses (Ebola and Marburg hemorrhagic fevers)
- Arenaviruses (Lassa fever, Argentine hemorrhagic fever)

Category B
- Coxiella burnetii (Q fever)
- Brucella species (brucellosis)
- Burkhoderia mallei (glanders)
- Alphaviruses (Venezuelan encephalomyelitis, eastern and western equine encephalomyelitis)
- Ricin toxin (Ricinus communis)
- Epilson toxin (Clostridiuym perfringerns)
- Staphylococcus enterotoxin B
- Foodborne and waterborne pathogens
  - Salmonella species
  - Shigella dysenteria
  - Escherichia coli O157:H7
  - Vibrio cholerae
  - Cryptosprodium parvum

Category C
- Nipah virus
- Hantaviruses
- Tickborne hemorrhagic fever viruses
- Tickborne encephalitis viruses
- Yellow fever
- Multi-drug resistant tuberculosis

Source: Centers for Disease Control and Prevention, 2003.

exist in nature, they would be completely unknown to public health and medical experts. Attacks related to biological or chemical threats initiated by a bioterrorist would not likely follow known epidemiological patterns, diminishing the value of using past experience with disease transmission and manifestation to identify the source or cause.

It is likely that bioterrorists would seek to be covert, expending great energy and attention to assure the delayed discovery of the disease to maximize the population's exposure. Intentional outbreaks may develop in multiple locations simultaneously, thereby straining local, state, and federal response efforts. With many emerging and re-emerging infectious disease threats (Ebola Virus, Sudden Acute Respiratory Syndrome, West Nile Virus, Hantavirus, etc.), it is increasingly difficult to predict the precise nature of the next public health emergency. It could result from a chance mutation of a microorganism or it could result from the intentional act of terrorists. Multiple

Exhibit 8–2 Chemical Agents with Bioterrorism Potential

- Albrin
- Adamsite (DM)
- Agent 15
- Ammonia
- Arsenic
- Arsine (SA)
- Benzene
- Bromobenzylcyanide (CA)
- BZ
- Cannabinoids
- Chlorine (CL)
- Chloroacetophenone (CN)
- Chloropicrin (PS)
- CNB (CN in Benzene and Carbon Tetrachloride)
- CNC (CN in Chloroform)
- CNS (CN and Chloropicrin in Chloroform)
- CR
- CS
- Cyanide
- Cyanogen Chloride (CK)
- Cyclohexyl Sarin (GF)
- Diphenylchloroarsine (DA)
- Diphenylcyanoarsine (DC)
- Diphosgene (DP)
- Distilled Mustard (HD)
- Ethyldichloroarsine (ED)
- Ethylene Glycol
- Fentanyls and Other Opioids
- Hydrafluoric Acid
- Hydrogen Chloride
- Hydrogen Cyanide (AC)
- Lewisite (L, L-1, L-2, L-3)
- LSD
- Mercury
- Methyldichloroarsine (MD)
- Mustard Gas (H) (Sulfur Mustard)
- Mustard/Lewisite (HL)
- Mustard/T
- Nitrogen Mustard (HN-1, HN-2, HN-3)
- Nitrogen Oxide (NO)
- Paraquat
- Perflurorisobutylene (PHIB)
- Phenodichloroarsine (PD)
- Phenothiazines
- Phosgene (CG)
- Phosgene Oxime (CX)
- Phosphine
- Potassium Cyanide (KCN)
- Red Phosphorous (RP)
- Ricin
- Sarin (GB)
- Sesqui Mustard
- Sodium Azide
- Sodium Cyanide (NaCN)
- Soman (GD)
- Strychnine
- Sulfur Trioxide-Chlorosulfonic Acid (FS)
- Tabun (GA)
- Teflon and Perflurorisobutylene (PHIB)
- Thallium
- Titanium Tetrachloride (FM)
- VX
- White Phosphorus
- Zinc Oxide (HC)

Source: Centers for Disease Control and Prevention, 2003.

threats are possible, necessitating preparedness and response systems that can address a wide variety of unknown and unanticipated hazards. This concept of multiple threats and unknown hazards has led many experts to advocate for a robust public health infrastructure capable of responding to many different forms of emergencies.

Workplace Preparedness

Public health emergencies, including those related to terrorism, have many different visages and many different venues. Yet most of the direct victims of terrorism in the United States in recent years have been people at work, including the victims of the bombing of the federal building in Oklahoma City, those who died in the World Trade Center and the Pentagon on September 11, 2001, and the victims who contracted anthrax transmitted through the mail later in that same year.

Acts of terrorism intend to make people feel powerless and believe that they cannot take steps to prevent such incidents or mitigate their consequences. But experience to-date in battling other workplace safety risks ("Public Health Achievements in Twentieth-Century America: Improvements in Workplace Safety" below) suggests that there are steps that can be taken by employers and employees. The workplace is, in effect, a key line of defense for homeland security. This is recognized formally in the formation and scope of responsibilities for the new federal Department of Homeland Security, as well as in the response of the business community after 2001 in taking tangible steps to enhance security.

Example

Public Health Achievements in Twentieth-Century America: Improvements in Workplace Safety

Public health interventions address priority health problems. Efforts to improve workplace safety demonstrate the importance of the workplace in both routine and public health emergency preparedness efforts.

At the beginning of this century, workers in the United States faced remarkably high health and safety risks on the job. Through efforts by individual workers, unions, employers, government agencies, scientists, and others, considerable progress has been made in improving these conditions. Despite these successes, much work remains, with the goal for all workers to have productive and safe working lives and retirements free from long-term consequences of occupational disease and injury. Using the limited data available, this report documents large declines in fatal occupational injuries during the 1900s, highlights the mining industry as an example of improvements in worker safety, and discusses new challenges in occupational safety and health.

Data from multiple sources reflect the large decreases in work-related deaths from the high rates and numbers of deaths among workers during the early twentieth century. The earliest systematic survey of workplace fatalities in the United States in this century covered Allegheny County, Pennsylvania, from July 1906 through June 1907; that year in the one county, 526 workers died in "work accidents"; 195 of these were steel workers. In contrast, in 1997, there were 17 steel worker fatalities nationwide. The National Safety Council estimated that in 1912, work-related injuries resulted in 18–21,000 deaths. In 1913 the Bureau of Labor Statistics documented approximately 23,000 industrial deaths among a workforce of 38 million, equivalent to a rate

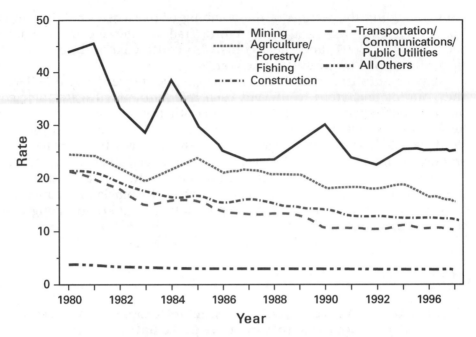

Figure 8–2 Occupational Injury Death Rates (per 100,000 Workers), by Industry Division and Year, United States, 1980–1995. *Source:* Reprinted from Achievements in Public Health, United States, 1900–1999: Improvements in Workplace Safety, *Morbidity and Mortality Weekly Report,* Vol. 48, No. 22, pp. 461–469, the Centers for Disease Control and Prevention, 1999.

of 61 deaths per 100,000 workers. Under a different reporting system, data from the National Safety Council from 1933 through 1997 indicate that deaths from unintentional work-related injuries declined 90 percent, from 37 per 100,000 workers to 4 per 100,000. The corresponding annual number of deaths decreased from 14,500 to 5,100; during this same period, the workforce more than tripled, from 39 million to approximately 130 million.

More recent and probably more complete data from death certificates were compiled from CDC's National Institute for Occupational Safety and Health (NIOSH) National Traumatic Occupational Fatalities (NTOF) surveillance system. These data indicate that the annual number of deaths declined 28 percent, from 7,405 in 1980 to 5,314 in 1995 (the most recent year for which complete NTOF data are available). The average rate of deaths from occupational injuries decreased 43 percent during the same time, from 7.5 to 4.3 per 100,000 workers. Industries with the highest average rates for fatal occupational injury during 1980–1995 included mining (30.3 deaths per 100,000 workers), agriculture/forestry/fishing (20.1), construction (15.2), and transportation/communications/public utilities (13.4) (Figure 8–2). Leading causes of fatal occupational injury during the period include motor vehicle-related injuries, workplace homicides, and machine-related injuries (Figure 8–3).

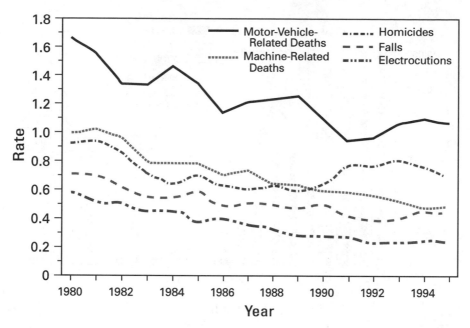

Figure 8–3 Rates (per 100,000 Workers) for Leading Causes of Occupational Injury Deaths, by Cause and Year, United States, 1980–1995. *Source:* Reprinted from Achievements in Public Health, United States, 1900–1999: Improvements in Workplace Safety, *Morbidity and Mortality Weekly Report,* Vol. 48, No. 22, pp. 461–469, the Centers for Disease Control and Prevention, 1999.

The decline in occupational fatalities in mining and other industries reflects the progress made in all workplaces since the beginning of the century in identifying and correcting the etiologic factors that contribute to occupational health risks. If today's workforce of approximately 130 million had the same risk as workers in 1933 for dying from injuries, an additional 40,000 workers would have died in 1997 from preventable events. The declines can be attributed to multiple, interrelated factors, including efforts by labor and management and by academic researchers to improve worker safety. Other efforts to improve safety were developed by state labor and health authorities and through the research, education, and regulatory activities undertaken by government agencies (e.g., the U.S. Bureau of Mines [USBM], the Mine Safety and Health Administration [established as the Mining Enforcement and Safety Administration in 1973], the Occupational Safety and Health Administration [OSHA, established in 1970], and NIOSH). Efforts by these groups led to physical changes in the workplace, such as improved ventilation and dust suppression in mines; safer equipment; development and introduction of safer work practices; and improved training of health and safety professionals and of workers. The reduction in workplace deaths has occurred in the context of extensive changes in U.S. economic activity, the U.S. industrial mix, and workforce demographics. Society-wide

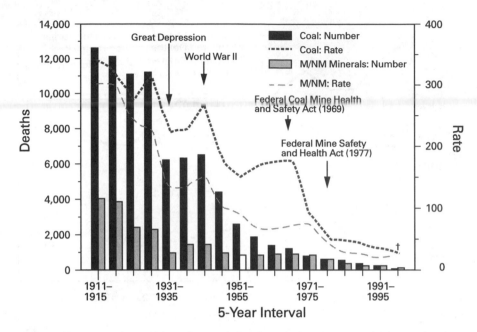

Figure 8–4 Number of Deaths and Fatality Rates (per 100,000 Workers) in Mining Coal and Metal/Nonmetallic (M/NM) Minerals, by 5-Year Interval, United States, 1911–1997. *Source:* Reprinted from Achievements in Public Health, United States, 1900–1999: Improvements in Workplace Safety, *Morbidity and Mortality Weekly Report,* Vol. 48, No. 22, pp. 461–469, the Centers for Disease Control and Prevention, 1999.

progress in injury control also contributes to safer workplaces—for example, use of safety belts and other safety features in motor vehicles and improvements in medical care for trauma victims.

Only in some instances do data permit association of declines in fatalities with specific interventions. Before 1920, using permissible explosives and electrical equipment (which can be operated in an explosive methane-rich environment without igniting the methane), applying a layer of rock dust over the coal dust (which creates an inert mixture and prevents ignition of coal dust), and improved ventilation, such as reversible fans, led to dramatic reductions in fatalities from explosions (Figure 8–4). New technologies in roof support and improved mine design reduced the number of deaths from roof falls. However, technology also introduced new hazards, such as fatalities associated with machinery. An approximately 50 percent decrease in coal mining fatality rates occurred from 1966–1970 to 1971–1975 (Figure 8–5); 1971–1975 is the period immediately following passage of the 1969 Federal Coal Mine Health and Safety Act, which greatly expanded enforcement powers of federal inspectors and established mandatory health and safety standards for all mines. The act also served as the model for the 1970 Occupational Safety and Health Act. Following the

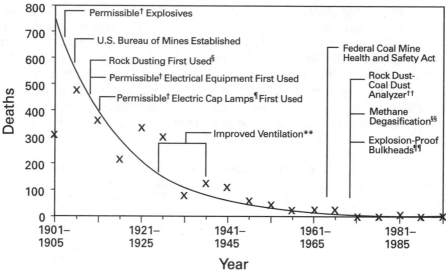

* Each X represents the 5-year average of the number of deaths resulting from explosions; the line is a smoothed regression line through the 5-year averages.
† Explosives and equipment that can be used in an explosive methane-rich environment without causing a methane explosion.
§ The process of applying a layer of rock dust over the coal dust, which creates an inert mixture and inhibits a coal dust explosion.
¶ Lamps worn on miners' caps.
** Ventilation improvements, including the use of reversible fans, reduce the concentration of methane and remove the explosive gas from the mine.
†† A hand-held monitor that provides instantaneous readings of the rock-to-coal dust mixture to ensure that it is inert.
§§ Techniques to remove methane from the coal bed before mining the coal.
¶¶ Explosion-proof walls used to seal abandoned (mined-out) areas to protect workers in active parts of the mine.

Figure 8–5 Five-Year Averages of Annual Number of Deaths Related to Coal Mine Explosions, United States, 1901–1995. *Source:* Reprinted from Achievements in Public Health, United States, 1900–1999: Improvements in Workplace Safety, *Morbidity and Mortality Weekly Report,* Vol. 48, No. 22, pp. 461–469, the Centers for Disease Control and Prevention, 1999.

1977 Federal Mine Safety and Health Act, a 33 percent decrease in fatalities occurred in metal and nonmetallic mineral mining (1976–1980, compared with 1981–1985).

Similarly, the impact of more recent targeted efforts to reduce workplace fatalities can be illustrated by data on work-related electrocutions. During the 1980s, there were concerted research and dissemination efforts by NIOSH, changes to the National Electrical Code and occupational safety and health regulations, and public awareness campaigns by power companies and others. During this decade, work-related electrocution rates declined 54 percent, from 0.7 per 100,000 workers per year in 1980 to 0.3 in 1989; the number of electrocutions decreased from 577 to 329.

Although the decline in injuries in general industry since 1970 seems to have resulted from a variety of factors, some sources point to the Occupational Safety and Health Act of 1970, which created NIOSH and OSHA. Since 1971, NIOSH has investigated hazardous work conditions, conducted research to prevent injury, trained health professionals, and developed educational materials and recommendations for worker protection. OSHA's regulatory authority for worksite inspection and development of safety standards has brought about safety regulations, mandatory workplace safety controls, and worker training. During 1980–1996, research findings indicated that training creates safer workplaces through increased worker knowledge of job hazards and safe work practices in a wide array of worksites.

Source: Adapted from Achievements in Public Health, United States, 1900–1999: Improvements in Workplace Safety, *Morbidity and Mortality Weekly Report,* Vol. 48, No. 22, pp. 461–469, the Centers for Disease Control and Prevention, 1999.

NATIONAL PUBLIC HEALTH PREPAREDNESS AND RESPONSE COORDINATION

The events of late 2001 resulted in the creation of a new federal Department of Homeland Security with extensive authority and powers related to domestic terrorism and security. In accord with the Homeland Security Act of 2002, several important public health functions were transferred into the new Department of Homeland Security in 2003, including the Strategic National Stockpile (SNS) of emergency pharmaceutical supplies and medical equipment. This new federal agency immediately became part of the American everyday experience through activities such as the national homeland security alert system summarized in Exhibit 8–3 with its color-coded levels of perceived threat.

Exhibit 8–3 Homeland Security Advisory System

1. Low Condition (Green)
  This condition is declared when there is a low risk of terrorist attacks. Federal departments and agencies should consider the following general measures in addition to agency-specific protective measures they develop and implement.
  • Refining and exercising as appropriate preplanned protective measures
  • Ensuring personnel receive proper training on the Homeland Security Advisory System and specific preplanned department or agency protective measures
  • Institutionalizing a process to assure that all facilities and regulated sectors are regularly assessed for vulnerabilities to terrorist attacks and that all reasonable measures are taken to mitigate these vulnerabilities.

continues

Exhibit 8–3 continued

2. Guarded Condition (Blue)

This condition is declared when there is a general risk of terrorist attacks. In addition to the protective measures taken in the previous threat condition, federal departments and agencies should consider the following general measures in addition to the agency specific protective measures that they will develop and implement.

- Checking communications with designated emergency response or command locations
- Reviewing and updating emergency response procedures
- Providing the public with any information that would strengthen its ability to act appropriately

3. Elevated Condition (Yellow)

An elevated condition is declared when there is a significant risk of terrorist attacks. In addition to the protective measures taken in the previous threat condition, federal departments and agencies should consider the following general measures in addition to the agency specific protective measures that they will develop and implement.

- Increasing surveillance of critical locations
- Coordinating emergency plans, as appropriate, with nearby jurisdictions
- Assessing whether the precise characteristics of the threat require the further refinement of preplanned protective measures
- Implementing, as appropriate, contingency and emergency response plans

4. High Condition (Orange)

A high condition is declared when there is a high risk of terrorist attacks. In addition to the protective measures taken in the previous threat condition, federal departments and agencies should consider the following general measures in addition to the agency-specific protective measures that they will develop and implement.

- Coordinating necessary security efforts with federal, state, and local law enforcement agencies or any National Guard or other appropriate armed forces organizations
- Taking additional precautions at public events and possibly considering alternative venues or even cancellation
- Preparing to execute contingency procedures, such as moving to an alternate site or dispersing their workforce
- Restricting threatened facility access to essential personnel only

5. Severe Condition (Red)

A severe condition reflects a severe risk of terrorist attacks. Under most circumstances, the protective measures for a severe condition are not intended to be sustained for substantial periods of time. In addition to the protective measures taken in the previous threat condition, federal departments and agencies should consider the following general measures in addition to the agency specific protective measures that they will develop and implement.

- Increasing or redirecting personnel to address critical emergency needs
- Assigning emergency response personnel and pre-positioning and mobilizing specially trained teams or resources
- Monitoring, redirecting, or constraining transportation systems
- Closing public and government facilities

Source: U.S. Department of Homeland Security, 2003.

The establishment of a new federal agency, however, did not substantially alter the configuration of public health responsibilities within the system of operational federalism described in Chapter 4. Federal agencies are significant contributors, but public health remains largely a state responsibility with the bulk of public health activity taking place at the local level. For public health emergencies, such as bioterrorism events or threats, preparedness and coordinated response across all levels of government are critical. Nonetheless there are significant issues related to intergovernmental relationships, resource deployment, and financing that make public health emergencies especially difficult challenges for the public health system. The following sections examine key aspects of the structure, operations, and problems in public health emergency preparedness and response at the national, state, and local levels.

Federal Agencies and Assets

More than 20 separate federal departments and agencies have roles in preparing for or responding to public health emergencies, including bioterrorist attacks. Within this constellation of agencies, the Departments of Health and Human Services (DHHS) and Homeland Security (DHS) play the most important public health roles.

Prior to 2003 the Department of Health and Human Services (DHHS) was the primary federal agency responsible for the medical and public health response to emergencies (including major disasters and terrorist events). Beginning in 2003 DHHS now shares center stage with the new Department of Homeland Security. DHHS discharges its responsibilities through several operating agencies, including the following:

- Centers for Disease Control and Prevention (CDC): CDC works with state public health agencies to detect, investigate, and prevent the spread of disease in communities. CDC provides support to state public health agencies in a variety of ways, including financial assistance, training programs, technical assistance and expert consultation, sophisticated laboratory services, research activities, and standards development. The Office of Terrorism Preparedness and Emergency Response coordinates efforts across the various CDC centers, institutes, and offices.
- Health Resources and Services Administration (HRSA): HRSA administers a state grant program to facilitate regional hospital preparedness planning and to upgrade the capacity of hospitals and other health care facilities to respond to public health emergencies. HRSA is also generally responsible for health care workforce development, including grant programs for curriculum development and continuing education for health professionals on bioterrorism preparedness and response.
- Food and Drug Administration (FDA): FDA has responsibilities both for ensuring the safety of the food supply and for assuring the safety and efficacy of pharmaceuticals, biologics, and medical devices. FDA fulfills its food safety responsibilities in partnership with the Department of Agriculture, which is responsible for the safety of meat, poultry, and processed egg products.

- National Institutes of Health (NIH): NIH conducts and supports biomedical research, including research targeted at the development of rapid diagnostics and new and more effective vaccines and anti-microbial therapies.
- Office of Public Health Emergency Preparedness: OPHEP sets policy direction and coordinates public health emergency preparedness and response activities across the various DHHS agencies.

In March 2003, 23 federal agencies, programs and offices were fashioned into a new federal Department of Homeland Security (DHS). The new agency sought to bring a coordinated approach to national security from emergencies and disasters, both natural and man-made. DHS actively promotes an "all-hazards" approach to disasters and homeland security issues. The Federal Emergency Management Agency (FEMA), formerly an independent agency, became one of the major branches of the new DHS responsible for Emergency Preparedness and Response, tasked with responding to, planning for, recovering from, and mitigating against disasters under authority provided by the Stafford Act (Exhibit 8–4).

Within DHS, the Emergency Preparedness and Response Directorate coordinates emergency medical response in the event of a public health emergency, including the National Disaster Medical System and the Metropolitan Medical Response Systems (these are described later in this chapter). Other major directorates (divisions) of the new DHS include Border and Transportation Security,

---

Exhibit 8–4 Robert T. Stafford Disaster Relief and Emergency Assistance Act (P.L. 93–288, as amended)

The Congress hereby finds and declares that (1) because disasters often cause loss of life, human suffering, loss of income, and property loss and damage; and (2) because disasters often disrupt the normal functioning of governments and communities, and adversely affect individuals and families with great severity; special measures, designed to assist the efforts of the affected States in expediting the rendering of aid, assistance, and emergency services, and the reconstruction and rehabilitation of devastated areas, are necessary.

It is the intent of Congress, by this Act, to provide an orderly and continuing means of assistance by the Federal Government to State and local governments in carrying out their responsibilities to alleviate the suffering and damage which result from such disasters by—

(1) revising and broadening the scope of existing disaster relief programs;
(2) encouraging the development of comprehensive disaster preparedness and assistance plans, programs, capabilities, and organizations by the States and by local government;
(3) achieving greater coordination and responsiveness of disaster preparedness and relief programs;
(4) encouraging individuals, States, and local governments to protect themselves by obtaining insurance coverage to supplement or replace governmental assistance;
(5) encouraging hazard mitigation measures to reduce losses from disasters, including development of land use and construction regulations; and
(6) providing Federal assistance programs for both public and private losses sustained in disasters.

Science and Technology, Information Analysis and Infrastructure Protection, and Management.

A variety of other federal agencies have organizational responsibilities related to bioterrorism and public health emergency preparedness. The Environmental Protection Agency (EPA) responds to emergencies involving chemicals and other hazardous substances. The Department of Defense indirectly supports public health preparedness through various research efforts on biologic and chemical weapons, intelligence gathering related to terrorism threats, and civil support functions in the event of an emergency that results in severe social unrest. The Department of Justice has lead responsibility for assessing and investigating terrorist threats, including those related to bioterrorism, and provides funds and assistance to emergency responders (police, fire, ambulance, and rescue personnel) at state and local levels. The Department of Veterans Affairs purchases drugs and other therapeutics for the Strategic National Stockpile and operates one of the nation's largest health care systems, which could provide critical surge capacity in the event of a mass casualty event. Several other federal agencies, including the Departments of Transportation, Commerce, and Energy also have potential roles to play in preparing for and responding to a public health emergency.

National Incident Management System

Prior to the establishment of the new Department of Homeland Security, the management of large scale health events was complicated by the involvement of so many different federal agencies. States have established a similar web of agencies to manage disasters and other emergencies with each developing its own form of an incident management system. In order to assure greater consistency across states and for interfaces between the federal government and states, a National Incident Management System (NIMS) was prescribed by a presidential directive in 2003 to cover all incidents (natural and unnatural) for which the federal government deploys emergency response assets. The Secretary of Homeland Security is responsible for the development and implementation of NIMS. Its success depends in large part on the establishment of consistent approaches within the states as to roles and responsibilities for both public health agencies and the hospital community (including their supporting health-care systems) in managing emergencies at the state and regional levels and developing and deploying incident management plans at sub-state levels.

Bioterrorism and other public health incidents fall within the scope of NIMS. To this end, the Department of Health and Human Services has the initial lead responsibility for the federal government and will deploy assets as needed within the areas of its statutory responsibility (such as the Public Health Service Act and the Federal Food, Drug, and Cosmetic Act) while keeping the Secretary of Homeland Security apprised regarding the course of the incident and nature of the response operations.

The Department of Homeland Security assumes responsibility for coordinating federal response operations, including those involving public health components, under certain conditions. DHS will coordinate the federal government's resources utilized in response to or recovery from terrorist attacks, major disasters, or other emergencies if and when any of the following four conditions applies:[3]

1. a federal department or agency acting under its own authority has requested the assistance,
2. the resources of state and local authorities are overwhelmed and federal assistance has been formally requested by state and local authorities,
3. more than one federal department or agency has become substantially involved in responding to the incident, or
4. DHS has been directed to assume responsibility for managing the domestic incident by the President.

For states and local governments to gain full benefit from the emergency response assets of the federal government, states must develop incident management systems that are interoperable with NIMS. Beginning in 2004, adherence to and compatibility with NIMS will be a condition of all grants and other awards from federal agencies for any aspect of state or local emergency preparedness and response.

Federal Emergency Medical Assets

Several national emergency response assets are available to state and local governments from the new DHS. These include the National Disaster Medical System (NDMS), the Metropolitan Medical Response Systems (MMRS), and the Strategic National Stockpile (SNS).

The NDMS now operates within the Emergency Preparedness and Response Directorate of DHS after being transferred from the Office of the Secretary of DHHS. NDMS brings together medical services from DHHS, DHS, Defense, and Veterans Affairs to augment local emergency medical services during a disaster or other large scale emergency. The NDMS has several operational components including Disaster Medical Assistance Teams (DMATs), Disaster Mortuary Teams (DMORTs), Federal Coordinating Centers, and Management Support Units.

DMATs are self-sustaining squads of licensed, actively practicing, volunteer professional and paraprofessional medical personnel who provide emergency medical care at the site of a disaster or other emergency. DMAT teams often triage, stabilize and prepare patients for evacuation in mass casualty situations. They are sent into these situations to supplement, rather than supplant or replace, local capacity. Once activated, these professionals are federalized, allowing them to practice with their current professional licenses in any jurisdiction. DMORTs include mortuary, dental, and forensic specialists who serve to augment the services of local coroners and medical examiners. Portable temporary mortuaries for mass casualty situations are provided when needed. Management support units provide command, coordination, and communication capabilities for DMATs and DMORTs and other federal assets. Federal Coordinating Centers recruit hospitals to participate in the NDMS and recruit health workers for the DMATs and DMORTs.

The Metropolitan Medical Response System, involving more than 100 metropolitan communities, integrates existing emergency response systems at the local level, including emergency management, medical and mental health providers, public health agencies, law enforcement, fire departments, emergency medical services, and the National Guard. The MMRS seeks to develop a unified regional response to mass casualty events. MMRS was transferred from DHHS when the new DHS was established in 2003.

The Strategic National Stockpile (formerly National Pharmaceutical Stockpile) ensures the availability and rapid deployment of life-saving pharmaceuticals, antidotes, other medical supplies, and equipment necessary to counter the effects of nerve agents, biological pathogens, and chemical agents. The SNS stands ready for immediate deployment to any U.S. location in the event of a terrorist attack using a biological toxin or chemical agent directed against a civilian population. In the event of possible bioterrorist attack, a 12-hour push package containing 50 tons of stockpile materials can be immediately dispatched to predetermined Receipt, Store, and Storage (RSS) sites identified in state bioterrorism response plans. There are twelve 12-hour push packages centrally located around the U.S. for immediate deployment. Detailed deployment activities for SNS materials are prescribed in state and local emergency response plans.

Federal Funding for Public Health Infrastructure

Although multiple agencies provide federal funding for emergency preparedness, federal support for the public health infrastructure at the state and local levels is provided largely from grants and cooperative agreements with CDC. In 1999, for the first time, CDC awarded more than $40 million for bioterrorism preparedness to states and cities for enhanced laboratory and electronic communication capacity and another $32 million to establish a national pharmaceutical stockpile to ensure availability of vaccines, prophylactic medicines, chemical antidotes, medical supplies, and equipment needed to support a medical response to a biologic or chemical terrorist incident. At the time, these appeared to be large sums. In the wake of September 11, 2001 and the anthrax attacks the following month, increased concerns regarding homeland security led to a $2.1 billion FY 2002 appropriation for CDC's anti-terrorism activities, over a twenty-fold increase from FY 1999 levels. The FY 2002 supplemental appropriations provided $917 million for grants to states and localities to upgrade state and local capacity. Similar levels of funding were provided in 2003. The state and local activities impacted by this funding are described in subsequent sections of this chapter.

STATE AND LOCAL PREPAREDNESS COORDINATION

State Agencies and Assets

Similar to the federal pattern, states rely on a variety of agencies to deliver public health emergency services. Also similar to the federal model, these functions tend to be concentrated within a limited number of agencies at the state level with the state health department and state emergency management agency playing the most significant roles. As described in Chapter 4, most state health departments are freestanding agencies (not part of a larger human services agencies), and most have responsibility for emergency medical service systems within the state. However, most states have an environmental health agency that is separate from the state health agency. Although these states may have a small environmental health section within the health agency, the environmental health agency is charged with monitoring environmental contaminants and remediation of hazardous conditions. Nearly all states have a separate emergency management agency (patterned after FEMA), although some states have established their own Departments of Homeland Security. In responding to a public health emergency, the state health agency works collaboratively with the state emergency management agency, as well as with the state environmental protection, law enforcement, public safety, and transportation agencies and, possibly, the National Guard.

States derive their powers and authority to act in public health emergencies from their public health laws as described in Chapter 4. There are concerns that existing public health laws may be inadequate in some states because they are obsolete and fragmented. A Model Public Health Emergency Powers Act has been used to assist states in examining and enhancing their legal framework for public health emergencies. The model act addresses key issues related to preparedness, surveillance, protection of persons, management of property, and public information and communications.[4]

Considerable differences exist among states in the breadth and depth of services provided within their jurisdictions and the degree to which public health service delivery responsibilities are delegated to local governments. In general, however, state governments are ultimately responsible for assuring adequate response to a public health emergency and tend to play certain key roles in preparedness and response, regardless of how decentralized a particular public health system might be. Except in the largest metropolitan local public health departments, local public health officials rely on state personnel and capacity for a number of key functions, including advanced laboratory capacity, epidemiological expertise, and serving as a conduit for federal assistance.

Incident Command Systems

In order to manage resources effectively and facilitate decision making during emergencies, incident command systems (ICS) are in wide use by police, fire, and emergency management agencies. Initially adopted for the fire service, ICS eliminates many common problems related to communication, terminology, organizational structure, span of control, and other difference across different disciplines and agencies in response to a critical incident. Critical incidents include any natural or manmade event, civil disturbance, or any other occurrence of unusual or severe nature that threatens to cause or actually causes the loss of life or injury to citizens and/or severe damage to property.

In managing critical incidents clear goals and objectives are established and communicated to responders, response plans are utilized, communications are effective, and resources are utilized in a timely and effective manner. ICS should not be considered an additional set of procedures; rather the system must become part of routine operations with personnel fully trained in its use and standard operating procedures reflective of the capabilities actually available.

One important key to effective ICS is the ability to size up the incident scene and make the initial call for resources. This allows responders to get control of the incident rather than playing catch-up for the rest of the incident. Appropriate initial size-up prevents unnecessary injury or loss of life, property or environmental damage, and negative perceptions on the responding agencies.

Key components of ICS include:

- Common terminology—Major organizational functions and units are named; in multiple incidents, each incident is named. Common names are used for personnel, equipment, and facilities. Clear terms are used in radio transmissions (for example, codes, such as "ten" codes, are not used).
- Modular organization—ICS develops "top down" from the first unit involved based on the specific incident's management needs. Each ICS is staffed with a designated incident commander (responsible for safety, liaison, and information) with other functions (operations, planning, logistics, finance/administration) staffed as needed.
- Integrated communications—ICS uses a common communications plan and redundant two-way communications.
- A unified command structure—This is necessary when the incident is within a single jurisdiction with multiple agencies involved, or the incident is multi-jurisdictional, or individuals representing different agencies or jurisdictions share common responsibilities. All agencies involved contribute to the unified command process by determining overall goals and objectives, planning jointly for tactical activities, conducting integrated tactical operations, and maximizing the use of assigned resources.
- Consolidated action plans—Written action plans are necessary when the incident is complex and/or when several agencies and/or jurisdictions are involved. Action plans include specific goals, objectives, and support activities.
- A manageable span of control—The number of subordinates one supervisor can manage effectively should be between 3 and 7, with 5 being optimal.
- Designated incident facilities—These include the command post from which all incident operations, direction, control, coordination, and resource management are directed. Command posts can be fixed or mobile, but need adequate communications capabilities.
- Comprehensive resource management—This maximizes resource use, consolidates control, reduces communications load, provides accountability, and reduces freelancing.

The emergency management team functions at the emergency operations center (EOC), managing strategic decisions through the incident command structure. Ideally the team should be isolated from the confusion, media, and weather during the incident. EOC participants must have adequate authority and decision-making capability. EOC decisions could include issuing curfews, circumventing normal bidding processes, emergency appointments, permanent or temporary relocation, emergency demolition of unsafe properties, or implementation of prophylaxis to populations. The EOC is supported operationally by incident command posts in the field, which are responsible for tactical decisions as well as oversight and command of responders at the scene.

Effective emergency operations plans and standard operating procedures simplify decision making during incidents. Training makes implementation of decisions easier for subordinates. When the level of preparation and practice exercises is inadequate, emergency operations plans can become overwhelmed by common incidents and unable to deal with those that are not fully anticipated. In such circumstances, decision making becomes complex and challenging. A comprehensively planned and frequently exercised organizational system is necessary to overcome these pitfalls.

As ICS became increasingly accepted as an effective framework for responding to incidents, its use has extended to other settings. For example, there has been much progress in development and deployment of hospital emergency incident command systems and table top exercises for hospitals. Several states have expanded on the ICS concept to develop standardized emergency management systems that formally incorporate ICS, mutual aid agreements, and multi-jurisdictional and inter-agency cooperation at the sub-state level resulting in coordinated and unified decisions throughout the state.

Local Agencies and Assets

The front line of response to public health emergencies is at the local level where local public health agencies (LPHAs) work collaboratively with other "first responders," such as fire and rescue personnel, emergency medical service providers, law enforcement officers, hazardous materials teams, physicians, and hospitals in preparing for and managing the consequences of health-related emergencies. Although the relationships between state and local public health agencies vary greatly from state-to-state, and even from local jurisdiction-to-local jurisdiction within the same state, local government has significant responsibilities for dealing with emergencies in virtually all states. First responders play key roles in:

- recognizing public health emergencies, including those that result from terrorist attacks,
- identifying unique personal safety implications associated the emergency situation,
- identifying security issues that are unique to the event or to the emergency medical system response, and
- understanding basic principles of patient care based upon the type of emergency event encountered.

Focusing on the services most directly related to emergency preparedness and response, the vast majority of LPHAs carry out activities related to epidemiology and surveillance (84 percent), communicable disease control (94 percent), food safety (85 percent), and restaurant inspections (80 percent).[5] (See Exhibit 7-1 in Chapter 7.) LPHAs are somewhat less likely to be directly involved in emergency medical response (61 percent), and less than half of LPHAs operate laboratory services (45 percent), air quality (44 percent), animal control (40 percent), or water inspections (44 percent).[5]

In those cases where the LPHA is not responsible for these services, they are typically delivered by another agency of local government agency (for example, a fire department or environmental services agency), by a private agency (hospital or ambulance service), or the state. Even when services are offered by an LPHA, they may be quite limited in terms of scope or hours of availability. For example, although nearly half of LPHAs report providing laboratory services, these services may be quite limited in nature (for example, to support TB and STD testing). Many LPHAs that report having laboratory services are likely to rely on state public health labs for more specialized diagnostic needs.

The state of readiness among LHPAs has increased since 2001 when only about one-fourth of LHPAs had completed a comprehensive emergency response plan with another one-fourth indicating their plans were at least 80 percent complete. LPHAs have tailored the national threat advisory guidelines for public health emergencies. In general, LPHA threat advisory guidelines describe a spectrum of activities that range from planning through implementation. The activities that are undertaken at each threat level are summarized in Exhibit 8–5 and roughly equate to the preparedness and response concepts listed below:

- Low threat (green)—creating, developing, identifying
- General threat (blue)—reviewing, updating, distributing
- Significant threat (yellow)—evaluating, testing, verifying
- High threat (orange)—preparing to implement and implementing partially
- Severe threat (red)—fully implementing

Deployment of LPHA staff to assist in emergencies is limited by the size and qualification of the agency's workforce. More than half of all LPHAs have 13 or fewer staff members.[5] Larger agencies generally have much higher staffing levels and a more comprehensive range of expertise, as was described in Chapters 4 and 6.

The configuration of LHPAs within a state or in a multi-state metropolitan area also varies across the country. Several states organize local public health activities at a regional or district level. Other states have virtually hundreds of LHPAs that serve towns or townships, some in counties or districts served by a larger LHPA. Some communities have no LPHA at all. Organizing preparedness and response efforts in these different circumstances present special problems in terms of multi-jurisdictional response, surge capacity, back-up, and mutual aid agreements. Several capacity assessment and enhancement tools are available from NACCHO and CDC to assist local assessment of readiness.[6-8]

Medical Reserve Corps are locally based volunteer response teams that can be deployed in emergency situations. These multi-disciplinary teams often have ongoing relationships with local public health agencies and other community medical care providers that may include volunteer work on health promotion and screening projects or assistance with mosquito control activities in communities where West Nile Virus presents a risk. During emergencies, Medical

Exhibit 8–5 Homeland Security Advisory System Guidelines for Local Public Health Agencies

	Key Activities for Each Threat Condition
Emergency Planning, Training, Staffing	**Green (Low)** • Ensure personnel receive proper training on Homeland Security Advisory and agency protective measures/disaster plans • Ensure employee emergency notification system is current • Develop and train staff on staffing modification plans including 24/7 duty assignments • Train staff on local and state disaster plans • Develop and review roles and responsibilities in an emergency situation for each employee in the agency (all hazards plan which includes bioterrorism) **Blue (guarded)** • Review and update disaster plans specific to the agency (local health department medication distribution plan, smallpox pre- and post-event plans) • Provide training to key personnel on handling inquiries from the media **Yellow (Elevated)** • Coordinate emergency plans with nearby jurisdictions and review mutual aid agreements • Conduct employee emergency notification system drill • Be aware of large scale community events (sports, concerts, etc.) and include these in emergency planning • Review technical information on chemical and biological agents with all staff **Orange (High)** • Prepare to staff the agency's emergency operations center (EOC) or provide staff at the city/county EOC • Activate the employee emergency notification system and place staff on full alert • Review medication dispensing plans and mass vaccination plans with all staff **Red (Severe)** • Staff the agency's EOC or provide staff at the city/county EOC • Activate the agency's disaster preparedness plan • Activate the employee emergency notification system and secure as many additional staff as necessary to implement the agency's disaster preparedness plan • Prepare to implement the medication dispensing and mass vaccination plans • Coordinate preparedness and response activities with all public health partners and local jurisdictions (hospitals, physicians, local law enforcement, neighboring local health departments, emergency management agencies, and state health department) • Conduct a comprehensive disaster plan review with all staff to ensure an effective response in the event of a terrorist attack

continues

Exhibit 8–5 continued

Communications	Green (Low) • Ensure all emergency communication systems are in operational condition (Health Alert Network, e-mail, fax, and pagers) • Ensure staff have the technical information on chemical and biological agents necessary to respond to inquiries from the public or the media (fact sheets) • Review procedure/protocol for disseminating information to the community and media during a public health emergency Blue (Guarded) • Alert all agency staff that the threat condition has been raised to Guarded (Blue) • Assign a staff person to routinely monitor for faxes, e-mails, and correspondence from the state health agency • Obtain technical information from the state health agency and the Centers for Disease Control and Prevention on biological and chemical weapons of mass destruction for possible dissemination to health care providers and the public Yellow (Elevated) • Alert all agency staff that the threat condition has been raised to Elevated (Yellow) • Review media protocols with key personnel • Brief key personnel at least weekly on threat status, changes in security, and potential action plans Orange (High) • Alert all agency staff that the threat condition has been raised to Elevated (Orange) • Ensure that all members of the jurisdiction-wide bioterrorism committee are aware that the threat condition has been raised to High (Orange) • Advise staff of shift modifications if the situation escalates • Test all emergency communication systems Red (Severe) • Alert all agency staff that the threat condition has been raised to Severe (Red) • Ensure that all members of the jurisdiction-wide bioterrorism committee are aware that the threat condition has been raised to Severe (Red) • Issue periodic news releases with factual information on chemical and biological agents to reduce the potential for public panic • Brief key personnel daily on threat status, changes in security, and potential action plans • Check all emergency communications equipment on a daily basis
Administration	Green (Low) • Maintain routine operations without security stipulations • Continue to include employee safety and common sense practices in daily routines • Report suspicious circumstances and/or individuals to law enforcement agencies

continues

Exhibit 8–5 continued

	• Ensure all staff have issued current security credentials (ID badges) • Build networking relationships with other agencies, inside and outside the health professions Blue (Guarded) • Increase liaison with local and state agencies to monitor the threat • Prohibit casual access by unauthorized personnel • Assess mail handling procedures Yellow (Elevated) • Ensure security of facility operations • Check all essential equipment for operational readiness • Check inventories of critical supplies and re-order if necessary Orange (High) • Ensure security of the agency's critical infrastructure • Have designated staff continuously monitor for emergency communications from state health agency • Have designated staff continuously monitor radio and TV stations for a possible change in threat condition Red (Severe) • Initiate or augment security staffing at department facilities • Control building access and implement positive identification of all persons, include inspection of all incoming packages, brief cases, and deliveries • Maintain continuous monitoring for emergency communications from state health agency, as well as continuous monitoring of radio and TV stations for breaking news concerning terrorist attacks within state or elsewhere in United States
Public Health Surveillance	Green (Low) • Review agency procedures for handling reportable infectious diseases in the state Blue (Guarded) • Ensure information concerning reportable infectious diseases is coming into the agency from the health care providers within the jurisdiction Yellow (Elevated) • Request that hospitals (infectious control nurses and emergency departments), local laboratories, outpatient clinics, managed care organizations, and physicians report significant increases or clusters of illness of unknown etiology and review mandatory reporting procedures Orange (High) • Contact all hospitals (infectious control nurses and emergency departments), local laboratories, outpatient clinics, managed care organizations, and physicians and emphasize the importance of timely reporting of significant increases or clusters of illness of unknown etiology and review mandatory reporting procedures

Source: Illinois Department of Public Health, 2003.

Reserve Corps teams play predetermined roles such as providing local surge capacity for triage and medical care or assisting with deployment of Strategic National Stockpile materials. By 2004 it is expected that several hundred communities will participate in the Medical Reserve Corps program, either through start-up funding from the Health Resources and Services Administration or through local resources.

Private Health-Care Providers and Other Partners

In nearly all communities, government agencies play a central role in preparing for and responding to public health emergencies. Often overlooked, however, is the critical contribution made by private-sector health-care providers, pharmaceutical manufacturers, agricultural producers, the food industry, and other private sector interests. An important example is the role played by alert health professionals who are trained to recognize potential emergency situations and report these suspicions to public health officials. Clinicians in Florida played a major role in first identifying and then linking anthrax cases with bioterrorism in 2001. Hospital emergency rooms and physicians' offices are where most individuals who have contracted an infectious disease or are exposed to dangerous chemicals encounter their community's emergency response system. That encounter should trigger an appropriate response if the condition is one that represents a threat to others. Every state has incorporated requirements in state statute that call for physicians, laboratories, and other health providers to notify public health officials when specific notifiable diseases or conditions are encountered. (See Exhibit 6–10, Chapter 6.) Some states include a general provision that physicians should report "unusual" infectious diseases. Despite these laws and regulations, compliance with disease reporting is well-documented to be low among physicians due to a variety of reasons. The requirements and the reporting procedures may not be understood by some physicians. Others believe reporting is not worth the time and effort. Reporting from laboratories is more complete, but concerns exist as to whether laboratories serving multiple jurisdictions are fully aware of differences in requirements among the jurisdictions served.

In addition to playing an important role in identifying potential public health emergencies, health care providers play a critical role in responding to the medical consequences of those emergencies, especially in mass casualty situations. For the relatively rare disease threats associated with bioterrorism, health care providers often have only limited experience dealing with these conditions and look to public health authorizes for clinical guidance. Through the development of community-wide emergency response plans, public health agencies, private sector delivery systems, hospitals, physicians, pharmacies, nursing homes, and others are mobilized in the event of an emergency to provide needed treatment to those affected by disease and to provide prophylactic care to those at risk for exposure to disease. State and federal laws that confer tax-exempt status on hospitals typically require those institutions to provide significant community benefit, including the provision of emergency medical services and participation in regional emergency medical service planning. Funds for hospital preparedness, including staff training and preparedness planning, are provided by HRSA and channeled through state health departments.

Other private sector interests also contribute to public health emergency preparedness. Although NIH makes significant investments in the development of new vaccines and antimicrobial agents, pharmaceutical manufacturers represent the primary source of funding for research and development. Efforts to encourage industry interest in the development of vaccines and other countermeasures include incentives such as liability protections, antitrust waivers, patent extensions, and long-term contracts. Similarly, activities to improve the safety and security of the food supply will rely on the agricultural and food production industries to make necessary upgrades to their processes and to seek innovative ways to minimize disease threats.

Public Perceptions

The flurry of activity to improve public health emergency preparedness and response capabilities is understandable. The public is highly concerned over the possibility of terrorist attacks of all types.[9] Fears of possible anthrax or smallpox attacks are nearly as high as concerns of conventional explosives, airline hijacking or bombings, and attacks using radioactive, toxic, or hazardous materials as weapons. Among these potential terrorist weapons, concern is growing that smallpox will be used, related in part to the attention placed on smallpox at the national level with the initiation of smallpox preparedness programs that include vaccinations for key medical and first responder personnel. Although the public believes that the country is better prepared for a biological or chemical attack than it was prior to 2002, the public perceives that the current level of preparedness is not high enough and more needs to be done. The public is also concerned that the emphasis on bioterrorism will reduce efforts on other public health problems and issues that are important to the public. The public rates bioterrorism preparedness and response high, but no higher than health alerts, immunizations, testing and monitoring for diseases, education, natural epidemics, and chronic diseases.[9]

STATE AND LOCAL BIOTERRORISM PREPAREDNESS GRANTS

With the public health infrastructure increasingly viewed as a front line defense against terrorism and homeland security priority, federal funding for public health purposes increased dramatically beginning in 2002. To put this increase into perspective, total governmental spending in 2000 for population-based public health services was $17.4 billion, with the federal government accounting for 29 percent of that total, or about $5 billion.[10] The federal share of total governmental public health spending has been under 30 percent since the mid-1980s after having been as high as 72 percent in 1970.

Beginning in 2002, federal funding increased by more than $2 billion, with about half that amount directed to state and local governments for public health infrastructure improvements. Similar levels were funded in 2003 and are expected for at least the next few years. The infusion of this magnitude of resources creates the opportunity to address serious and longstanding gaps in public health protection and foster greater consistency and enhanced quality throughout the national network of governmental public health agencies at the federal, state, and local levels.

Public health infrastructure funding, approximately $1 billion annually, is channeled to the states and several large cities (including New York, Chicago, Los Angeles, and Washington, DC) through CDC. Each state receives a minimum award of $5 million plus an additional amount based on a population formula.

State Proposals and Workplans

Activities supported by these funds must be consistent with federal guidance. For funding from CDC for public health preparedness, grantees must undertake activities that increase capacity in seven focus areas, identified as Focus Areas A through G. HRSA funding for hospital preparedness can be considered an additional focus area and is included below with those supported by CDC funding.

A. Preparedness planning and readiness assessment—These activities establish strategic leadership, direction, assessment, and coordination of activities (including Strategic National Stockpile response) to ensure statewide readiness, interagency collaboration, local and regional preparedness (both intrastate and interstate) for bioterrorism, other outbreaks of infectious disease, and other public health threats and emergencies.

B. Surveillance and epidemiology capacity—Surveillance and epidemiologic capacities enable state and local health departments to enhance, design, and develop systems for rapid detection of unusual outbreaks of illness that may be the result of bioterrorism, other outbreaks of infectious disease, and other public health threats and emergencies. These activities assist state and local health departments in establishing expanded epidemiologic capacity to investigate and mitigate such outbreaks of illness as part of a National Electronic Disease Surveillance System (NEDSS). NEDSS is an initiative that promotes the use of data and information system standards to advance the development of efficient, integrated, and interoperable surveillance systems at federal, state, and local levels. NEDSS-based systems can be used by states for the surveillance and analysis of notifiable diseases providing a platform upon which modules can be built to meet state and program area data needs, as well as providing a secure, accurate, and efficient way for collecting and processing data.

C. Laboratory capacity for biologic agents—These activities ensure that core diagnostic capabilities for bioterrorist agents are available at all state and major city/county public health laboratories in order to conduct rapid and accurate diagnostic and reference testing for select biologic agents likely to be used in a terrorist attack. Given the myriad forms that terrorism might take, emergency preparedness requires not only a variety of different types of analytical laboratories, but also well defined operational relationships among them, especially with respect to routing of samples and sharing of test results. The national Laboratory Referral Network (LRN) provides this connectivity.

D. Laboratory capacity for chemical agents—These activities ensure that all state public health laboratories have the capacity to measure chemical threat agents in human specimens (e.g., blood, urine) or to appropriately collect and ship specimens to qualified LRN partner laboratories for analysis and further the establishment of a network of public laboratories for analysis of chemical threat agents.

E. Health alert network/communications and information technology—Activities for this focus area enable state and local public health agencies to establish and maintain a network that will support exchange of key information and training over the Internet by linking public health and private partners on a 24/7 basis, provide for rapid dissemination of public health advisories to the news media and the public at large, ensure secure electronic data exchange between public health partners' computer systems, and ensure protection of data, information, and systems, with adequate backup, organization, and surge capacity to respond to bioterrorism and other public health threats and emergencies.

F. Health risk communication and health information dissemination—Activities for this focus area ensure that state and local public health organizations develop an effective risk communications capacity that provides for timely information dissemination to citizens during a bioterrorist attack, bioterrorism, outbreak of infectious disease, or other public health threat and emergency. This includes training for key individuals in communications skills, the identification of key spokespersons (particularly those who can deal with infectious diseases), printed materials, timely reporting of critical information, and effective interaction with the media.

G. Education and training—Activities for this focus area ensure that state and local health agencies have the capacity to assess the training needs of key public health professionals, infectious disease specialists, emergency department personnel, and other healthcare (including mental health) providers in preparedness for and response to bioterrorism, other outbreaks of infectious disease, and other public health threats and emergencies, and ensure effective provision of needed education and training to key target audiences through multiple channels, including schools of public health, schools of medicine, other academic institutions, healthcare professionals, CDC, HRSA, and other sources. Emergency preparedness competencies (Exhibit 8–6) for all public health workers serve as the focal point for these assessment, enhancement, and recognition efforts. A more extensive panel of bioterrorism and emergency readiness competencies for various categories of public health workers is also in wide use.[11]

Exhibit 8–6 Emergency Preparedness Core Competencies for All Public Health Workers

All Public Health Workers must be competent to:
- Describe the public health role in emergency response in a range of emergencies that might arise (e.g., "The department provides surveillance, investigation and public information in disease outbreaks and collaborates with other agencies in geological, environmental, and weather emergencies.").
- Describe the chain of command in emergency response.
- Identify and locate the agency emergency response plan (or the pertinent portion of the plan).
- Describe his/her functional role(s) in emergency response and demonstrate his/her role(s) in regular drills.
- Demonstrate correct use of all communication equipment used for emergency communication (phone, fax, radio, etc.).
- Describe communication role(s) in emergency response: within the agency using established communication systems; with the media; with the general public; and personal (with family, neighbors).
- Identify limits to own knowledge/skill/authority and identify key system resources for referring matters that exceed these limits.
- Recognize unusual events that might indicate an emergency and describe appropriate action (e.g., communicate clearly within chain of command).
- Apply creative problem solving and flexible thinking to unusual challenges within his/her functional responsibilities and evaluate effectiveness of all actions taken.

Public Health Leaders/Administrators must also be competent to:
- Describe the chain of command and management system ("incident command system" or similar protocol for emergency response in the jurisdiction.
- Communicate the public health information, roles, capacities, and legal authority to all emergency response partners—such as other public health agencies, other health agencies, other governmental agencies—during planning, drills, and actual emergencies. (This includes contributing to effective community-wide response through leadership, team building, negotiation, and conflict resolution.)
- Maintain regular communication with emergency response partners. (This includes maintaining a current directory of partners and identifying appropriate methods for contacting them in emergencies.)
- Assure that the agency (or the agency unit) has a written, regularly updated plan for major categories of emergencies that respects the culture of the community and provides for continuity of agency operations.
- Assure that the agency (or agency unit) regularly practices all parts of emergency response.
- Evaluate every emergency response drill (or actual response) to identify needed internal and external improvements.
- Assure that knowledge and skill gaps identified through emergency response planning, drills, and evaluation are addressed.

Public Health Professionals must also be competent to:
- Demonstrate readiness to apply professional skills to a range of emergency situations during regular drills. (For example: access, use, and interpret surveillance data; access and use lab resources; access and use science-based investigation and risk assessment protocols; identity and use appropriate personal protective equipment.)

continues

Exhibit 8–6 continued

- Maintain regular communication with partner professionals in other agencies involved in emergency response. (This includes contributing to effective community-wide response through leadership, team building, negotiation, and conflict resolution.)
- Participate in continuing education to maintain up to date knowledge in areas relevant to emergency response. (For example: emerging infectious diseases, hazardous materials, and diagnostic tests.)

Public Health Technical and Support Staff must also be competent to:

- Demonstrate the use of equipment (including personal protective equipment) and skills associated with his/her functional role in emergency response during regular drills.
- Describe at least one resource for backup support in key areas of responsibility.

Source: Bioterrorism & Emergency Readiness Competencies for All Public Health Workers, Centers for Disease Control and Prevention, 2003.

H. Hospital Preparedness—Not a focus area funded by CDC, hospital preparedness is the primary category of activity supported by HRSA funding to states and large cities. Activities that are supported include: development of regional hospital preparedness and response plans; identification of hospital capacity for isolation, quarantine, and decontamination; procedures for receipt and distribution of materials from the Strategic National Stockpile; personal protective equipment; communications capabilities; biological disaster drills; and training.

Critical benchmarks identify those grantee activities that should be prioritized and fully achieved during the current budget period. For the 2002/2003 funding cycle, federal guidance identified 17 critical benchmarks (14 for the CDC funded state bioterrorism preparedness and 3 for the HRSA funded hospital preparedness program) to be accomplished by September 2003. Each focus area has one or more critical capacities associated with it. Critical capacities are the core expertise and infrastructure to enable a public health system to prepare for and respond to bioterrorism, other infectious disease outbreaks, and other public health threats and emergencies. These must be fully addressed by state and local grantees. Enhanced capacities represent additional expertise and infrastructure over and beyond the critical capacities. These should be addressed only after critical capacities have been achieved or are well along in development. As conveyed by the critical and enhanced capacities, federal expectations were broad and general. Exhibit 8–7 identifies the critical and enhanced capacities for each focus area for funding awarded in 2003.

As conveyed by the critical and enhanced capacities, expectations were unclear. In effect, responsibility for defining and operationalizing the capacities was left to the states, posing the risk of little consistency and standardization of approaches from state-to-state. CDC plans to transition critical capacities to readiness goals and readiness indicators in the future in order to establish an operational definition of preparedness, something that has been lacking in the early years of funding.

Exhibit 8–7 Critical and Enhanced Capacities for State Bioterrorism Project Grants, 2003

Critical Capacities

Enhanced Capacities

Focus Area A: Preparedness Planning and Readiness Assessment

- Establishment of a process for strategic leadership, direction, coordination, and assessment of activities to ensure state and local readiness, interagency collaboration, and preparedness for bioterrorism, other outbreaks of infectious disease, and other public health threats and emergencies
- Conducting integrated assessments of public health system capacities related to bioterrorism, other infectious disease outbreaks, and other public health threats and emergencies to aid and improve planning, coordination, and implementation
- Responding to emergencies caused by bioterrorism, other outbreaks of infectious disease, and other public health threats and emergencies through the development, exercise, and evaluation of a comprehensive public health emergency preparedness and response plan
- Effective management of the CDC Strategic National Stockpile (SNS), should it be deployed, translating SNS plans into firm preparations, periodic testing of SNS preparedness, and periodic training for entities and individuals that are part of SNS preparedness

- Ensuring public health emergency preparedness and response through the development of necessary public health infrastructure
- Recruiting, retaining, and fully developing public health leaders and managers with current knowledge and expertise in advanced management and leadership principles who will play critical roles in responding to bioterrorism, other outbreaks of infectious disease, and other public health threats and emergencies
- Ensuring that public health systems have optimal capacities to respond to bioterrorism, other outbreaks of infectious disease, and other public health threats and emergencies

Focus Area B: Surveillance and Epidemiology Capacity

- Rapidly detection of terrorist events through a highly functioning, mandatory reportable disease surveillance system, as evidenced by ongoing timely and complete reporting by providers and laboratories in the jurisdiction, especially of illnesses and conditions possibly resulting from bioterrorism, other outbreaks of infectious disease, and other public health threats and emergencies
- Rapid and effective investigation and response to potential terrorist events as evidenced by a comprehensive and exercised epidemiologic response plan

- Rapid detection and compilation of additional information about bioterrorism, other outbreaks of infectious disease, and other public health threats and emergencies through other core, cross-cutting health department surveillance systems such as vital record death reporting; medical examiner reports; emergency department, provider, or hospital discharge reporting; or ongoing population-based surveys
- Rapid detection and compilation of additional information about bioterrorism, other outbreaks of infectious dis-

continues

Exhibit 8–7 continued

that addresses surge capacity, delivery of mass prophylaxis and immunizations, and pre-event development of specific epidemiologic investigation and response needs

- Rapid and effective investigation and response to potential terrorist events, as evidenced by ongoing effective state and local response to naturally occurring individual cases of urgent public health importance, outbreaks of disease, and emergency public health interventions such as emergency chemoprophylaxis or immunization activities.

ease, and other public health threats and emergencies by accessing potentially relevant pre-existing datasets outside the health department, or through the development of new active or sentinel surveillance activities

- Creation or strengthening of pre-event, ongoing working links between health department staff and key individuals and organizations engaged in health care, public health, and law enforcement

Focus Area C: Laboratory Capacity, Biologic Agents

- Development and implementation of a jurisdiction-wide program to provide rapid and effective laboratory services in support of the response to bioterrorism, other outbreaks of infectious disease, and other public health threats and emergencies
- Ensuring, as a member of the Laboratory Response Network (LRN), adequate and secure laboratory facilities, reagents, and equipment to rapidly detect and correctly identify biological agents likely to be used in a bioterrorist incident

Focus Area D: Laboratory Capacity, Chemical Agents

- Development and implementation of a jurisdiction-wide program for Level One Laboratories that provides rapid and effective laboratory response for chemical terrorism by establishing competency in collection and transport of clinical specimens to laboratories capable of measuring chemical threat agents

- Establish adequate and secure Level Two laboratory facilities, reagents, and equipment (e.g., ICP-MS, CG-MSD) to rapidly detect and measure in clinical specimens for chemical agents (such as cyanide-based compounds, heavy metals, and lewisites). Currently, CDC methods for Level Two chemical agents use analytical techniques of inductively coupled plasma mass spectrometry and gas chromatography mass spectrometry. The list of Level Two chemical agents may expand as better methods are developed. Tandem mass spectrometry methods are not required for Level Two chemical agents.

continues

Exhibit 8–7 continued

- Establish adequate and secure Level Three laboratory facilities, reagents, and equipment (e.g., tandem mass spectrometer) to rapidly detect and measure in clinical specimens Level Three chemical agents (such as nerve agents, mustards, mycotoxins, and selected toxic industrial chemicals). Level Three Laboratories also provide surge capacity to CDC and serve as referral laboratories for Level One and Level Two laboratories.

Focus Area E: Health Alert Network/ Communications and Information Technology

- Effective communication connectivity among public health departments, health care organizations, law enforcement organizations, public officials, and others (e.g., hospitals, physicians, pharmacists, fire departments, 911 centers)
- Methods of emergency communication for participants in public health emergency response that are fully redundant with standard telecommunications (telephone, e-mail, Internet, etc.)
- Ongoing protection of critical data and information and capabilities for continuity of operations
- Electronic exchange of clinical, laboratory, environmental, and other public health information in standard formats between the computer systems of public health partners

- Provision of or participation in an emergency response management system to aid the deployment and support of response teams, the management of response resources, the facilitation of inter-organizational communication and coordination
- Ensuring full information technology and support services

Focus Area F: Communicating Health Risks and Health Information Dissemination

- Provision of needed health/risk information to the public and key partners during a terrorism event by establishing critical baseline information about the current communication needs and barriers within individual communities, and identifying effective channels of communication for reaching the general public and special populations during public health threats and emergencies

- Identifying, developing, and pre-testing communications concepts, messages, and strategies to ensure that state and local public health agencies prepare in advance and produce effective and culturally appropriate public information for terrorism, other infectious disease outbreaks, and other public health threats and emergencies

continues

Exhibit 8–7 continued

Focus Area G: Education and Training

- Ensure the delivery of appropriate education and training to key public health professionals, infectious disease specialists, emergency department personnel, and other healthcare (including mental health) providers in preparedness for and response to bioterrorism, other outbreaks of infectious disease, and other public health threats and emergencies, either directly or through the use (where possible) of existing curricula and other sources, including schools of public health, schools of medicine, academic health centers, CDC training networks, and other providers

- Ensure that public and private health professionals and other members of the community are identified in advance and can be effectively trained to mobilize and respond during a public health emergency
- Ongoing systematic evaluation of the effectiveness of training, and the incorporation of lessons learned form performance during bioterrorism drills, simulations, other exercises, events, and evaluations of those exercises would also enhance this focus area

Source: Centers for Disease Control and Prevention, 2003.

Several new emphases were injected into guidance for the 2003 awards, reflecting actual and perceived issues encountered in the previous year. These include laboratory capacity for chemical agents, integration of mental health services into preparedness planning and response activities, coordination of CDC funding with HRSA-funded hospital preparedness activities, and concurrence of local public health authorities with state spending plans. Finally, the 2003 guidance incorporates specific smallpox preparedness and response capacities and allows for costs associated with smallpox preparedness to be covered by grant funds. These and several other issues arose in many states during early implementation of bioterrorism preparedness activities.

Early Lessons

Comprehensive preparedness programs require hazard and vulnerability analyses, forecasts of the probable health effects, analyses of the availability of needed resources, identification of vulnerable populations, and development of detailed plans for both preparedness and response. Many factors influence a state's ability to complete these tasks. Public health preparedness is particularly challenging because public health and public safety roles differ for federal, state, and local governments. The federal government has primary responsibility for national security, while state and local governments carry the responsibility and financial burden for most other public health responsibilities. Some of the early lessons from the states reflect these themes.

Early experience with the infusion of federal support for public health emergency preparedness and response activities indicates that considerable progress has occurred (although much remains to be done), consistent with apparently conflicting conclusions of an ASTHO assessment of progress through December 2002, on the one hand, and that from the Independent Task Force on Emergency Responders, on the other. The ASTHO report found that states are making significant progress in the enterprise of building the capacity to respond quickly and effectively to bioterrorism, outbreaks of infectious diseases, and other public health threats and emergencies.[12] The Independent Task Force on Emergency Responders summarized its conclusions in its report's title, "Emergency Responders: Drastically Underfunded, Dangerously Unprepared."[13]

An early start does not guarantee success. Many states had a head start on public health preparedness and stood ready to benefit from and effectively deploy the substantial resources received beginning in 2002. Some states had already received as much as three years of funding, often for development of statewide health alert networks. States with a solid pre-existing statewide public health infrastructure were particularly well positioned to move ahead rapidly. Yet despite a head start and other positive influences, a variety of intergovernmental, political, bureaucratic, and economic forces slowed progress. Some of these influences were unique to specific states, while others reflect circumstances existing in many other states. Still others reflect a long-standing pattern of intergovernmental relationships, the operational aspects of federalism and public health.

Political influences included shifts in the political balance of power within state government, such as occurs when a new governor takes office. Discord between the state and its local health jurisdictions over fairness of past state funding of public health infrastructure and current plans for allocating public health preparedness resources represents another political influence. The concept of regional health consortia controlling resources for public health preparedness merits consideration and appears to be successful in several states.

Local jurisdictions deal with public expectations as well as with state and federal directives, while attempting to meet a wide variety of health needs at the local level. West Nile Virus hit many states hard in 2002 and 2003, forcing local health agencies to redeploy staff and resources. Smallpox vaccination activities resulted in similar redeployments in early 2003. One local health officer reported that smallpox preparedness activities required 80 percent of the time for 20 percent of his agency's staff over a four-month period.

Critical in many states was a state budget in heavy deficit mode, making significant reductions in state general revenue funding for the public health department and other state agencies necessary. State budget crises often prompted the enactment of early retirement programs that resulted in the displacement of many middle and senior level staff within the state health agency. Reduced staffing levels, decimated leadership ranks, and greater control over hiring created a management crisis to accompany the financial crisis. Bargaining unit provisions further complicated the hiring process in some states as workers previously laid off by other state agencies bumped workers in similar titles within the state health agency and were given priority for some newly funded positions.

The net effect was an environment conducive to supplanting state and local resources with federal funds. Federal guidance specifically prohibits supplanting state and local resources, meaning that funds under this program may not be used to replace or supplant any current state or local expenditures. Supplanting had become an issue in several states, including Connecticut where public health organizations fought efforts by the state to pull $2.3 million out of infrastructure grants to local health jurisdictions while the state was developing a new $2.3 million bioterrorism grant program for locals.[14] Boston and Seattle have also witnessed reduced state and local appropriations for public health services while ramping up bioterrorism preparedness-related activities.[15] The evidence to-date in most states does not indicate that widespread and explicit supplanting has occurred, but a continuing state fiscal crisis could make federal bioterrorism resources look even more attractive a year or two further down the road. In any event, state and local cutbacks in funding for public health infrastructure coupled with increased federal funds ultimately results in lower total funding levels than envisioned. Although this may not violate the letter of the prohibition against supplanting, it certainly challenges its spirit.

The degree to which these factors are operative in the 50 states varies. Changes in governorships and state administrations are a regular occurrence in virtually all states. Nearly all states have shared in the economic plight. Hiring and procurement policies seem to be problems everywhere, even in good economic times. State-local tensions are the rule rather than the exception for public health in states with relatively independent local health jurisdictions. West Nile Virus may not have hit all states yet, but almost certainly will emerge as a community health risk, and the smallpox redeployment affects local health jurisdictions throughout the U.S. In any event, political, bureaucratic, economic, and intergovernmental factors control the speed with which progress toward public health preparedness occurs.

Systems take time and need sustained support. The early experience also demonstrates that systems take time and need sustained support. Even for those states with three years of early work to develop the health alert network and upgrade disease surveillance systems, it will be several more years until these systems are completed, fully functional, and integrated into a national network. The development of a comprehensive public health workforce preparedness system will also take several years, as will true multi-state planning. It is unrealistic to believe that these systems can be up-and-running after only a year or two of funding.

ASTHO and NACCHO have recognized this in arguing for coordinated surveillance systems, development of a fully trained workforce, and sustained support of the public health infrastructure. The Independent Task Force on Emergency Responders (convened by the Council on Foreign Relations, a respected think tank organization) concluded that public health preparedness and response will require $6.7 billion more than projected funding for 2004–2008.[13] A Government Accounting Office (GAO) report concluded that it will take $1 billion per year for five years for there to be a national impact on state/local preparedness.[16]

Workforce is a particularly difficult and important systems issue. Funding alone will not ensure that competent staff can be recruited and hired in a timely manner. A myriad of factors related to political and fiscal control, as well as others related to bureaucratic processes and labor relations, can derail hiring plans. Effective public health workforce development systems that ensure the appropriate quantity, composition, distribution, and competency of public health workers lag far behind the development of other preparedness systems.

Spending on ongoing activities, such as workers, training, surveillance, and communications systems requires sustained levels over many years—not one or two shots. For this to occur, public health preparedness must remain a national priority, and federal leadership must be strong.

Federal leadership is essential. Federal health agencies are at risk of criticism from both sides. At times they provide too much direction and guidance in categorical programs. At other times they are criticized for providing too little. Aspects of both critiques are apparent in CDC's bioterrorism grant relationships with the states. Focus areas are well defined, but expectations within these focus areas are not. Within CDC separate units provide program support and review for each focus area with inadequate prioritization and integration across all focus areas. States tend to mimic federal structures and develop separate staff and budgets for each focus area, again without adequate coordination across all focus areas for priorities and cross cutting needs (training, equipment, hiring, etc.). Separate units within states run the hospital preparedness program, mimicking the less than optimal coordination between CDC and HRSA over their separate bioterrorism preparedness priorities.

Federal guidance for public health preparedness provides a framework of critical and enhanced capacities and critical benchmarks. Needed is a better approach to setting standards that would include both functional and operational performance in preparedness activities. Currently, states are not clear on what is meant by preparedness and how it can be measured and recognized. In this vacuum, states are left to fend for themselves, resulting in uneven, inconsistent, and unstandardized approaches from state-to-state, and from locality-to-locality within states.

Several of these themes derive from the history of federalism and public health in America, which has left the federal government in a precarious situation of weakened leadership capacity at a time when leadership is most badly needed. The federal decline is evident in the federal agencies' shrinking percent of total public health spending, the reduction in the federal public health workforce, and several decades of active devolution of health responsibilities back to the states.[17] Only one percent of total federal spending on health supports population-based public health activities.[10]

Needed are explicit national preparedness standards as an operational definition of national, state, and local readiness. One such effort is already underway with 12 local health jurisdictions participating as pilot sites for NACCHO's project, Public Health Ready.[18] In order to be certified as "ready" local health jurisdictions must meet standards for workforce training, establishment of an agency response plan linked to a communitywide response plan, and exercising of that plan.

Another hallmark of federalism and public health in the U.S., the lack of coordination between and among federal agencies, has long been a concern for state and local public health agencies. With HRSA funding relatively small in comparison with CDC funds for the 2002/2003 funding cycle, this may not have appeared to represent a significant problem. However, HRSA funding for 2003/2004 increased four-fold while CDC funds remained at the same level as the previous year, increasing the scope and possible repercussions of problems due to lack of coordination. Early experience and reactions from the states resulted in strengthened guidance for the 2003/2004 funding cycle related to coordination of CDC and HRSA funding. Rather than each state having two separate advisory committees, one for the CDC funded activities and one for HRSA funded activities, the latest guidance calls for a joint advisory committee for CDC and HRSA cooperative agreements. More than 25 entities/interests must be included on the unified advisory committee and/or its subcommittees.

Preparedness is primarily local. Preparedness, like public health and politics, is primarily local. In that light, careful attention must be paid to identifying and addressing local needs for public health preparedness and response. Local health officials in many states have raised concerns over the distribution of funding in 2002, perceiving that local health jurisdictions should have received more than the share allotted to them. In future years, the proportion of funding shared with local health jurisdictions may need to increase as state level needs are addressed. Some local health jurisdictions would prefer that CDC directly fund local jurisdictions in a manner similar to what is now done for only a handful of the largest U.S. cities. They argue that political whims at the state level too often result in poor priorities, state money grabs, and inefficient reimbursement mechanisms. States, on the other hand, argue that state control and decision making promotes interoperable equipment, complementary resources across jurisdictions, and avoidance of gaps in coverage. It is not possible to draw conclusions as to the wisdom of separate grants to states and localities within that state. Some differences in approach are apparent for surveillance systems, hospital relationships, and training. But none appear, as yet, to be major. Strong leadership within state and local health agencies should minimize the potential for problems. Further, strong federal leadership and assurance of consistency across jurisdictions could also serve to avert problems. However, federal guidance for inter-jurisdictional (city-state), multi-jurisdictional (multi-state) regional preparedness has been minimal to date, at least in comparison to that for statewide and sub-state regional preparedness. The impact on local public health practice should ultimately be positive as better systems and workforce development advance. However, preparedness competes with other local priorities and may have suffered in the past year due to the need for West Nile virus and smallpox focused activities. Ongoing community health priorities may have fared even worse.

Notable in the latest federal guidance for bioterrorism preparedness grants is the requirement for evidence of consensus, approval, or concurrence between state and local public health officials for the proposed use of the funds. States must provide assurance that both state and local capacity development is to be achieved and local public health officials, especially those serving a significant portion of the state's population, concur with the proposed use of funds. The intent of this guidance is to shift the focus of funding to the benefit achieved rather than the level of government spending the dollars. Whether it will serve to constructively engage state and local public health interests remains to be seen. In states with a long history of collaboration around public health improvement initiatives, it could serve to upset the delicate balance that has evolved over time.

At the local level, public health preparedness must be well coordinated with hospital preparedness. The experience to date suggests that hospitals feel isolated from much of the communitywide planning that is taking place. Yet hospitals are key players in response to actual events. Lessons from several large scale national exercises substantiate this concern. States have identified a need for exercises and drills similar to the TOPOFF 2 exercise (see Exhibit 8–8) involving Washington State and Illinois in 2003.[19]

Ideally, the infusion of resources to shore up the sagging public health infrastructure would foster positive structural changes in public health systems at the state and local level. The impact on core public health practice activities should be measurable and, ultimately, there is a need to assess this impact as preparedness efforts advance. Preparedness should be viewed as an important quality or attribute of an effective public health system rather than as a categorical end in itself. This is the essence of the philosophy that has become to be known as the "dual use," "multiple use," or "all hazards" strategy. Although this has been the public position of federal officials since late 2001, federal actions have not always been consistent with federal rhetoric.

Indeed, credibility is one theme that constantly reemerges from the early experience of the states with preparedness funding. CDC's emphasis on small-pox preparedness has both helped and hurt its credibility with the state and local public health community. It hurt in several ways, including the lack of information related to the hazard and risk assessment process. States and localities were to accept the risk assessment undertaken by the federal government based on undisclosed intelligence information. Many public health officials questioned whether a terrorist-generated smallpox attack represents enough of a real risk to justify the harm associated with smallpox vaccination strategies. Secondly, federal directives on smallpox undermine the credibility of an all hazards approach through the enormous emphasis placed on one specific threat at the expense of all others. This nurtures the fear that the federal preparedness program may be little more than another federal categorical program. Countering these concerns is the perception that the implementation steps for smallpox provide useful practical experience that may assist future responses to other threats and actual events. In any event, all sides recognize the need to take full advantage of federal funding increases to leverage overall infrastructure improvements. How this can be done when states and localities are tempted to cut back on their own support of public health infrastructure will require vision, leadership, and follow-through beyond anything seen to date.

CONCLUSION

Preparing for and responding to emergencies is a well established role for public health agencies and their workers. This role, highlighted in the Public Health in America statement[1] as one of six critical responsibilities, has often been viewed as one of responding to an occasional natural disaster such as an earthquake, hurricane, or flood. Large scale events that threaten public health

Exhibit 8–8 National TOPOFF2 Exercise, 2003

Terrorism drill unfolds this week

The Department of Homeland Security will stage a weeklong series of simulated disasters in Chicago and Seattle May 10-16 to test the government's ability to respond to terrorist attacks.

THE SCENARIO

A fictional terrorist group releases pneumonic plague in the Chicago area and explodes a "dirty bomb" in Seattle. Local and state agencies in both cities coordinated their responses with federal agencies in Washington, D.C. and the American Red Cross. In Canada, agencies coordinate with U.S. officials after the plague spreads from Chicago to Vancouver.

SATURDAY

The scenario begins in Chicago when pneumonic plague is supposedly released into the environment at three spots, spreading undetected throughout Cook, DuPage, Kane and Lake Counties.

Chicago
☐ Affected counties

Sources: Department of Homeland Security, City of Chicago, City of Seattle, Department of the Solicitor General of Canada Chicago Tribune

MONDAY AND TUESDAY

SEATTLE
CHICAGO

SEATTLE

MONDAY
• At about noon, a fake radiological dispersion device, or "dirty bomb," is detonated.

TUESDAY
• A public shelter is opened, using high school students as mock victims. Meanwhile, a "safe house" for terrorists is located.

CHICAGO

TUESDAY
• A growing number of mock patients show up at hospitals complaining of flulike symptoms.

WEDNESDAY

CHICAGO
• More mock patients show up at hospitals.
• Five sites are prepared to distribute mock antibiotics.
• Taylor Street from Clinton to Jefferson Streets is scheduled to be closed from 3-7 p.m. A police motorcade is expected to travel the Kennedy Expressway to the downtown area.

THURSDAY

★ At 10 a.m., heath officials act as though they are administering drugs to crowds at five sites.

After 6 p.m., a simulated aircraft crash generates a loud sound and smoke at Midway Airport.

After 9 a.m., officials respond to a mock "hazardous materials incident" and a building collapse in Bedford Park.

After 9 p.m., Police raid a mock bioterrorism lab at 1700 W. 39th St.

Lake Bluff ★

Lake Michigan

5 MILES

LAKE CO.

COOK CO.

1400 N. Larrabee ★
Chicago ★
Bridgeview ★

DUPAGE CO.

Wheaton ★

KANE CO.

Aurora ★

WHAT YOU MIGHT SEE

• Traffic delays, emergency vehicles and equipment in southwest Chicago.

• Helicopters, flash grenades and simulated gunshots near 1700 W. 39th St.

• Parking will be prohibited in the 1400 block of North Larrabee Street for several hours beginning at 8 a.m. CTA buses and drill volunteers will be lined up along the street.

• Officials will close 55th Street from Laramie to Central Avenues for several hours starting at about 5 p.m. At Midway Airport, mock victims will wear makeup to resemble injuries. Rescue teams will be present.

Source: Chicago Tribune, May 11, 2003.

355

and safety have seldom been intentionally inflicted, despite recent examples to the contrary such as the bombing of the federal building in Okalahoma City in the 1990s. Events in the international theater raised the specter of increased risk for terrorist acts, including bioterrorism, directed against the American population and prompted interest in preparedness and response capacities within the federal government in the mid-1990s.

The cycle of progress in public health preparedness has been remarkably consistent over several centuries in the U.S. A terrible epidemic or another form of health-related disaster or threat occurs. Public expectations call for such an event to never occur again. Significant new resources are deployed to raise the level of preparedness and protection. The threat seems to dissipate over time. Preparedness, though still important, becomes relatively less important. Eventually, a new threat or event appears, and the cycle repeats itself. This recurring scenario raises the question as to whether current preparedness efforts represent a new and different strategy that could short circuit this chain of events. Past preparedness efforts focused on a specific threat and diminished as that specific threat diminished. Perhaps a more broadly focused preparedness campaign, one that is valued because it battles many different threats, will fare differently. Although still early in the process, some things are clear.

The price for public health preparedness will be high, regardless of how it is calculated. In crude dollar terms, its costs reflect a 20 percent increase in the federal investment in governmental public health services provided through governmental public health agencies. This increase will need to be sustained indefinitely since it primarily supports information, communications, and workforce development systems that are ongoing in nature. And it will require commensurate commitment and investment on the part of state and local governments. Otherwise supplanting will occur in one form or another, and the opportunity for federal preparedness funds to leverage other resources will be lost.

If the price is to be calculated in terms of federalism and intergovernmental relationships, it will also be high. States will need to encourage and accept stronger federal leadership on the one hand and generate a better understanding of local needs and priorities on the other. These will need to be fashioned into effective local, regional, state, and multi-state efforts in ways that will challenge states to live up to their primary responsibility for the health of its citizens. All this must be done while navigating through a treacherous obstacle course laden with political, economic, and bureaucratic impediments to sustained progress.

The federal government must avoid the pitfall of merely throwing money at the problem, without fostering a national vision of public health preparedness and nurturing the state-local public health systems that must carry out that vision. This will require the federal agencies to be accountable for meaningful capacity and performance standards, consistent credibility as to both ends and means, integration both across focus areas and across federal agencies, and leadership rather than either regulatory or advisory approaches to dealing with state-local public health system issues.

Although these are formidable challenges, the opportunities (and the opportunity costs) are unprecedented. The boost in federal funding and potential for federal leadership provide a unique opportunity to fashion a more coordinated national public health system. Certainly, the public now expects this,[9] and the price of not being prepared will be high. But progress often comes at a high price. The history of public health preparedness reflects this lesson. Ironically, failure to seize this opportunity will increase the likelihood that another cycle will occur. We can either learn the lessons of the past, the lessons of public health threats and responses, and the lessons of public health operated within a federalist form of government, or we can relive this history over and over again.

DISCUSSION QUESTIONS AND EXERCISES

1. What constitutes vulnerability in populations who live in disaster prone areas? Give a concrete example from a disaster that has drawn media attention in recent years (several media web sites are provided in the Course Resources catalog).
2. Choose a public health discipline or occupational group (either your own or one that you are somewhat familiar with) and describe the range of tasks that group of public health practitioners may be asked to perform in disaster preparedness and response. Why is public health participation important?
3. Why should public health organizations take a leadership role in emergency and disaster planning?
4. Why is the process of planning more important than the written plan itself? Describe the "paper plan" syndrome and how it can detract from public health emergency preparedness. Identify factors contributing to disaster and other public health emergency planning apathy.
5. What is meant by the term *surge capacity* and how is this addressed in public health emergency response plans?
6. Describe three or more elements of public health statues that are important elements of public health emergency response plans.
7. Describe the role of your agency and at least four other agencies that work in conjunction with your agency in public health emergencies.
8. Describe your own specific role for several different public health emergency situations.
9. What are the basic functions that a health department should perform in response to an emergency or disaster? When should a health department identify these functions?
10. What public health resources are available at the federal, state, or local level in an emergency or disaster? How would you go about requesting these resources?

REFERENCES

1. Public Health Functions Steering Committee. *Public Health in America.* Washington, DC: PHS; 1995.
2. Landesmann LY. Public Health Management of Disasters: The Practice Guide. Washington, DC: APHA, 2001.
3. Presidential Homeland Security Directive No. 3, February 28, 2003.
4. The Center for Law and the Public's Health. The Model State Emergency Health Powers Act Emergencies Act. Georgetown and Johns Hopkins Universities; 2001.
5. National Association of County and City Health Officials. Local Public Health Infrastructure: A Chartbook. Washington, DC: NACCHO; 2001.
6. Elements of Effective Local Bioterrorism Preparedness: A Planning Primer for Local Public Health Agencies. NACCHO; 2001 (PDF document)
7. Local Centers for Public Health Preparedness: Models for Strengthening Local Public Health Capacity. National Association of County and City Health Officials; 2001 (PDF document)
8. Local Emergency Preparedness and Response Inventory: A Tool for Rapid Assessment of Local Capacity to Respond to Bioterrorism, Outbreaks of Infectious Disease, and Other Public Health Threats and Emergencies. The Centers for Disease Control and Prevention; 2001 (PDF document).
9. Lake, Snell, Perry & Associates. Americans Speak Out on Bioterrorism and U.S. Preparedness to Address Risk. Robert Wood Johnson Foundation, December 2002.
10. Centers for Medicare and Medicaid Services, National Health Accounts, 1960–2000.
11. Bioterrorism & Emergency Readiness Competencies for All Public Health Workers (in PDF format). Public Health Ready (CDC/NACCHO/Columbia).
12. Association of State and Territorial Health Officials. *Public Health Preparedness: A Progress Report.* Washington, DC: ASTHO, 2003.
13. Independent Task Force on Emergency Responders. Emergency Responders: Drastically Underfunded, Dangerously Unprepared. Council on Foreign Relations, June 2003.
14. Randall TJ. Advocates in Action: Connecticut Local Health Officials Go to Battle to Save State Funding. *NACCHO Exchange.* 2003 (Summer):18–19.
15. Smith S. Anthrax vs. the Flu: As State Governments Slash Their Public Health Budgets, Federal Money is Pouring in for Bioterror Preparedness. *Boston Globe.* July 29, 2003.
16. Government Accounting Office. Bioterrorism Preparedness Varied across State and Local Jurisdictions. Washington, DC: GAO-03-373, April 2003.
17. National Association of County and City Health Officials. Public Health Ready. Washington, DC: NACCHO; 2003.
18. Turnock BJ and Atchison C. Governmental Public Health in the United States: The Implications of Federalism. *Health Affairs.* 2002:6:68–72.
19. Dizon NZ. Terrorism Drill Comes to Chicago. *Chicago Tribune.* May 13, 2003.

Chapter 9

Future Challenges for Public Health in America

This text approaches what public health is and how it works from a unified conceptual framework. Key dimensions of the public health system are examined, including its purpose, functions, capacity, processes, and outcomes. Although this is a simple framework, many of the concepts addressed are anything but simple. As a result, much has been left unsaid, and many important issues and problems facing the public health system have been addressed only in passing. This may serve to whet the appetite of those eager to move beyond the basics and ready to tackle emerging and more complex issues in greater depth. The basic concepts included in this text seek to facilitate that process and encourage thinking "outside the book." Delving into these other issues without the benefit of a broad understanding of the system and how it works, however, can be an occupational hazard in any field of endeavor. For public health workers, continuously fighting off alligators remains the major deterrent to draining the swamp in order to prevent the problem in the first place.

Each chapter highlights one or more public health achievements of the twentieth century, telling the story of how we got where we are today. Together, these stories demonstrate that the problems facing public health have changed over the past century and suggest that we can expect them to continue to change throughout the current one. In retrospect, many past problems appear relatively easy to solve in comparison with those on the public health agenda at the beginning of the twenty-first century. However, we often forget that last century's problems appeared to be quite formidable to public health advocates back in 1900. Although formidable, they were deemed unacceptable, initiating the chain of events that resulted in an impressive catalog of accomplishments.

Each of these achievements has provided valuable lessons and insights into the obstacles to achieve even further gains that lie ahead. Challenges reside at many levels, especially at the level of preparedness for unforeseen, and previously unanticipated, threats to the public's health. Melding the expectations for addressing ongoing health problems in the community with those for preparing and responding to new threats leads us to the three key questions addressed in this chapter:

- What are the lessons learned from the threats and challenges faced by public health in twentieth-century America?
- What are the limitations and challenges facing public health in the twenty-first century?
- How can these limitations and challenges be overcome?

LESSONS FROM A CENTURY OF PROGRESS IN PUBLIC HEALTH

The remarkable achievements of the twentieth century did not completely eradicate the public health problems faced in 1900. Many of these continue to threaten the health of Americans and impede progress toward realizing the life span projections presented in Figure 9–1. New faces for old enemies have appeared in the form of challenges and obstacles to be overcome in the early decades of the twenty-first century. Infectious diseases, tobacco, maternal and infant mortality, unintentional injuries, cardiovascular diseases, food safety, and occupational health remain high on the list of leading threats to the public's health. Each presents special challenges, not unlike those recounted by the young public health physician in Exhibit 9–1.

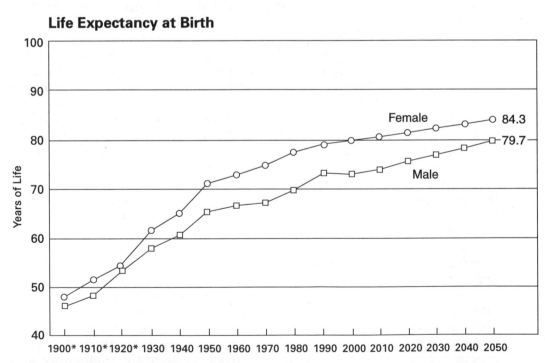

Life Expectancy at Birth

Figure 9–1 Past and Projected Female and Male Expectancy at Birth, United States, 1900–2050. *Source:* Reprinted from *Healthy People 2010: Understanding and Improving Health*, U.S. Department of Health and Human Services, Public Health Service, 2000.

Exhibit 9-1 A Young Public Health Physician's Story

In 1940 I left private practice to accept a position as a local health officer in Kentucky. After a three month course at the University of Kentucky which included the principles of epidemiology and law, I was assigned to Breckenridge, Hancock and Meade counties—three rural counties with a county seat as the only town in each and a combined population of approximately 45,000. The staff in each county consisted of a public health nurse, a sanitarian and a clerk.

During my two years in this assignment here were outbreaks of poliomyelitis, smallpox, typhoid fever, diphtheria, scarlet fever, measles, and whooping cough. Tuberculosis, syphilis, and gonorrhea were widely prevalent. Rabies was endemic in the wild animal and dog populations. Very few women received prenatal care and most were delivered in the home. Most of the wells were polluted. Disposal of human waste was haphazard and privies were unsanitary. Practically all the milk consumed was raw and restaurants were not inspected.

To raise immunity levels quickly, the nurses and I visited every school in the three counties and vaccinated every child we could hold still long enough to give the immunizations. If you were to do today what we did then, you would be sued. Also, I am sure the Food and Drug Administration would not approve the antigens we used.

Weekly venereal disease clinics were set up in each county. Treatment was a year of weekly injections of arsenicals intravenously and bismuth intramuscularly. Keeping patients in treatment was a problem and I frequently sent the sheriff to bring in patients who missed treatments.

For tuberculosis patients, we set up the best isolation we could achieve in their own homes. Pregnant women were referred by their physicians to the nurses for prenatal nursing care. A sterile pack of sheets and instruments was developed; the nurses accompanied the doctors to assist in home deliveries.

Well deficiencies were corrected and a system of bacterial testing of well water was instituted. The privy program was a problem because the county court had to set up a procedure to collect for building the privies. Instituting the use of pasteurized milk was a problem because a vocal minority predicted all manner of medical problems that would result from the use of processed milk. They exhibited the same mind-set we see today in those who rail against the radiation of foods and fluoridation of water supplies.

Restaurant inspection and food handler instruction posed few problems. The transfer of vital records from the county clerk to the health department required a high order of diplomacy, but was achieved and we were able to hand tabulate a report of births and deaths.

These were primitive programs, but that was public health in the early 1940s. Probably more important than the specific program activities was the public health process. The staff gathered information, then made decisions as to what was needed, gave priorities to the problems and planned the various programs. This is still a hallmark of the public health method.

Source: Paul Q. Peterson MD, MPH. Public Health: Its Program Evolution and Future Challenges. Convocation Address, School of Public Health, University of Illinois at Chicago, May 1994.

Infectious Diseases

The continuing battle against infectious diseases will be fought on several fronts due to the emergence of new infectious diseases and the reemergence of old enemies, often in drug-resistant forms. Infections due to *Escherichia coli* *O157:H7* have emerged as a frequent and frightening risk to the public. Initially identified as the cause of hemorrhagic conditions in the early 1980s, this pathogen was increasingly associated with food-borne illness outbreaks in the 1990s, including a major outbreak in the Pacific Northwest related to *E. coli*-contaminated hamburgers distributed through a national fast food chain.[1] The source of the *E. coli* was cattle. Other outbreaks of this pathogen involved swimmers in lake water contaminated by bathers infected with the organism (Figure 9–2). Because many of the illnesses are minor and both medical and public health practitioners fail to perform the tests necessary to diagnose *E. coli* infections properly, current surveillance efforts greatly underreport the extent of this condition.

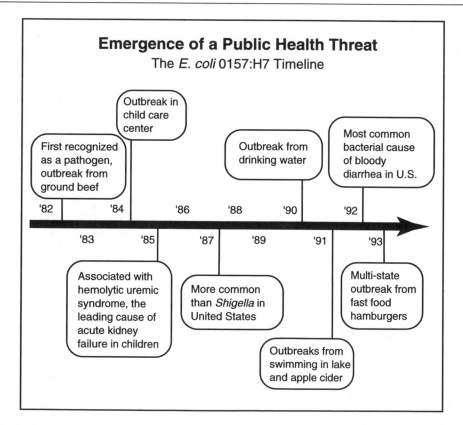

Figure 9–2 Emergence of a Public Health Threat: The *Escherichia coli* O157:H7 Timeline. *Source:* Reprinted from *Addressing Emerging Infectious Disease Threats: A Prevention Strategy for the United States,* 1994, U.S. Centers for Disease Control and Prevention, Atlanta, GA.

Multi-drug-resistant pathogens represent another emerging infectious disease problem for the public health system. The widespread and, at times, indiscriminate use of antibiotics in agricultural and health-care settings produces strains of bacteria that are resistant to these drugs. Antimicrobial agents have been increasingly deployed throughout the second half of the twentieth century. Slowly, over this period, the consequences of these "miracle drugs" have been experienced in the community, as well as in health facilities. The emergence of drug-resistant strains has reduced the effectiveness of treatment for several common infections, including tuberculosis, gonorrhea, pneumococcal infections, and hospital-acquired staphylococcal and enterococcal infections. For tuberculosis, drug resistance played a substantial role in its resurgence in the early 1990s.

Pathogens, both old and new, have devised ingenious ways of adapting to and thwarting the weapons used to control them. Many factors in society, the environment, and global interconnectedness continue to increase the risk of emergence and spread of infectious diseases. Heightened concerns over the risk of acts of bioterrorism add a new dimension to the threats posed by infectious diseases. As noted in the previous chapter, these concerns have raised expectations for public health to serve both national security and personal safety roles.

The role of infectious diseases in the development of chronic diseases such as diabetes, heart disease, and some cancers further argues that infectious diseases will continue as important health risks in the new century. To battle infectious diseases, the development and deployment of new methods, both in laboratory and epidemiologic sciences, are needed to better understand the interactions among environmental factors as contributors to the emergence and reemergence of infectious disease processes. Also, despite the successes realized in the development and use of vaccines over the past century, substantial gaps persist in the infrastructure of the vaccine delivery system, including parents, providers, information technology, and biotech and pharmaceutical companies. Improving the coordination of these elements holds the promise of reducing the toll from infectious diseases in the twenty-first century.

Tobacco Use

The potential gains to be realized from further reduction of tobacco usage are also apparent. Despite the overall decline in tobacco use among adults over the second half of the twentieth century, an alarmingly high prevalence of tobacco use among teens persists, and rates among adults are no longer declining, as they did prior to 1980. These trends suggest that concerns over risks related to exposure to environmental tobacco smoke will continue for many years to come. Disparities in tobacco use by race and ethnicity, together with the growth of demographic groups with high use rates, add yet another dimension to the war against tobacco. New approaches and new products will raise new issues of safety, whereas the increase in tobacco use across the globe will transport old and new challenges around the world.

Maternal and Child Health

Even as maternal and child health outcomes have improved dramatically, there has been little change in the prime determinants of perinatal outcomes—the rate of low birth weight and pre-term deliveries. This situation must be addressed to even partially replicate the gains realized in the twentieth century. Another important risk factor moving in the wrong direction is the rate of unintended pregnancies. Together, these challenges call for improved understanding of the biologic, social, economic, psychological, and environmental factors that influence maternal and infant health outcomes and in the effectiveness of intervention strategies designed to address these causative factors.

Injuries

The impressive gains realized in reducing motor vehicle injuries have uncovered gaps in our understanding of comprehensive prevention. Challenges include expanding surveillance to monitor nonfatal injuries, detect new problems, and set priorities. Greater research into emerging and priority problems, as well as intervention effectiveness, is also needed, as are more effective collaborations and interagency partnerships. Injuries to pedestrians and from vehicles other than automobiles will also challenge public health in the twenty-first century. The effects of age, alcohol use, seat belt use, and interventions targeting these risks will require greater attention for progress to continue in the battle against motor vehicle injuries.

Cardiovascular Disease

An aging population less threatened by infectious disease and injury will place even more people at risk of ill health related to cardiovascular diseases. Greater attention to research to understand the various social, psychological, environmental, physiologic, and genetic determinants of cardiovascular diseases is needed in the new century. Reducing disparities that exist in terms of burden of disease, prevalence of risk factors, and ability to reach high-risk populations represents another mega-challenge. Identifying new and emerging risk factors and their relationships, including genetic and infectious disease factors, will be necessary in both developed and developing parts of the world.

Food Safety

Our understanding of food safety and nutrition made great strides in the 1900s, but both old and new risks will need to be addressed in the new century. Iron and folate deficiencies continue, and many of the advantages related to breastfeeding remain unrealized. The emergence of obesity as an increasingly prevalent condition throughout the population is one of the most startling developments of the late twentieth century. Persistent challenges include applying new information about nutrition, dietary patterns, and behavior that promote health and reduce the risk of chronic diseases.

Oral Health

One of the most overlooked achievements of public health in the twentieth century was the dramatic decline in dental caries due to fluoridation of drinking water supplies. Ironically, these advances in oral health have contributed to the perception that dental caries are no longer a significant public health problem and that fluoridation is no longer needed. These battles are likely to be fought in political, rather than scientific, arenas, presenting a substantial challenge to public health in the twenty-first century.

Workplace Safety

Workplaces are now safer than ever before, yet challenges remain on this front, as well. Improved surveillance of work-related injuries and illnesses and better methods of conducting field investigations in high-risk occupations and industries remain formidable challenges. Applying new methods of risk assessment to improve assessment of injury exposures and intervention outcomes, as well as improved research into intervention effectiveness, surveillance methods, and organization of work represent additional challenges for public health practice in the twenty-first century.

Unfinished Agenda

It is clear that much remains to be done. Healthy People 2010 articulates this unfinished agenda by identifying important targets and leading indicators of health status for the United States.[2] Various chapters of this text identify some of these leading indicators and targets, including tobacco use (Chapter 2), access to care (Chapter 3), physical activity (Chapter 5), and immunizations (Chapter 7). Targets for six other leading indicators have also been established, including substance abuse (Figure 9–3), obesity, sexual behavior, mental health, environmental quality, and injuries/violence (Table 9–1). Many of these represent health problems that are new to the public health agenda. In recent decades, medical care issues, substance abuse, mental health, long-term care, and, today, violence have been categorized as public health problems and have taken their rightful place on the public health agenda. Applying the lessons learned from the recent century of progress in public health to both new and persisting health threats will be necessary to increase the span of healthy life and eliminate the huge disparities in health outcomes that are the overarching goals of the year 2010 national health objectives. The public health challenges of both centuries call for the application of sound science in an environment that supports social justice in health. This remains the most formidable challenge facing public health practice in the twenty-first century.

LIMITATIONS OF TWENTY-FIRST-CENTURY PUBLIC HEALTH

Despite the remarkable achievements of the twentieth century, there is much for public health to do in the early years of the new century. Continued progress is by no means assured due to a new constellation of problems and

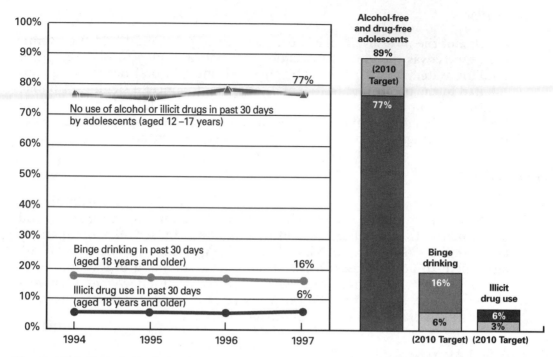

Figure 9–3 Use of Alcohol and/or Illicit Drugs, United States, 1994–1997. *Source:* Reprinted from *Healthy People 2010: Understanding and Improving Health,* U.S. Department of Health and Human Services, Public Health Service, 2000.

Table 9–1 Year-2010 Targets for Selected Health Indicators

Indicator	Reference Year	Reference Level	Year-2010 Target
Overweight or obese children & adolescents	1988–94	11%	5%
Obese adults >20 years of age	1988–94	23%	15%
Motor vehicle death rate (per 100,000)	1997	15.8	9
Homicide death rate (per 100,000)	1995	7.2	3.2
Exposed to ozone above EPA standard	1997	43%	0%
Exposed to environmental tobacco smoke	1988–94	65%	45%
Sexually active unmarried women ages 18–44 who use condoms	1995	23%	50%
Adolescents in grades 9–12 not sexually active or sexually active who use condoms	1997	85%	95%
Adults with depression who receive treatment	1997	23%	50%

Source: Adapted from *Healthy People 2010: Understanding and Improving Health,* U.S. Department of Health and Human Services, Public Health Service, 2000.

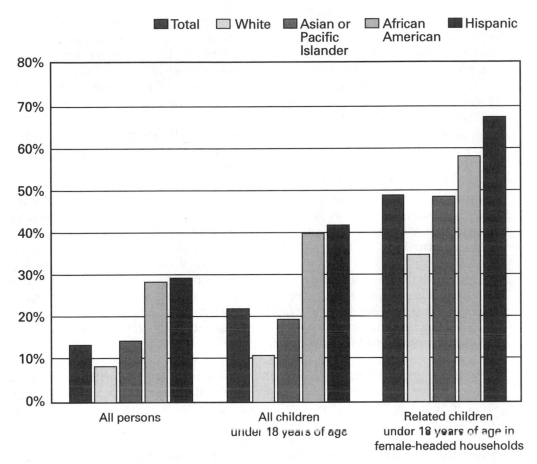

Figure 9–4 Percentage of Persons Below the Poverty Level by Race/Ethnic Group and Type of Household, United States, 1996. *Source:* Reprinted from *Healthy People 2010: Understanding and Improving Health,* U.S. Department of Health and Human Services, Public Health Service, 2000.

important limitations of conventional public health efforts. Global environmental threats, the disruption of vital ecosystems, global population overload, persistent and widening social injustice and health inequalities, and lack of access to effective care add to the list of health problems left over from the twentieth century.[3] Consider, for example, the implications of Figure 9–4, in terms of the link between income and health, and a nation growing more and more diverse, with a disproportionate burden of poverty falling on children, minorities, and one-parent families. Further gains in health status may be less related to science than to social policies. For some public health professionals, the limitations of conventional public health are difficult to accept because, in large part, they represent the supporting pillars of the public health enterprise. This reluctance to critically self-assess makes future progress less certain. It is useful to examine these limitations in terms of their relationship to the two major forces shaping public health responses—science and social values.

Among the limitations affecting the science of public health is an undue emphasis on reductionist thinking that seeks molecular-level explanations for social and structural phenomena. Identification of risk factors has been useful for public health efforts, but the emphasis on individual risk factors often obscures patterns that call for multi-level responses. The persistent identification of the association of social deprivation with many of the important health problems of the last century is a case-in-point. Approaches for reducing coronary heart disease provide another example. Health interventions targeting a reduction in coronary heart disease frequently focus on risk factors at the physiologic level, such as blood pressure control, cholesterol, and obesity and on lifestyle factors at the individual level, including smoking, nutrition, physical activity, and psychosocial factors. However, there are also environmental influences, such as geographic location, housing conditions, occupational risks, and social structure influences, such as social class, age, gender, and race/ethnicity. In this multi-level view of coronary heart disease, interventions that focus on primary and secondary prevention (those addressing the physiologic and individual levels) need to be supplemented by organization and community-level interventions (addressing environmental influences) and healthy public policy (addressing the social structure level).

Another limitation of public health's scientific heritage is the penchant for dichotomous thinking and the failure to view health phenomena as continuous. Using coronary heart disease as an example, dichotomous thinking draws attention to individual and physiologic level factors, whereas viewing this condition as continuous encourages a population-wide view and development of interventions that reduce overall incidence and prevalence by affecting frequency distributions in the entire population. A view of health problems as continuous phenomena suggests that efforts be made throughout the population to move the entire frequency distribution for coronary heart disease "to the left," rather than to reduce disease burden only among those groups most heavily impacted. Here it is apparent that science and social values are not pure and mutually exclusive forces.

Discussion and debate over scientific approaches to public health problems are not, however, purely scientific in nature. At the heart of collective actions are collective values as to whether issues affecting individuals are more important than issues affecting communities of individuals and as to the meaning of health itself. Should public health emphasize the health of individuals or the health of communities? In part, these reflect the different perspectives of health described in Chapters 2 and 3. On one hand is a mechanistic view of health as the absence of disease, promoting health interventions that emphasize curative treatment for afflicted individuals. On the other hand is a more holistic view of health that sees health as a complex equilibrium of forces and factors necessary for optimal functioning of that individual. This latter view emphasizes health maintenance and health promotion, often through broad social policies affecting the entire community. Differences in public health systems among societies are largely described by these differences. Some societies, like the United States, focus on individuals using a largely medical treatment approach. Others are more heavily influenced by collectivism and a holistic view of health. At the core of what can be accomplished, however, are basic values and social philosophies that guide the use of the scientific knowledge available at any point in time.

These differences in social values also affect perceptions as to what is expected of government and, as a result, the form and leadership of public health efforts. To a large extent, these forces have hastened the development of community public health practice in the United States, a phenomenon described in previous chapters.

THE FUTURE OF PUBLIC HEALTH IN 1988 AND 15 YEARS LATER

In many respects, the limitations of modern public health are as apparent as its achievements. Persisting, emerging, reemerging, and newly assigned problems will forever challenge public health as a social enterprise. Success will depend on both the structure and the content of the public health response. A continuous, critical, and comprehensive self-examination of the public health enterprise offers the greatest chance for continued success. A series of such self-examinations began with the 1988 report of Institute of Medicine (IOM), The Future of Public Health.[4] A comprehensive re-examination, The Future of the Public's Health in the 21st Century, was completed in 2002.[5] A complementary study of issues related to educating public health professionals was also completed by the IOM in 2002.[6] These examinations outlined the limitations of public health efforts in the twentieth century, but cast these failings as lessons, challenges, and opportunities for public health in the twenty-first century.

The Future of Public Health, 1988

The IOM's landmark report, completed in 1988, found much of value in the nation's public health efforts, but it also identified a long list of problems. The most serious problem of all was that Americans were taking their public health system for granted. The nation had come to believe that epidemics of communicable diseases were a thing of the past and that food and water would forever be free of infectious and toxic agents. Americans assumed that workplaces, restaurants, and homes were safe and that everyone had access to the information and skills needed to lead healthy lives. They also assumed that all of this could occur even while public health agencies were being increasingly called upon to provide health services to more than 40 million Americans who had no health insurance or were underinsured. However, across the nation, states and localities were failing to provide the resources that would allow both the traditional public health and more recent health service roles to be carried out successfully. When future benefits compete with immediate needs, the results are predictable.

These circumstances fostered the image of a public health system in disarray. Within this system, neither the public nor those involved in the work of public health appreciated the scope and content of public health in modern America. There was little consensus as to the specific responsibilities to be expected from the various levels of government and even less interest in securing such consensus.

Previous chapters document that several formulations in the IOM report have been widely embraced by the public health community. These include statements of the mission, substance, and core functions of public health. The mission has been described simply as assuring conditions in which people can be healthy. The substance consists largely of organized community efforts to promote health and prevent disease. The IOM report identified an essential role for government in public health in organizing and assuring that the mission gets addressed. An expanded view of the fundamental functions of governmental public health was articulated in the three core functions of assessment, policy development, and assurance. These represent a more comprehensive view of public health efforts than that conveyed by earlier views that public health primarily furnished services and enforced statutes. The new public health differed in its emphasis on problem identification and resolution as the basis of rational interventions and on working with and through other stakeholders, rather than intervening unilaterally.

But perhaps the most motivating aspect of the IOM report was its characterization of the disarray of public health and the significance of that disarray. The IOM report painted a picture of disjointed efforts in the 1980s to deal with immediate crises, such as the epidemic of human immunodeficiency virus (HIV) infections and an increasing lack of access to health services; and enduring problems with significant social impacts, such as injuries, teen pregnancy, hypertension, and tobacco and drug use. With impending crises on the horizon in the form of toxic substances, Alzheimer's disease, and public health capacity, the IOM report found the situation to be grimmer still.

The report found a wide gap between the capabilities of the public health system of the 1980s and those of a public health system capable of rising to modern challenges. It charted a course to move ever closer to an optimally functioning system. Several enabling steps were identified:[4]

- improving the statutory base of public health
- strengthening the structural and organizational framework
- improving the capacity for action, including technical, political, management, programmatic, and fiscal competencies of public health professionals
- strengthening linkages between academia and practice

In the end, the report concluded that working through a multitude of society's institutions, rather than through only traditional public health organizations, is the key to improving the public health system. It is also a daunting task, calling for entering into partnerships with sectors such as education, law enforcement, media, faith, corrections, and business, and fostering change through leadership and influence, rather than through command and control. The barriers to effecting these collaborations are the major obstacles to achieving the aspirations outlined in Healthy People 2010's national health objectives. These barriers come in all sizes and shapes and from many different sources. Some are perceived as external barriers; others appear to be more internal.

The IOM report identified important barriers inhibiting effective public health action:[4]

- Lack of consensus on the content of the public health mission
- Inadequate capacity to carry out the essential public health functions of assessment, policy development, and assurance of services
- Disjointed decision making without necessary data and knowledge
- Inequities in the distribution of services and the benefits of public health
- Limits on effective leadership, including poor interaction among the technical and political aspects of decisions, rapid turnover of leaders, and inadequate relationships with the medical profession
- Organizational fragmentation or submersion
- Problems in relationships among the several levels of government
- Inadequate development of necessary knowledge across the full array of public health needs
- Poor public image of public health, inhibiting necessary support
- Special problems that unduly limit the financial resources available to public health

The Future of Public Health, 2003

The IOM advanced these themes through several other reports published in the 1990s and early years of the new century. A brief status report on progress in implementing the 1988 report's major recommendations was completed in the mid-1990s, and a report promoting community health improvement processes (see Chapter 5) appeared later in the decade. A full scale re-examination of the public health enterprise, titled The Future of the Public's Health in the 21st Century, was undertaken after the turn of the century and completed in late 2002. That report focused more extensively on multisectoral partnerships with government than had the 1988 report, which emphasized government's role in achieving public health goals.

The 2002 IOM report (although not published until 2003) restated the unique responsibility that government has for promoting and protecting the health of its people. It noted, however, that four factors argue that government alone should not bear full responsibility for the health of the public:[5]

- Public resources are limited, and public health spending must compete with other valid causes
- Democratic societies expressly limit the powers of government and reserve many activities for private institutions
- Determinants affecting health derive from multiple sources and sectors, including many social determinants that cannot be addressed by government alone
- There is growing evidence that multi-sectoral collaborations are more powerful and effective than government acting alone

In light of these factors, the 2002 IOM report examined both the governmental contributions to the public's health and those from other sectors of

American society. Recommendations for the governmental enterprise were complemented by recommendations for health-care providers, business, media, the faith community, and academia. The report proposed six major areas for action:[5]

- Adopting a population health approach that considers the multiple determinants of health
- Strengthening the governmental public health infrastructure, which forms the backbone of the public health system
- Building a new generation of intersectional partnerships that also draw on the perspectives and resources of diverse communities and actively engages them in health actions
- Developing systems of accountability to assure the quality and availability of public health services
- Making evidence the foundation of decision making and the measure of success
- Enhancing and facilitating communication within the public health system (e.g., among all levels of the governmental public health infrastructure, between public health professionals and community members)

Barriers to Progress

The barriers to future progress are apparent in both IOM reports. Foremost is the lack of an ecological view of health that attempts to understand good and ill health in terms of the multiple factors that interact with each other at the personal, family, community, and population level. Another set of important barriers affecting public health are the prevailing values of the American public—in particular, those restricting the ability of government to identify and address factors that influence health. Social values determine the extent to which government can regulate human behavior, such as through controlling the production and use of tobacco products or requiring bicycle or motorcycle helmet use. These values also determine whether and to what extent family planning or school-based clinic services are provided in a community and determine the content of school health education curricula. Some of these social values find strange bedfellows. For example, many Americans oppose control of firearms on the basis of principles of self-protection embodied in the U.S. Constitution; gun companies also oppose control, although on the basis of more direct economic considerations.

Economic and resource considerations are common themes, as well. One obvious issue is that most public health activities remain funded from the discretionary budgets of local, state, and federal government. At all levels, discretionary programs have been squeezed by true entitlement programs, such as Medicaid and Medicare, as well as by some governmental responsibilities that have become near-entitlements, such as public safety, law enforcement, corrections, and education. Funding one set of health-related services from governmental discretionary funds while other health services are financed through a competitive marketplace widens the imbalance between treatment and prevention as investment strategies for improved health status. There are powerful economic interests among health sector industries, as well as among industries whose products affect health, such as the tobacco, alcohol, pesticide, and firearms industries. One can only dream that equally powerful lobbies might develop for hepatitis or drug-resistant tuberculosis.

All too often, the complex problems and issues of public health, with causes and contributing factors perceived to lie outside its boundaries, lead public health professionals to believe that they should not be held accountable for failure or success. However, many facets of public health practice itself could be further improved. These include relationships with the private sector and medical practice, and some internal reengineering of public health processes. Fear and suspicion of the private sector can lead to many missed opportunities. Just as the three most important factors determining real estate values are location, location, and location, it can be argued that the three most important factors for health are jobs, jobs, and jobs. If this is anywhere near true, suspicions of the private sector need to be put to rest. There is little question that employment is a powerful preventive health intervention, in terms of both individual and community health status. Community development activities that bring new businesses and jobs to a community can affect health status more positively than a public health clinic on every corner. Further, businesses have been major forces behind the growth of managed care systems in the United States. Their partnership with public health interests will be essential to secure new resources or to shift the balance between treatment and prevention strategies. Increased partnerships with medical care interests will also be necessary. Unfortunately, there is widespread ignorance of the medical care sector among public health workers.

Among barriers internal to public health agencies is one that often goes unnoticed—the widespread use of categorical approaches to program management, which often fragments and isolates individual programs, one from another. In addition to the unnecessary proliferation of information, management, and other administrative processes, each program tends to develop its own assortment of interest and constituency groups, including those involving program staff members, who often work to oppose meaningful consolidation and integration of programs.

Another limiting factor is the generalized inability to prioritize and focus public health efforts, despite the wealth of information as to which factors most affect health at the national, state, or even local levels. Time and time again, tobacco, alcohol, diet, and violence have been shown to lie at the root of most preventable mortality and years of potential life lost. Ideally, resource allocation decisions would be made on the basis of the most important attributable risks, rather than being spread around to address, ineffectively, risks both large and small. With scores of priorities, there are really none, and without clear priorities, accountability is seldom expected. Public health has always operated at the confluence of science and politics; political issues and compromises are natural. Still, inconsistencies between stated public health priorities and actual program priorities, as demonstrated through funding, are themselves barriers to public understanding and support for public health work.

Other factors that influence public understanding and support for public health relate to the transition from conditions caused by microorganisms to those caused by human behaviors. It is more difficult for the public to appreciate the scientific basis for public health interventions when social, rather than physical sciences, guide strategies. This occurs at a time when government is increasingly portrayed as both incompetent and overly intrusive. Largely because governmental processes are considered by the public to be intensely political, the public view of public health processes, including programs and regulations, is that of highly politicized and partly scientific exercises.

There has been considerable debate as to whether the 1988 IOM report accurately captured the problems and needs of the American public health system. In many respects, the report restated the fundamental values and concepts underlying public health in terms of its emphasis on prevention, professional diversity, collaborative nature, community problem solving, loosely attached constituencies, assurance functions, need to draw other sectors into the solution of public health problems, and lack of an identifiable constituency. Taken together, these features appear to represent disarray. However, the cause of this disarray may not lie with public health but rather with our social and governmental institutions, more generally. Posing solutions that restructure the system's components may do little more than rearranging the deck chairs on the Titanic.

It may be necessary to more broadly restructure the tasks and functions of public health to deal with modern public health problems. The larger work of public health is to get the prevention job done right, rather than to get it done through a traditional structuring of roles and responsibilities. Preventing disease and promoting health must be embraced throughout society and its health institutions, rather than existing in a parallel subsystem. There is no evidence to support the contention that public health activities are best organized through public health agencies of government. It is the mission and the effort that are important and not necessarily the organization from which those efforts are generated.

CONCLUSION: THE NEED FOR A MORE EFFECTIVE PUBLIC HEALTH SYSTEM

The perpetual frustration for public health is the gap between what has been achieved and what could have been achieved. The unfulfilled promise of public health should not be viewed as some unfortunate accident but as a direct result of a series of past decisions and actions undertaken quite purposefully. Sadly, they reflect both a history of disregard and the consequences of battles over the legitimacy, scope, professional authority, and political reach of public health.[7] A recent example is the use of tobacco settlement funds.

The various settlements in 1998 with a group of the major tobacco companies will provide $250 billion to the states over a 25-year period. These settlements were initially viewed as a colossal success for public health over one of its most important enemies. Although still in the early years of this possible quarter-century windfall, state legislative and executive branch leaders have opted to use these funds for a variety of purposes, some for health purposes but much for other ends. It was expected that approaches would vary from state-to-state, with most using some portion of the money to support tobacco cessation and prevention interventions. But early indications are that as little as one-third of the settlement funds were earmarked for health programs through 2002, and that the health share declined rapidly in the face of state budget deficits after 2002.

The tobacco company settlement can be viewed as a success story or as part of a full accounting of the massive failure of public health efforts in the battle against tobacco use. Why did it take three decades to change public perceptions and values to the point that settlement became inevitable? Without attention to the lessons of this saga and to strengthening the public health system, tobacco will be the first of many health hazards that are inadequately addressed and for which a negotiated settlement will eventually occur. If we look at the tobacco settlement as a signal of the failure of public health and evidence of a weak public health infrastructure, this windfall becomes, at best, a bittersweet victory. Perhaps the tobacco settlement windfall would best be directed toward averting the next tobacco-like settlement. Difficult questions arise, even in otherwise good times!

In any event, the settlement offered the possibility of a sustained increase in public health resources to the tune of about $10 billion annually for 25 years. Considering that only about $17 billion was expended for governmental public health activities in 2000, the tobacco funds represented a possible 70 percent increase. Additional funding to governmental public health agencies for bioterrorism preparedness on top of the tobacco settlement funds provided for a possible doubling of governmental public health activities in the early years of the twenty-first century. As we have seen, however, this was an illusion that never materialized.

These circumstances and other key issues and challenges facing the future of public health defy simple summarization. This chapter has examined several, including those offered by the achievements and limitations of public health practice in the twentieth century and others offered by the IOM reports; earlier chapters presented many more. Which of these are most important remains a point of contention. It would be useful to have an official list that represents the consensus of policy makers and the public alike. However, because an official list is lacking, several general conclusions as to the critical challenges and obstacles facing the future of public health in the United States are presented. They summarize some of the important themes of this text in describing why we need more effective public health efforts.

The Easy Problems Have Already Been Solved

Major successes have been achieved through public health efforts over the past 150 years, largely related to massive reductions in infectious diseases but also involving substantial declines in death rates for injuries and several major chronic diseases since about 1960. The list of current problems for public health includes the more difficult chronic diseases, new and emerging conditions, including bioterrorism, and broader social problems with health effects (teen pregnancy and violence are good examples) that have identifiable risk and contributing factors that can be addressed only through collective action. The days of command-and-control approaches to relatively simple infectious risks are behind us. In the past, environmental sanitation and engineering could collaborate with communicable disease control expertise to address important public health problems. The collaborations needed for violence prevention or bioterrorism preparedness require very different skills and relationships.

To a Hammer, the Entire World Looks Like a Nail

Behind this aphorism is the perception that common education and work experiences foster common professional perspectives. The danger lies in believing that one's own professional tools are adequate to the task of dealing with all of the problems and needs that are served by the profession. Each profession has its own scientific base and jargon. Problems are given labels or diagnoses, using the profession's specialized language, so that the tools of the profession can be brought to bear on those problems. All too often, however, the problems come to be considered as the domain of that profession, and the potential contributions of other professions and disciplines are underappreciated. Although public health professionals are remarkably diverse in terms of their educational and experiential backgrounds, we can also fall into this trap. When we do, bridges to other partners are not built, and collaborations do not take place. As a result, problems that can be addressed only through collaborative inter-sectoral approaches flourish unabated.

A Friend in Need Is a Friend Indeed

Finding means to build such bridges can be difficult, but some key collaborations appear to be absolutely essential for the work of public health to succeed. Certainly, links between public health and medical care must be improved for both to prosper in a reforming health system. Links with businesses also represent another avenue for mutually successful collaborations. The key is to find major areas of common purpose. For medical care interests, the common denominator is that prevention saves money and rewards those who use it as an investment strategy. For business interests, the bottom line has to be improved, and businesses must accept the premise that improving health status in the community serves their bottom lines through healthier, more productive workers and healthier and wealthier consumers.

You Get What You Pay For

There is good cause to question the current national investment strategy as it relates to health. The excess capacity that has been established in the American health system is becoming increasingly unaffordable, and the results are nothing to write home about. Still, the competition for additional dollars is intense among the major interests that dominate the health industry, and there is little movement to alter the current balance between treatment and prevention strategies. With less than 5 percent of all health expenditures supporting public health's core functions and essential services and only about one percent supporting population-based prevention, even small shifts could reap substantial rewards. The argument that resources are limited and that there simply are not adequate resources to meet treatment, as well as prevention purposes, is uniquely American and quite inimical to the public's health. More disconcerting yet are the lost opportunities in securing and utilizing recent tobacco settlement and bioterrorism preparedness funding to shore up a sagging public health infrastructure.

It's Not My Job?

The job description of public health has never been clear. As a result, public health has become quite proficient in delivering specific services, with less attention paid to mobilizing action toward those factors that most seriously affect community health status. Among traditional health-related factors, tobacco, alcohol, and diet are factors responsible for much of modern America's mortality and morbidity. Nonetheless, the resources supporting interventions directed toward these factors are minuscule. Similarly, the primary cause of America's relatively poor health outcomes, in comparison with other developed nations, as well as the most likely source for further health gains in the United States, resides in the huge and increasing gaps between racial and ethnic groups. The public health system, from national to state and local levels, must recognize these circumstances and move beyond them to advocate and build constituencies aggressively for efforts that target the most important of the traditional health risk factors and that promote social policies that will both minimize and equalize risks throughout the population. The task is as simple as following the Golden Rule and doing for others what we want done for ourselves because efforts to improve the health of others make everyone healthier. This does not constitute a new job description for public health in the United States, but rather a recommitment to an old, successful, and necessary one.

DISCUSSION QUESTIONS AND EXERCISES

1. What was the most important achievement of public health in the twentieth century? Why?
2. What will be the most important achievement of public health in the twenty-first century? Why?
3. If randomized clinical trials are considered the gold standard of research, why is there not more emphasis on this approach in assessing community-based interventions?
4. Using a scale from 1 to 10, how effective is the public health system in the United States? How did you arrive at this rating?
5. Do you agree with the IOM assertion that public health is in disarray or with the counter-assertion that it is government, not public health, that is in disarray?
6. What impact did The Future of Public Health have on the public health community during the 1990s?
7. What impact has The Future of the Public's Health in the 21st Century had on the public health community since 2003?

8. What do you think are the most important new or expanded roles for public health in the twenty-first century?
9. Your state has $100 million from tobacco settlement funds. What strategies and programs should receive funding? Why?
10. How has your understanding of what public health is and how it works changed after examining the topics in this book?

REFERENCES

1. Centers for Disease Control and Prevention (CDC). *Addressing Emerging Infectious Disease Threats: A Prevention Strategy for the United States.* Atlanta, GA: U.S. Public Health Service (PHS); 1994.

2. U.S. Department of Health and Human Services (DHHS). Healthy People 2010: Understanding and Improving Health. Washington, DC: DHHS-PHS; 2000.

3. McKinlay JB, Marceau LD. To boldly go . . . *Am J Public Health.* 2000;90:25–33.

4. Institute of Medicine. *The Future of Public Health.* Washington, DC: National Academy Press; 1988.

5. Institute of Medicine. *The Future of the Public's Health in the 21st Century.* Washington, DC: National Academy Press, 2003.

6. Institute of Medicine. *Who Will Keep the Public Healthy? Educating Public Health Professionals for the 21st* Century. Washington, DC: National Academy Press, 2003.

7. Fee E and Brown TM. The Unfulfilled Promise of Public Health: Déjà vu All Over Again. *Health Affairs* 2002;21(6):31–43.

Glossary

ACCESS

The potential for or actual entry of a population into the health system. Entry is dependent on the wants, resources, and needs that individuals bring to the care-seeking process. Ability to obtain wanted or needed services may be influenced by many factors, including travel distance, waiting time, available financial resources, and availability of a regular source of care.

ACTIVITIES

Specific tasks that must be completed for a program's processes to achieve their targets.

ACTIVITY MEASURES

Indicators of whether a program's activities are successfully completed.

ACTUAL CAUSE OF DEATH

A primary determinant or risk factor associated with a pathologic or diagnosed cause of death. For example, tobacco use would be the actual cause for deaths from many lung cancers.

ADJUSTED RATE

The adjustment or standardization of rates is a statistical procedure that removes the effect of differences in the composition of populations. Because of its marked effect on mortality and morbidity, age is the variable for adjustment used most commonly. For example, an age-adjusted death rate for any cause permits a better comparison between different populations and at different times because it accounts for differences in the distribution of age.

ADMINISTRATIVE LAW

Rules and regulations promulgated by administrative agencies within the executive branch of government that carry the force of law. Administrative law represents a unique situation in which legislative, executive, and judicial powers are carried out by one agency in the development, implementation, and enforcement of rules and regulations.

AGE-ADJUSTED MORTALITY RATE

The expected number of deaths that would occur if a population had the same age distribution as a standard population, expressed in terms of deaths per 1,000 or 100,000 persons.

APPROPRIATENESS

Health interventions for which the expected health benefit exceeds the expected negative consequences by a wide enough margin to justify the intervention.

ASSESSMENT

One of public health's three core functions. Assessment calls for regularly and systematically collecting, analyzing, and making available information on the health of a community, including statistics on health status, community health needs, and epidemiologic and other studies of health problems.

ASSESSMENT PROTOCOL FOR EXCELLENCE IN PUBLIC HEALTH (APEXPH)/MOBILIZING FOR ACTION THROUGH PLANNING AND PARTNERSHIPS (MAPP)

See Mobilizing for Action through Planning and Partnerships (MAPP)

ASSETS

Resources available to achieve a specific end, such as community resources that can contribute to community health improvement efforts or emergency response resources, including human, to respond to a public health emergency.

ASSOCIATION

The relationship between two or more events or variables. Events are said to be associated when they occur more frequently together than one would expect by chance. Association does not necessarily imply a causal relationship.

ASSURANCE

One of public health's three core functions. It involves assuring constituents that services necessary to achieve agreed-upon goals are provided by encouraging actions on the part of others, by requiring action through regulation, or by providing services directly.

ATTRIBUTABLE RISK

The theoretical reduction in the rate or number of cases of an adverse outcome that can be achieved by elimination of a risk factor. For example, if tobacco use is responsible for 75 percent of all lung cancers, the elimination of tobacco use will reduce lung cancer mortality rates by 75 percent in a population over time.

BEHAVIORAL RISK FACTORS SURVEILLANCE SYSTEM

A national data collection system funded by the Centers for Disease Control and Prevention (CDC) to assess the prevalence of behaviors that affect health status. Through individual state efforts, CDC staff coordinate the collection, analysis, and distribution of survey data on seat belt use, hypertension, physical activity, smoking, weight control, alcohol use, mammography screening, cervical cancer screening, and AIDS, as well as other health-related information.

BIOTERRORISM

The threatened or intentional release of biological agents (viruses, bacteria, or their toxins) for the purpose of influencing the conduct of government or intimidating or coercing a civilian population to further political or social objectives. These agents can be released by way of the air (as aerosols) food, water, or insects.

CAPACITY

The capability to carry out the core functions of public health. (Also see Infrastructure.)

CAPITATION

A method of payment for health services in which a provider is paid a fixed amount for each person served, without regard to the actual number or nature of services provided to each person in a set period of time. Capitation is the characteristic payment method in health maintenance organizations.

CASE DEFINITION

Standardized criteria for determining whether a person has a particular disease or health-related condition. Criteria often include clinical and laboratory findings, as well personal characteristics (age, sex, location, time period, etc.) Case definitions are often used in investigations and for comparing potential cases.

CASE MANAGEMENT

The monitoring and coordinating of services rendered to individuals with specific problems or who require high-cost or extensive services.

CASUALTY

Any person suffering physical and/or psychological damage that leads to death, injury, or material loss.

CAUSALITY

The relationship of causes to the effects they produce; several types of causes can be distinguished. A cause is termed necessary when a particular variable must always precede an effect. This effect need not be the sole result of the one variable. A cause is termed sufficient when a particular variable inevitably initiates or produces an effect. Any given cause may be necessary, sufficient, neither, or both.

CAUSE OF DEATH

For the purpose of national mortality statistics, every death is attributed to one underlying condition, based on the information reported on the death certificate and utilizing the international rules for selecting the underlying cause of death from the reported conditions.

CENTERS FOR DISEASE CONTROL AND PREVENTION (CDC)

The Centers for Disease Control and Prevention, based in Atlanta, Georgia, is the federal agency charged with protecting the nation's public health by providing direction in the prevention and control of communicable and other diseases and responding to public health emergencies. CDC's responsibilities as the nation's prevention agency have expanded over the years and will continue to evolve as the agency addresses contemporary threats to health, such as injury, environmental and occupational hazards, behavioral risks, and chronic diseases; and emerging communicable diseases, such as the Ebola virus.

CERTIFICATION

A process by which an agency or association grants recognition to another party who has met certain predetermined qualifications specified by the agency or association.

CHRONIC DISEASE

A disease that has one or more of the following characteristics: it is permanent, leaves residual disability, is caused by a nonreversible pathologic alteration, requires special training of the patient for rehabilitation, or may be expected to require a long period of supervision, observation, or care.

CLINICAL PRACTICE GUIDELINES

Systematically developed statements that assist practitioner and patient decisions about appropriate health services for specific clinical conditions.

CLINICAL PREVENTIVE SERVICES

Clinical services provided to patients to reduce or prevent disease, injury, or disability. These are preventive measures (including screening tests, immunizations, counseling, and periodic physical examinations) provided by a health professional to an individual patient.

COMMUNITY

A group of people who have common characteristics; communities can be defined by location, race, ethnicity, age, occupation, interest in particular problems or outcomes, or other common bonds. Ideally, there should be available assets and resources, as well as collective discussion, decision making, and action.

COMMUNITY HEALTH IMPROVEMENT PROCESS

A systematic effort that assesses community needs and assets, prioritizes health-related problems and issues, analyzes problems for their causative factors, develops evidence-based intervention strategies based on those analyses, links stakeholders to implementation efforts through performance monitoring, and evaluates the effect of interventions in the community.

COMMUNITY HEALTH NEEDS ASSESSMENT

A formal approach to identifying health needs and health problems in the community. A variety of tools or instruments may be used; the essential ingredient is community engagement and collaborative participation.

COMMUNITY PREVENTIVE SERVICES

Population-based interventions to reduce or prevent disease, injury, or disability. These are preventive interventions targeting the entire population, rather than individuals.

COMPREHENSIVE EMERGENCY MANAGEMENT

A broad style of emergency management, encompassing prevention, preparedness, response, and recovery.

CONDITION

A health condition is a departure from a state of physical or mental well-being. An impairment is a health condition that includes chronic or permanent health defects resulting from disease, injury, or congenital malformations. All health conditions except impairments are coded according to an international classification system. Based on duration, there are two types of conditions—acute and chronic.

CONSEQUENCE MANAGEMENT

An emergency management function includes measures to protect public health and safety, restore essential government services, and provide emergency relief to governments in the event of terrorism.

CONTAMINATION

An accidental release of hazardous chemicals or nuclear materials that pollute the environment and place humans at risk.

CONTRIBUTING FACTOR

A risk factor (causative factor) that is associated with the level of a determinant. Direct contributing factors are linked with the level of determinants; indirect contributing factors are linked with the level of direct contributing factors.

CORE FUNCTIONS

Three basic roles for public health for assuring conditions in which people can be healthy. As identified in the Institute of Medicine's landmark report, The Future of Public Health; these are assessment, policy development, and assurance.

COST-BENEFIT ANALYSIS

An economic analysis in which all costs and benefits are converted into monetary (dollar) values, and results are expressed as dollars of benefit per dollars expended.

COST-EFFECTIVENESS ANALYSIS

An economic analysis assessed as a health outcome per cost expended.

COST-UTILITY ANALYSIS

An economic analysis assessed as a quality-adjusted outcome per net cost expended.

COVERT RELEASES

For biologic agents, an unannounced release of a biologic agent that causes illness or other effects. If undetected, a covert release has the potential to spread widely before it is detected.

CRISIS MANAGEMENT

Administrative measures that identify, acquire, and plan the use of resources needed to anticipate, prevent, and/or resolve a threat to public safety (such as terrorism).

CRUDE MORTALITY RATE

The total number of deaths per unit of population reported during a given time interval, often expressed as the number of deaths per 1,000 or 100,000 persons.

CULTURAL COMPETENCE

The ability to communicate with and provide services to an individual or a group with full respect for the culturally associated values, preferences, language, and experiences of the group.

DECISION ANALYSIS

An analytic technique in which probability theory is used to obtain a quantitative approach to decision making.

DECONTAMINATION

The removal of hazardous chemicals or nuclear substances from the skin and/or mucous membranes by showering or washing the affected area with water or by rinsing with a sterile solution.

DEMOGRAPHICS

Characteristic data, such as size, growth, density, distribution, and vital statistics, which are used to study human populations.

DEMONSTRATION SETTINGS

A population- or clinic-based environment in which prevention strategies are field-tested.

DETERMINANT

A primary risk factor (causative factor) associated with the level of health problem, i.e., the level of the determinant influences the level of the health problem.

DISABILITY LIMITATION

An intervention strategy that seeks to arrest or eradicate disease and/or limit disability and prevent death.

DISASTER

Any event, typically occurring suddenly, that causes damage, ecological disruption, loss of human life, or deterioration of health and health services and which exceeds the capacity of the affected community on a scale sufficient to require outside assistance.

DISASTER SEVERITY SCALE

A scale that classifies disasters by the following parameters: the radius of the disaster site, the number of dead, the number of wounded, the average severity of the injuries sustained, the impact time, and the rescue time. By attributing a numeric score to each of the variables from 0 to 2, with 0 being the least severe and 2 the most severe, a scale with a range of 0 to 18 can be created.

DISCOUNTING

A method for adjusting the value of future costs and benefits. Expressed as a present dollar value, discounting is based on the time value of money (i.e., a dollar today is worth more than it will be a year from now, even if inflation is not considered).

DISTRIBUTIONAL EFFECTS

The manner in which the costs and benefits of a strategy affect different groups of people in terms of demographics, geographic location, and other descriptive factors.

EARLY CASE FINDING AND TREATMENT

An intervention strategy that seeks to identify disease or illness at an early stage so that prompt treatment will reduce the effects of the process.

EFFECTIVENESS

The improvement in health outcome that a strategy can produce in typical community-based settings. Also, the degree to which objectives are achieved.

EFFICACY

The improvement in health outcome effect that a strategy can produce in expert hands under ideal circumstances.

EMERGENCY

Any natural or manmade situation that results in severe injury, harm, or loss to humans or property.

EMERGENCY MANAGEMENT AGENCY

The agency, under the authority of the governor's office, coordinates the efforts of the state's health department, housing and social service agencies, and public safety agencies (such as state police) during an emergency or disaster. The emergency management agency also coordinates federal resources made available to the states, such as the National Guard, Centers for Disease Control and Prevention, and the Public Health Service.

EMERGENCY MEDICAL SERVICES (EMS) SYSTEM

The coordination of the pre-hospital system (including public access, 911 dispatch, paramedics, and ambulance services) and the in-hospital system (including emergency departments, hospitals, and other definitive care facilities and personnel) to provide emergency medical care.

EMERGENCY OPERATIONS CENTER (EOC)

The site from which civil governmental officials (such as municipal, county, state, or federal) direct emergency operations in a disaster.

EPIDEMIC

The occurrence of a disease or condition at higher than normal levels in a population.

EPIDEMIOLOGY

The study of the distribution of determinants and antecedents of health and disease in human populations; the ultimate goal is to identify the underlying causes of a disease, then apply findings to disease prevention and health promotion.

ESCHERICHIA COLI (*E. COLI*) O57:H7

A bacterial pathogen that can infect humans and cause severe bloody diarrhea (hemorrhagic colitis) and serious renal disease (hemolytic uremic syndrome).

ESSENTIAL PUBLIC HEALTH SERVICES

A formulation of the processes used in public health to prevent epidemics and injuries, protect against environmental hazards, promote healthy behaviors, respond to disasters, and ensure quality and accessibility of health services. Ten essential services have been identified:

1. monitoring health status to identify community health problems
2. diagnosing and investigating health problems and health hazards in the community
3. informing, educating, and empowering people about health issues
4. mobilizing community partnerships to identify and solve health problems
5. developing policies and plans that support individual and community health efforts
6. enforcing laws and regulations that protect health and ensure safety
7. linking people to needed personal health services and ensuring the provision of health care when otherwise unavailable
8. ensuring a competent public health and personal health care work force
9. evaluating effectiveness, accessibility, and quality of personal and population-based health services
10. conducting research for new insights and innovative solutions to health problems

EVACUATION

The organized removal of civilians from a dangerous or potentially dangerous area.

FEDERAL RESPONSE PLAN

The plan that coordinates federal resources in disaster and emergency situations in order to address the consequences when there is need for federal assistance under the authorities of the Stafford Disaster Relief and Emergency Assistance Act.

FEDERALLY FUNDED COMMUNITY HEALTH CENTER

An ambulatory health care program (defined under Section 330 of the Public Health Service Act), usually serving a catchment area that has scarce or nonexistent health services or a population with special health needs; sometimes known as a neighborhood health center. Community health centers attempt to coordinate federal, state, and local resources in a single organization capable of delivering both health and related social services to a defined population. Although such a center may not directly provide all types of health care, it usually takes responsibility to arrange all medical services for its patient population.

FIELD MODEL

A framework for identifying factors that influence health status in populations. Initially, four fields were identified: biology, lifestyle, environment, and health services. Extensions of this approach have also identified genetic, social, and cultural factors and have related these factors to a variety of outcomes, including disease, normal functioning, well-being, and prosperity.

FOODBORNE ILLNESS

Illness caused by the transfer of disease organisms or toxins from food to humans.

GENERAL WELFARE PROVISIONS

Specific language in the Constitution of the United States that empowers the federal government to provide for the general welfare of the population. Over time, these provisions have been used as a basis for federal health policies and programs.

GOALS

For public health programs, goals are general statements expressing a program's aspirations or intended effect on one or more health problems, often stated without time limits.

GOVERNMENTAL PRESENCE AT THE LOCAL LEVEL

A concept that calls for the assurance that necessary services and minimum standards are provided to address priority community health problems; this responsibility ultimately falls to local government, which may utilize local public health agencies or other means for its execution.

HARM REDUCTION

Harm reduction represents a set of practical strategies reflecting individual and community needs that meet individuals with risk behaviors where they are to help them reduce any harms associated with their risk behaviors.

HAZARD

A possible source of harm or injury.

HEALTH

The state of complete physical, mental, and social well-being and not merely the absence of disease or infirmity. It is recognized, however, that health has many dimensions (anatomic, physiologic, and mental) and is largely cultur ally defined The relative importance of various disabilities will differ, depending on the cultural milieu and on the role of the affected individual in that culture. Most attempts at measurement have been assessed in terms of morbidity and mortality.

HEALTH CARE FINANCE ADMINISTRATION

The government agency within the U.S. Department of Health and Human Services that directs the Medicare and Medicaid programs (Titles XVIII and XIX of the Social Security Act) and conducts the research to support those programs.

HEALTH DISPARITY

Difference in health status between two groups, such as the health disparity in mortality between men and women, or the health disparity in infant mortality between African-American and white infants.

HEALTH EDUCATION

Any combination of learning opportunities designed to facilitate voluntary adaptations of behavior (in individuals, groups, or communities) conducive to good health. Health education encourages positive health behavior.

HEALTH MAINTENANCE ORGANIZATIONS

Entities that manage both the financing and provision of health services to enrolled members; fees are generally based on capitation, and health providers are managed to reduce costs through controls on utilization of covered services.

HEALTH PLANNING

Planning concerned with improving health, whether undertaken comprehensively for an entire community or for a particular population, type of health services, institution, or health program. The components of health planning include data assembly and analysis, goal determination, action recommendation, and implementation strategy.

HEALTH POLICY

Social policy concerned with the process whereby public health agencies evaluate and determine health needs and the best ways to address them, including the identification of appropriate resources and funding mechanisms.

HEALTH PROBLEM

A situation or condition of people (expressed in health outcome measures such as mortality, morbidity, or disability) that is considered undesirable and is likely to exist in the future.

HEALTH PROBLEM ANALYSIS

A framework for analyzing health problems to identify their determinants and contributing factors so that interventions can be targeted rationally toward those factors most likely to reduce the level of the health problem.

HEALTH PROMOTION

An intervention strategy that seeks to eliminate or reduce exposures to harmful factors by modifying human behaviors. Any combination of health education and related organizational, political, and economic interventions designed to facilitate behavioral and environmental adaptations that will improve or protect health. This process enables individuals and communities to control and improve their own health. Health promotion approaches provide opportunities for people to identify problems, develop solutions, and work in partnerships that build on existing skills and strengths.

HEALTH PROTECTION

An intervention strategy that seeks to provide individuals with resistance to harmful factors, often by modifying the environment to decrease potentially harmful interactions. Those population-based services and programs control and reduce the exposure of the population to environmental or personal hazards, conditions, or factors that may cause disease, disability, injury, or death. Health protection also includes programs that ensure that public health services are available on a 24-hour basis to respond to public health emergencies and coordinate responses of local, state, and federal organizations.

HEALTH REGULATION

Monitoring and maintaining the quality of public health services through licensing and discipline of health professionals, licensing of health facilities, and enforcement of standards and regulations.

HEALTH STATUS INDICATORS

Measurements of the state of health of a specified individual, group, or population. Health status may be measured by proxies such as people's subjective assessments of their health; by one or more indicators of mortality and morbidity in the population, such as longevity or maternal and infant mortality;

or by the incidence or prevalence of major diseases (communicable, chronic, or nutritional). Conceptually, health status is the proper outcome measure for the effectiveness of a specific population's health system, although attempts to relate effects of available medical care to variations in health status have proved difficult.

HEALTH SYSTEM

As used in this text, the health system is the sum total of the strategies designed to prevent or treat disease, injury, and other health problems. The health system includes population-based preventive services, clinical preventive and other primary medical care services, and all levels of more sophisticated treatment and chronic care services.

HEALTHY COMMUNITIES 2010

A framework for developing and tailoring community health objectives so that these can be tracked as part of the initiative to achieve the year 2010 national health objectives included in Healthy People 2010.

HEALTHY PEOPLE 2010

The national disease prevention and health promotion agenda that includes 476 national health objectives to be achieved by the year 2010, addressing improved health status, risk reduction, and utilization of preventive health services.

IMPACT OBJECTIVE

The level of a determinant to be achieved through the processes and activities of an intervention strategy. Impact objectives are generally intermediate in term (2–5 years) and must be measurable and realistic.

INCIDENCE

A measure of the disease or injury in the population, generally the number of new cases occurring during a specified time period.

INCIDENT COMMAND SYSTEM (ICS)

The model for command, control, and coordination of a response to an emergency providing the means to coordinate the efforts of multiple agencies and organizations.

INDICATOR

A measure of health status or a health outcome.

INFANT MORTALITY RATE

The number of live-born infants who die before their first birthday per 1,000 live births; often broken into two components, neonatal mortality (deaths before 28 days per 1,000 live births) and postneonatal mortality (deaths from 28 days through the rest of the first year of life per 1,000 live births).

INFECTIOUS DISEASE

A disease caused by the entrance into the body of organisms (such as bacteria, protozoans, fungi, or viruses) that then grow and multiply there; often used synonymously with communicable disease.

INFRASTRUCTURE

The systems, competencies, relationships, and resources that enable performance of public health's core functions and essential services in every community. Categories include human, organizational, informational, and fiscal resources.

INPUTS

Sometimes referred to as capacities; human resources, fiscal and physical resources, information resources, and system organizational resources necessary to carry out the core functions of public health.

INTERVENTION

A generic term used in public health to describe a program or policy designed to have an impact on a health problem. For example, a mandatory seat belt law is an intervention designed to reduce the incidence of automobile-related fatalities. Five categories of heath interventions are: (1) health promotion, (2) specific protection, (3) early case finding and prompt treatment, (4) disability limitation, and (5) rehabilitation.

LEADING CAUSES OF DEATH

Those diagnostic classifications of disease that are most frequently responsible for deaths; often used in conjunction with the top 10 causes of death.

LEADING HEALTH INDICATORS

A panel of health-related measures that reflect the major public health concerns in the United States; they were selected to track progress toward achievement of Healthy People 2010 goals and objectives. They address 10 public health concerns: physical activity, overweight and obesity, tobacco use, substance abuse, responsible sexual behavior, mental health, injury and violence, environmental quality, immunizations, and access to health care.

LIFE EXPECTANCY

The number of additional years of life expected at a specified point in time, such as at birth or at age 45.

LOCAL HEALTH JURISDICTION (LHJ)

A unit of local government (county, multi-county, municipal, town, other), often with oversight and direction from a local board of health and with an identifiable local health department, that carries out public health's core functions throughout a defined geographic area.

LOCAL PUBLIC HEALTH AGENCY (LPHA)

Functionally, a local (county, multi-county, municipal, town, other) health agency, operated by local government, often with oversight and direction from a local board of health, that carries out public health's core functions throughout a defined geographic area. A more traditional definition is an agency serving less than an entire state that carries some responsibility for health and has at least one full-time employee and a specific budget.

LOCAL PUBLIC HEALTH AUTHORITY

The agency charged with responsibility for meeting the health needs of the community. Usually this is the policy/governing body and its administrative arm, the local health department. The authority may rest with the policy/ governing body, may be a city/county/regional authority, or may consist of a legislative mandate from the state. Some local public health authorities have independence from all other governmental entities, whereas others do not.

LOCAL PUBLIC HEALTH SYSTEM

The collection of public and private organizations having a stake in and contributing to public health at the local level; it involves far more than the local public health agency.

MANAGED CARE

A system of administrative controls intended to reduce costs through managing the utilization of services. Managed care can also mean an integrated system of health insurance, financing, and service delivery that focuses on the appropriate and cost-effective use of health services delivered through defined networks of providers and with allocation of financial risk.

MEASURE

An indicator of health status or a health outcome, used synonymously with *indicator* in this text.

MEDICAID

A federally aided, state-operated and administered program that provides basic medical services to eligible low-income populations; established through amendments as Title XIX of the Social Security Act in 1965. It does not cover all of the poor, however, but only persons who meet specified eligibility criteria. Subject to broad federal guidelines, states determine the benefits covered, program eligibility, rates of payment for providers, and methods of administering the program.

MEDICAL RESERVE CORPS

Locally-based teams of health professionals and other personnel who provide surge capacity for emergencies.

MEDICARE

A national health insurance program for elderly persons established through amendments to the Social Security Act in 1965 that were included in Title XVIII of that act.

META-ANALYSIS

A systematic, quantitative method for combining information from multiple studies to derive the most meaningful answer to a specific question. Assessment of different methods or outcome measures can increase power and account for bias and other effects.

MIDLEVEL PRACTITIONERS

Non-physician health care providers, such as nurse practitioners and physician assistants.

MISSION

For public health, assuring conditions in which people can be healthy.

MITIGATION

Measures taken to reduce the harmful effects of a disaster or emergency by attempting to limit the impact on human health and economic infrastructure.

MOBILIZING FOR ACTION THROUGH PLANNING AND PARTNERSHIPS (MAPP)/ASSESSMENT PROTOCOL FOR EXCELLENCE IN PUBLIC HEALTH (APEXPH)

A voluntary process for organizational and community self-assessment, planned improvements, and continuing evaluation and reassessment. The process focuses on community-wide public health practice, including a health department's role in its community and the community's actual and perceived problems. It provides for a community health improvement process to assess health needs, sets priorities, develops policy, and ensures that health needs are met.

MORBIDITY

A measure of disease incidence or prevalence in a given population, location, or other grouping of interest.

MORTALITY

Expresses the number of deaths in a population within a prescribed time. Mortality rates may be expressed as crude death rates (total deaths in relation to total population during a year) or as death rates specific for diseases and sometimes for age, sex, or other attributes (e.g., the number of deaths from cancer in white males in relation to the white male population during a given year).

NATIONAL HEALTH EXPENDITURES

The amount spent for all health services and supplies and health-related research and construction activities in the United States during the calendar year.

OBJECTIVES

Targets for achievement through interventions. Objectives are time-limited and measurable in all cases. Various levels of objectives for an intervention include outcome, impact, and process objectives.

OUTCOME OBJECTIVE

The level to which a health problem is to be reduced as a result of an intervention. Outcome objectives are often long-term (2–5 years), measurable, and realistic.

OUTCOMES

Sometimes referred to as results of the health system; these are indicators of health status, risk reduction, and quality-of-life enhancement. Outcomes are long-term objectives that define optimal, measurable future levels of health status; maximum acceptable levels of disease, injury, or dysfunction; or prevalence of risk factors.

OUTPUTS

Health programs and services intended to prevent death, disease, and disability, and to promote quality of life.

PERSONAL HEALTH SERVICES

Diagnosis and treatment of disease or provision of clinical preventive services to individuals or families in order to improve individual health status.

POLICE POWER

A basic power of government that allows for restriction of individual rights to protect the safety and interests of the entire population.

POLICY DEVELOPMENT

One of public health's three core functions. Policy development involves serving the public interest by leading in developing comprehensive public health policy and promoting the use of the scientific knowledge base in decision making.

POPULATION-BASED PUBLIC HEALTH SERVICES

Interventions aimed at disease prevention and health promotion that affect an entire population and extend beyond medical treatment by targeting underlying risks, such as tobacco, drug, and alcohol use; diet and sedentary lifestyles; and environmental factors.

POSTPONEMENT

A form of prevention in which the time of onset of a disease or injury is delayed to reduce the prevalence of a condition in the population.

PREPAREDNESS

All measures and policies taken before an event occurs that allow for prevention, mitigation, and readiness.

PREVALENCE

A measure of the burden of disease or injury in a population, generally the number of cases of a disease or injury at a particular point in time or during a specified time period. Prevalence is affected by both the incidence and the duration of disease in a population.

PREVENTED FRACTION

The proportion of an adverse health outcome that has been eliminated as a result of a prevention strategy.

PREVENTION

Anticipatory action taken to prevent the occurrence of an event or to minimize its effects after it has occurred. Prevention aims to minimize the occurrence of disease or its consequences. It includes actions that reduce susceptibility or exposure to health threats (primary prevention), detect and treat disease in early stages (secondary prevention), and alleviate the effects of disease and injury (tertiary prevention). Examples of prevention include immunizations, emergency response to epidemics, health education, modification of risk-prone behavior and physical hazards, safety training, workplace hazard elimination, and industrial process change.

PREVENTIVE STRATEGIES

Frameworks for categorizing prevention programs, based on how the prevention technology is delivered—provider to patient (clinical preventive services), individual responsibility (behavioral prevention), or alteration in an individual's surroundings (environmental prevention)—or on the stage of the natural history of a disease or injury (primary, secondary, tertiary).

PRIMARY MEDICAL CARE

Clinical preventive services, first-contact treatment services, and ongoing care for commonly encountered medical conditions. Basic or general health care focuses on the point at which a patient ideally seeks assistance from the medical care system. Primary care is considered comprehensive when the primary provider takes responsibility for the overall coordination of the care of the patient's health problems, whether these are medical, behavioral, or social. The appropriate use of consultants and community resources is an important part of effective primary health care. Such care is generally provided by physicians, but can also be provided by other personnel, such as nurse practitioners or physician assistants.

PRIMARY PREVENTION

Prevention strategies that seek to prevent the occurrence of disease or injury, generally through reducing exposure or risk factor levels. These strategies can reduce or eliminate causative risk factors (risk reduction).

PROCESS MEASURES

Steps in a program logically required for the program to be successful.

PROCESS OBJECTIVE

The level to which a contributing factor is to be reduced as a result of successfully carrying out a program's activities.

PUBLIC HEALTH

Activities that society undertakes to assure the conditions in which people can be healthy. These include organized community efforts to prevent, identify, and counter threats to the health of the public.

PUBLIC HEALTH AGENCY

A unit of government (federal, state, local, or regional) charged with preserving, protecting, and promoting the health of the population through assuring delivery of essential public health services.

PUBLIC HEALTH IN AMERICA

A document developed by the Core Functions Project that characterizes the vision, mission, outcome aspirations, and essential services of public health. See also *essential public health services* and Exhibit 1–5.

PUBLIC HEALTH ORGANIZATION

A nongovernmental entity (not-for-profit agency, association, corporation, etc.) participating in activities designed to improve the health status of a community or population.

PUBLIC HEALTH PRACTICE

The development and application of preventive strategies and interventions to promote and protect the health of populations.

PUBLIC HEALTH PRACTICE GUIDELINES

Systematically developed statements that assist public health practitioner decisions about interventions at the community level.

PUBLIC HEALTH PRACTICES

Those organizational practices or processes that are necessary and sufficient to assure that the core functions of public health are being carried out effectively. Ten public health practices have been identified: (1) assess the health needs of the community; (2) investigate the occurrence of health risks and hazards in the community; (3) analyze identified health needs for their determinants and contributing factors; (4) advocate and build support for public health; (5) establish priorities from among identified health needs; (6) develop comprehensive policies and plans for priority health needs; (7) manage resources efficiently; (8) ensure that priority health needs are addressed in the community; (9) evaluate the effects of programs and services; and (10) inform and educate the public.

PUBLIC HEALTH PROCESSES

Those collective practices or processes that are necessary and sufficient to assure that the core functions and essential services of public health are being carried out effectively, including the key processes that identify and address health problems and their causative factors and the interventions intended to prevent death, disease, and disability, and to promote quality of life.

PUBLIC HEALTH SERVICE

U.S. Public Health Service, as reorganized in 1996; now includes the Office of Public Health and Science (which is headed by the Assistant Secretary for Health and includes the Office of the Surgeon General), eight operating agencies (Health Resources and Services Administration; Indian Health Service; Centers for Disease Control and Prevention; National Institutes of Health; Food and Drug Administration; Substance Abuse and Mental Health Services Administration; Agency for Toxic Substances and Disease Registry; and Agency for Health Care Policy and Research); and the Regional Health Administrators for the 10 federal regions of the country.

PUBLIC HEALTH SYSTEM

That part of the larger health system that seeks to assure conditions in which people can be healthy by carrying out public health's three core functions. The system can be further described by its inputs, practices, outputs, and outcomes.

PUBLIC HEALTH WORKFORCE

The public health workforce includes individuals:

- employed by an organization engaged in an organized effort to promote, protect, and preserve the health of a defined population group. The group may be public or private, and the effort may be secondary or subsidiary to the principal objectives of the organization;
- performing work made up of one or more specific public health services or activities; and
- occupying positions that conventionally require at least one year of postsecondary specialized public health training and that are (or can be) assigned a professional occupational title.

QUALITY-ADJUSTED LIFE YEARS (QALYs)

A measure of health status that assigns to each period of time a weight, ranging from 0 to 1, corresponding to the health-related quality of life during that period; these are then summed across time periods to calculate QALYs. For each period, a weight of 1 corresponds to optimal health, and a weight of 0 corresponds to a health state equivalent to death.

QUALITY OF CARE

The degree to which health services for individuals increase the likelihood of desired health outcomes and are consistent with established professional standards and judgments of value to the consumer. Quality also may be seen as the degree to which actions taken or not taken maximize the probability of beneficial health outcomes and minimize risk and other undesired outcomes, given the existing state of medical science and art.

RAPID NEEDS ASSESSMENT

A variety of epidemiologic, statistical, anthropological techniques designed to provide information about an affected community's needs following a disaster or other public health emergency.

RATE

A mathematical expression for the relation between the numerator (number of deaths, diseases, disabilities, services, etc.) and denominator (population at risk), together with specification of time. Rates make possible a comparison of the number of events between populations and at different times. Rates may be crude, specific, or adjusted.

RECOVERY

Actions of responders, government, and victims that help return an affected community to normal by stimulating community cohesiveness and governmental involvement. The recovery period falls between the onset of an emergency and the reconstruction period.

REHABILITATION

An intervention strategy that seeks to return individuals to the maximum level of functioning possible.

RESPONSE

The phase in a disaster or public health emergency when relief, recovery, and rehabilitation occur.

RISK

The probability that exposure to a hazard will lead to a negative consequence.

RISK ASSESSMENT

A determination of the likelihood of adverse health effects to a population after exposure to a hazard.

RISK FACTOR

A behavior or condition that, on the basis of scientific evidence or theory, is thought to influence susceptibility to a specific health problem.

RISK RATIO/RELATIVE RISK

The ratio of the risk or likelihood of the occurrence of specific health outcomes or events in one group to that of another; risk ratios provide a measure of the relative difference in risk between the two groups. Relative risk is an example of a risk ratio in which the incidence of disease in the exposed group is divided by the incidence of disease in an unexposed group.

SCREENING

The use of technology and procedures to differentiate those individuals with signs or symptoms of disease from those less likely to have the disease. Then, if necessary, further diagnosis and, if indicated, early intervention and treatment can be provided.

SECONDARY MEDICAL CARE

Specialized attention and ongoing management for common and less frequently encountered medical conditions, including support services for people with special challenges due to chronic or long-term conditions. Services provided by medical specialists who generally do not have their first contact with patients (e.g., cardiologists, urologists, dermatologists). In the United States, however, there has been a trend toward self-referral by patients for these services, rather than referral by primary care providers.

SECONDARY PREVENTION

Prevention strategies that seek to identify and control disease processes in their early stages before signs and symptoms develop (screening and treatment).

SPAN OF HEALTHY LIFE

A measure of health status that combines life expectancy with self-reported health status and functional disabilities to calculate the number of years in which an individual is likely to function normally.

SPECIFIC RATE

Rates vary greatly by race, sex, and age. A rate can be made specific for sex, age, race, cause of death, or a combination of these.

STATE HEALTH AGENCY

The unit of state government that has leading responsibility for identifying and meeting the health needs of the state's citizens. State health agencies can be freestanding or units of multipurpose health and human service agencies.

STRATEGIC NATIONAL STOCKPILE

Formerly known as the National Pharmaceutical Stockpile, a collection of pharmaceuticals, medical supplies, and equipment that can be immediately deployed to meet state and local needs during a public health emergency.

STRATEGIC PLANNING

A disciplined process aimed at producing fundamental decisions and actions that will shape and guide what an organization is, what it does, and why it does what it does. The process of assessing a changing environment to create a vision of the future; determining how the organization fits into the anticipated environment, based on its mission, strengths, and weaknesses; then setting in motion a plan of action to position the organization.

SURVEILLANCE

Systematic monitoring of the health status of a population through collection, analysis, and interpretation of health data in order to plan, implement, and evaluate public health programs, including determining the need for public health action.

TERTIARY MEDICAL CARE

Sub-specialty referral care requiring highly specialized personnel and facilities. Services provided by highly specialized providers (e.g., neurologists, neurosurgeons, thoracic surgeons, intensive care units). Such services frequently require highly sophisticated equipment and support facilities. The development of these services has largely been a function of diagnostic and therapeutic advances attained through basic and clinical biomedical research.

TERTIARY PREVENTION

Prevention strategies that prevent disability by restoring individuals to their optimal level of functioning after a disease or injury is established and damage is done.

TRIAGE

The selection and categorization of victims of a disaster or other public health emergency as to their need for medical treatment according to the degree of severity of illness or injury as well as the availability of medical and transport facilities.

VULNERABILITY

The susceptibility of a population to a specific type of event, generally associated with the degree of possible or potential loss from a risk that results from a hazard at a given intensity. Vulnerability can be influenced by demographics, the age and resilience of the environment, technology, social differentiation and diversity as well as regional and global economics and politics.

WAIVER

States must obtain waivers of current federal Medicaid law provisions from the Health Care Financing Administration to enroll their Medicaid population in managed care plans or to deviate otherwise from law.

WEAPONS OF MASS DESTRUCTION

Any device, material, or substance used in a manner, in a quantity or type, or under circumstances evidencing intent to cause death or serious injury to persons or significant damage of property.

YEARS OF POTENTIAL LIFE LOST (YPLL)

A measure of the impact of disease or injury in a population that calculates years of life lost before a specific age (often age 65 or age 75). This approach places additional value on deaths that occur at earlier ages.

Index